The Complete Mediterranean Diet Cookbook:

Create and Follow Your Own Mediterranean Diet Plan with More Than 470 Recipes

Nadine Massri

Contents

The Fundamentals 1
    What is the Mediterranean Diet? 1
    The Mediterranean Diet Pyramid 2
    The Mediterranean Flavours 3
    Know the Ingredients 5
    The Mediterranean Way of Life 8
Benefits of the Mediterranean Diet 11
Planning Your Meals 18
Buying the Ingredients 21
Setting up Your Pantry 22
Mediterranean Spice Blends and Pastes 26
    Dukkah 26
    Green Zhoug 27
    Harissa 28
    Herbes de Provence 29
    Ras el Hanout 29
    Za'atar 30
    Pomegranate Molasses 30
    Preserved Lemons 31
Snacks and Appetizers 34
    Baba Ghanoush 34
    Brown Feta 35
    Bruschetta with Artichoke Hearts and Parmesan 36
    Bruschetta with Arugula Pesto and Goat Cheese 37
    Bruschetta with Black Olive Pesto, Ricotta, and Basil 37
    Bruschetta with Ricotta, Tomatoes, and Basil 38
    Caponata 39

- Classic Hummus 41
- Dolmathes 42
- Easy Toasted Almonds 43
- Fiery Red Whipped Feta 44
- Flavourful Calamari with Oranges 45
- Flavourful Green-Black Olives 46
- Flavourful Saffron Caulipeas 47
- Garmary White Bean Dip 48
- Giardiniera 49
- Infused Artichokes 50
- Labneh 51
- Lavash Crackers 52
- Muhammara 53
- Mussels Escabèche 54
- Olive Oil–Sea Salt Pita Chips 55
- Packed Sardines 56
- Provençal Anchovy Dip 57
- Rich Turkish Nut Dip 58
- Searing Garlic Shrimp 59
- Skordalia 60
- Soft and Crispy Halloumi 62
- Stuffed Dates Wrap 62
- Toasted Bread for Bruschetta 63
- Tzatziki 64

Soups 65
- Artichoke-Mushroom Soup 65
- Classic Chicken Broth 66
- Classic Croutons 67
- Classic Gazpacho 68

Cold Cucumber-Yogurt Soup 69
Fiery Moroccan Chicken Lentil Soup 70
French Lentil Soup 71
Greek White Bean Soup 72
Green Pea Soup 73
Italian Pasta e Fagioli 75
Libyan Lamb-Mint Sharba 76
Moroccan Chickpea Soup 77
Moroccan Spicy Fava Bean Soup 78
Provençal Vegetable Soup 79
Provene Fish Soup 81
Red Pepper Roast Soup with Sides 82
Shellfish Soup 84
Sicilian Chickpea-Escarole Soup 85
Spanish Lentil-Chorizo Soup 87
Spanish Meatball-Saffron Soup 88
Spicy Moroccan Lamb Lentil Soup 90
Spicy Red Lentil Soup 91
Tomato Soup with Eggplant Roast 92
Traditional Greek Avgolemono 94
Turkish Tomato Grain Soup 95
Vegetable Broth Base 96
White Gazpacho 97

Salad and Salad Dressings 99
Salad Dressings 99
Balsamic-Mustard Vinaigrette 99
Classic Vinaigrette 100
Herb Vinaigrette 100
Lemon Vinaigrette 101

    Tahini-Lemon Dressing 102

    Walnut Vinaigrette 103

Green Salads... 103

    Arugula Fennel Parmesan Salad 103

    Arugula Mix Salad 104

    Arugula Sweet Salad 105

    Asparagus Arugula Cannellini Salad 106

    Asparagus-Red Pepper-Spinach-Goat Cheese Salad 107

    Bitter Greens Olive Feta Salad.. 108

    Fiery Tuna-Olive Salad 109

    Fundamental Green Salad 110

    Green Artichoke Olive Salad 111

    Green Marcona Manchego Salad 112

    Kale-Sweet Potato Salad.. 112

    Mâche-Cucumber-Mint Salad 114

    Salade Niçoise.. 114

    Spinach-Feta-Pistachio Salad... 116

    Tangy Salad 117

    Tri-Balsamic Salad 118

Vegetable Salads 119

    Algerian Mix Salad 119

    Asparagus Mix Salad 120

    Brussels Pecorino Pine Salad 121

    Cauliflower Chermoula Salad 122

    Cherry Tomato Mix Salad 123

    Classic Greek Salad 124

    Crunchy Mushroom Salad 125

    Cucumber Sesame-Lemon Salad 126

    Cut Up Salad 127

Fattoush 128

French Potato Dijon Herb Salad 129

Green Bean Cilantro Salad 130

Halloumi-Veg Salad 131

Italian Panzanella Mix Salad 132

Mackerel-Fennel-Apple Salad 133

Moroccan Carrot Salad.. 134

Radish-Fava Salad... 135

Roasted Beet-Carrot Salad with 136

Scorched Beet Almond Salad 137

Sweet Nut Winter Squash Salad... 138

Tomato Mix Salad 139

Tomato-Burrata Mix Salad 140

Tomato-Tuna Mix Salad 141

Yogurt-Mint Cucumber Salad 142

Zucchini Parmesan Salad 143

Rice and Grain Recipes 144

Aromatic Baked Brown Rice 144

Aromatic Barley Pilaf 145

Basmati Rice Pilaf Mix 146

Brown Rice Salad with Asparagus, Goat Cheese, and Lemon 147

Carrot-Almond-Bulgur Salad 148

Chickpea-Spinach-Bulgur.. 149

Classic Baked Brown Rice 150

Classic Italian Seafood Risotto... 150

Classic Stovetop White Rice 152

Classic Tabbouleh 153

Farro Cucumber-Mint Salad 153

Farro Salad Mix... 154

Farrotto Mix 155

Fennel-Parmesan Farro 157

Feta-Grape-Bulgur Salad with Grapes and Feta 158

Greek Style Meaty Bulgur 159

Hearty Barley Mix 160

Hearty Barley Risotto 161

Hearty Freekeh Pilaf 162

Herby-Lemony Farro 163

Italian Paniscia 164

Italian Parmesan Farrotto 166

Lebanese Herbed Basmati Rice 167

Mushroom-Bulgur Pilaf 168

Mushroom-Thyme Farro 169

North African Spiced Baked Rice 170

Nutty Freekeh Salad 172

Nutty Wheat Berry Salad 173

Rich Italian Parmesan Polenta 174

Rich Spanish Vegetable Paella 176

Spanish Broth Rice 178

Spanish Paella 179

Spanish Style Brown Rice 181

Spiced Basmati Rice Mix 183

Tangy Rice Salad 184

Tangy Wheat Berry Salad 185

Ultimate Barley Mix 186

Vibrant Egyptian Barley Salad 187

Vibrant Spanish Grilled Paella 188

Wheat Berry Mix 190

Pasta and Couscous 192

Pasta Sauces 192

    Classic Marinara Sauce 192

    Fresh & Raw Tomato Sauce 193

    Quick Tomato Sauce 194

Pesto Sauces 195

    Classic Basil Pesto 195

    Green Olive and Orange Pesto 196

    Roasted Red Pepper Pesto 197

    Tomato and Almond Pesto 197

Pasta 198

    Briny Italian Spaghetti 198

    Cheesy Penne with Roasted Cherry Tomatoes 200

    Classic Clammed Italian Spaghetti 201

    Classic Italian Linguine ai Frutti di Mare 202

    Classic Italian Spaghetti al Limone 204

    Colourful & Nutty Farfalle 205

    Flavourful Italian Spaghetti Mix 206

    Flavourful Italian Tagliatelle 207

    Flavourful Toasted Orzo Mix 209

    Greek Crunchy Orzo Salad 210

    Greek Manestra 211

    Greek Spicy Orzo 213

    Green Penne and Fresh Tomato Sauce 214

    Lemony Shrimp Orzo 215

    Nutty Penne with Roasted Cherry Tomatoes 216

    Penne with Cherry Tomato Sauce 217

    Puglia-Style Orecchiette 218

    Rustic Italian Whole-Wheat Spaghetti 219

    Spanish Toasted Shrimpy Pasta 221

Spicy Beefy Rigatoni ... 222

Tangy Penne with Fresh Tomato Sauce ... 224

Whole-Wheat Spaghetti Mix ... 225

Zucchini-Tomatoes Farfalle ... 226

Couscous ... 228

Basic Couscous ... 228

Basic Couscous with Carrots, Raisins, and Pine Nuts ... 229

Basic Couscous with Dates and Pistachios ... 229

Basic Pearl Couscous ... 229

Basic Pearl Couscous Wholesome Mix ... 230

Basic Pearl Couscous with Peas, Feta, and Pickled Shallots ... 232

Basic Pearl Couscous with Radishes and Watercress ... 233

Basic Pearl Couscous with Tomatoes, Olives, and Ricotta Salata . 234

Lemony Sujuk Couscous ... 235

Moroccan Chickpea Couscous ... 237

Spicy Vegge Couscous ... 238

Tangy Lamb-Chickpea Couscous ... 239

Beans ... 241

Chickpea Mix 1 ... 241

Chickpea Mix 2 ... 242

Chickpea Mix 3 ... 242

Chickpea Mix 4 ... 242

Chickpea Salad 1 ... 243

Chickpea Salad 2 ... 243

Chickpea Salad 3 ... 244

Classis Levantine Mujaddara ... 244

Eastern Mediterranean Falafel ... 246

Egyptian Black-Eyed Pea Salad Mix ... 248

Egyption Koshari ... 249

- Flavourful Winter Squash Lentil Salad 251
- French Lentils with Carrots and Parsley 252
- French Lentils with Swiss Chard 253
- Greek Chickpea Cakes 253
- Greek Gigante Bean Mix 254
- Greek Stewed 256
- Italian Sweet and Sour Cranberry Bean Sauce 257
- Lentil Salad Mix 1 258
- Lentil Salad Mix 2 259
- Lentil Salad Mix 3 259
- Lentil Salad Mix 4 259
- Lentils with Spinach and Garlic Chips 260
- Moroccan Loubia 261
- North African Veggie Bean Stew 262
- Sicilian White Beans with Escarole 264
- Spanish Espinacas 265
- Spiced Cranberry Beans 266
- Squashed Fava Beans Basic Mix 267
- Squashed Fava Beans Mix 2 268
- Squashed Fava Beans Mix 3 268
- Squashed Fava Beans with Sautéed Escarole and Parmesan 269
- Tunisian Chickpea Spice 270
- Turkish Fasulye piyazi Salad 271
- White Bean Salad Basic 272
- White Bean Salad Mix 1 273
- White Bean Salad Squid-Pepperoncini Mix 274
- Wholesome Tuscan Bean Stew 275

Vegetable Recipes 277
- Braised Asparagus Mix 277

Braised Cauliflower Mix 1	278
Braised Cauliflower Mix 2	279
Braised Cauliflower Mix 3	279
Braised Green Beans Mix 3	280
Broiled Eggplant	280
Ciambotta	281
Classic French Vegetable Gratin	282
Eastern Cauliflower Cakes	284
Enhanced Pan-Roasted Asparagus Mix 1	285
Enhanced Pan-Roasted Asparagus Mix 2	286
Fava Beans Mix	287
Flavourful Grilled Radicchio	288
Garlic-flavoured Braised Kale	289
Greek Garlic-Lemon Potatoes Basic	290
Greek Garlic-Lemon Potatoes Mix 1	291
Greek Grilled Zucchini	291
Greek Marinated Eggplant	292
Greek Stewed Zucchini	293
Grilled Eggplant	294
Grilled Portobello Mushrooms and Shallots	296
Hearty North-African Tagine	297
Italian Broccoli Rabe Mix 1	298
Italian Broccoli Rabe Mix 2	299
Italian Broccoli Rabe Mix 3	300
Lamb-Stuffed Zucchini	300
Lemony Roasted Artichokes	301
Ratatouille	303
Roasted Asparagus Basic	304
Roasted Asparagus Mix 1	305

Roasted Asparagus Mix 2 305

Roasted Carrot Cilantro Spice 306

Roasted Celery Root 307

Roasted Greek Winter Squash 308

Roasted Green Beans Mix 1 309

Roasted Green Beans Mix 2 310

Roasted Mushrooms Mix 1 310

Roasted Mushrooms Mix 2 311

Roasted Mushrooms Mix 3 312

Roasted Tomatoes... 312

Sautéed Cabbage Mix 1... 313

Sautéed Cabbage Mix 2... 314

Sautéed Cherry Tomatoes Basic.. 314

Sautéed Cherry Tomatoes Mix 1 315

Sautéed Swiss Chard Mix 1.. 315

Sautéed Swiss Chard Mix 2.. 316

Sautéed Swiss Chard Mix 3.. 317

Sautéed Zucchini Ribbons Basic 317

Sautéed Zucchini Ribbons Mix 318

Simmered Braised Green Beans... 318

Skillet-Roasted Cauliflower Basic 319

Skillet-Roasted Cauliflower Mix 1 321

Skillet-Roasted Cauliflower Spicy Mix 321

Slow Cooked Braised Fennel 322

Slow-Cooked Whole Carrots Basic 323

Slow-Cooked Whole Carrots Mix 1 323

Slow-Cooked Whole Carrots Mix 2 324

Slow-Cooked Whole Carrots Mix 3 324

Stuffed Bell Peppers Beef Mix.. 324

Stuffed Bell Peppers Lamb Mix 326

Stuffed Tomato Mix 1 326

Stuffed Tomato Mix 2 328

Stuffed Tomatoes Mix 3 328

Tangy & Tender Sautéed Spinach 328

Tangy Grilled Vegetable Kebabs 329

Tomato-Thyme Braised Artichokes 331

Tunisian Mechouia 332

Turkish Stuffed Eggplant 334

Zesty Roasted Radicchio, Fennel, and Parsnips 335

Zesty Roasted Root Vegetables 336

Zucchini-Feta Fritters 337

Vegetable Sauces 338

Cucumber-Yogurt Sauce 338

Garlic Aïoli 338

Lemon-Yogurt Sauce 339

Tahini Sauce 340

Tahini-Yogurt Sauce 341

Yogurt-Herb Sauce 341

Seafood 343

Fish 343

Aromatic Grilled Swordfish Skewers 343

Aromatic Provençal Braised Hake 345

Aromatic Sicilian Fish Stew 346

Braised Halibut 347

Broiled Grouper Wrap 348

Charred Whole Sardines 349

Classic Provençal Bouillabaisse 350

Easy-Roasted Halibut with Chermoula 352

Easy-Roasted Monkfish 353

French Swordfish en Cocotte 354

Grilled Swordfish Salad 355

Grilled Swordfish with Italian Salsa Verde 357

Grilled Tuna Steaks 358

Grilled Whole Mackerel Variation 1 359

Grilled Whole Mackerel Variation 2 360

Grilled Whole Mackerel with Lemon and Marjoram 360

Italian Grilled Whole Sea Bass 361

Poached Snapper 363

Quick-Roasted Sea Bass 365

Quick-Roasted Sea Bass with Orange Relish 365

Quick-Roasted Sea Bass with Thyme Relish 366

Quick-Roasted Sea Bass with Wild Mushrooms 366

Sautéed Sole 367

Spanish Smokey Hake 369

Tangy Baked Stuffed Mackerel 370

Tangy Broiled Bluefish 371

Tangy Grilled Sea Bass 372

Tangy Whole Roasted Snapper 373

Traditional North African Monkfish Tagine 375

Zesty Hake Fillets 376

Shellfish 377

Citric Seared Scallops 377

Greek-Style Shrimp 378

Grilled Scallop-Zucchini Skewers 379

Italian Shrimp & White Beans 381

Moroccan Grilled Marinated Shrimp Skewers 382

Oven-Steamed Mussels 384

    Oven-Steamed Mussels Variation 385

    Roasted Garlic Shrimp 385

    Spanish Clams Mix 386

    Spanish Shellfish Stew 387

    White Wine Steamed Clams 389

  Squid and Octopus 389

    Classic Calamari Stew 389

    Greek Stuffed Squid 390

    Greek Tangy Grilled Squid 392

    Greek-Style Octopus Braised in Red Wine 393

    Spanish Grilled Octopus Salad 395

    Spanish Grilled Octopus Variation 397

Poultry and Meat 398

  Beef Recipes 398

    Beefy Grilled Flank Steak 398

    Braised Beef Short Ribs 400

    Braised Oxtails 401

    Italian Flank Steak Peperonata 403

    Kibbeh 404

    Tangy Grilled Beef Kebabs 406

  Poultry 408

    Sautéed Chicken Cutlets Alongside Romesco Sauce 408

    Sautéed Chicken Cutlets Variation 1 409

    Sautéed Chicken Cutlets Variation 2 410

    Sautéed Chicken Breasts Veggie Blast 410

    Tangy Pan-Seared Chicken Breasts Salad 411

    Circassian Chicken 412

    Spanish Pollo en pepitoria 414

    Classic chicken cacciatore 415

- Moroccan B'stilla 417
- Tangy Roasted Chicken Thighs 418
- Za'atar-Coated Chicken 419
- Italian alla Diavola 421
- Dressed & Grilled Chicken Kebabs 422
- Greek Souvlaki 423
- French Bouillabaisse 425
- North African Exotic Chicken Tagine 428
- Glazed Roasted Quail 429

Pork Recipes 430
- Fiery Braised Greek Sausages 431
- French-Style Sausage 432
- Greek Braised Pork 433
- North African Spice Grilled Pork Skewers 434
- Spicy Pork Tenderloin 436

Lamb Recipes 437
- Braised Lamb Shanks 437
- Braised Lamb Shoulder Chops 438
- Grilled Greek Gyro 439
- Grilled Lamb Kofte 441
- Grilled Lamb Shish Kebabs 442
- Grilled Lamb Shoulder Chops 444
- Lamb Meatballs 446
- Roast Butterflied Leg of Lamb 447

Egg Recipes 449
- Classic Greek Baked Eggs 449
- Crunchy Meaty Poached Eggs 450
- Egyptian Eggah 452
- Fried Eggs with Sides 453

Frittata 1: Broccoli-Feta 455

Frittata 2: Asparagus and Goat Cheese 456

Frittata 3: Mushroom and Pecorino Frittata 456

Israeli Sabich Eggplant and Egg Sandwiches 457

Ratatouille with Poached Eggs 458

Scrambled Eggs Mix 1 459

Scrambled Eggs Mix 2 460

Scrambled Eggs Mix 3 462

Spanish Tortilla 463

Traditional Greek Sfougato 464

Tunisian Shakshuka 466

Breads 468

Catalan Red Pepper Coques 468

French Socca 470

French Socca Variation 1 471

French Socca Variation 2 471

Greek Pita Bread 472

Greek Spanakopita 473

Italian Rosemary Focaccia 475

Italian Tart 1: Mushroom 477

Italian Tart 2: Tomato 479

Italian Tart 3: Zucchini 479

Lahmacun 480

Lavash With Veggies Mix 1 482

Lavash With Veggies Mix 2 483

Moroccan Chicken B'stilla 483

Palestinian Mushroom Musakhan 485

Phyllo Hand Pies 488

Pissaladière 490

  Pumpkin Borek 492

  Turkish Pide 494

  Za'atar Bread 496

Pizzas 499

  Thin-Crust Pizza 499

  Toppings For Thin-Crust Pizza 501

    Mushroom and Fennel Pizza Topping 501

    Olive, Caper, and Spicy Garlic Pizza Topping 502

    Prosciutto and Arugula Pizza Topping 502

  Whole-Wheat Crust Pizzas 502

    Pizza 1: Feta, Figs, Honey 502

    Pizza 2: Artichokes, Ricotta, Parmesan 505

    Pizza 3: Pesto, Goat Cheese 505

Fruit and Sweets 506

  Almond Cake 506

  Apricot Spoon Sweets 507

  Baklava 508

  Classic French Poached Pears 510

  Classic Greek Lemon Rice Pudding 511

  Dried Fruit Compote 512

  Fruit & Wine Dessert 512

  Fruit and Nut Roasted Pears 513

  Greek Pasteli 514

  Honey Biscotti 515

  Honey-Glazed Peaches 517

  Icy Delight 1: Lemon 518

  Icy Delight 2: Minted Lemon 518

  Icy Delight 3: Orange 519

  Italian Orange Polenta Cake 519

- Italian Pignoli 520
- Italian Vinegar Strawberries 521
- Italian Zabaglione & Berry Mix 522
- Lemon Yogurt Mousse 523
- Lemon-Anise Biscotti 525
- Mediterranean Berry Mix 526
- Poached Peaches and Cherries 527
- Raspberry Sorbet 527
- Semolina Pudding 528
- Sicilian Fig Phyllo Cookies 529
- Spanish Olive Oil–Yogurt Cake 531
- Spicey Biscotti 532
- Sweet Fruit Salad 534
- Sweet Warm Figs 534
- Turkish Stuffed Apricots 535

Endnote 536

The Fundamentals

What is the Mediterranean Diet?

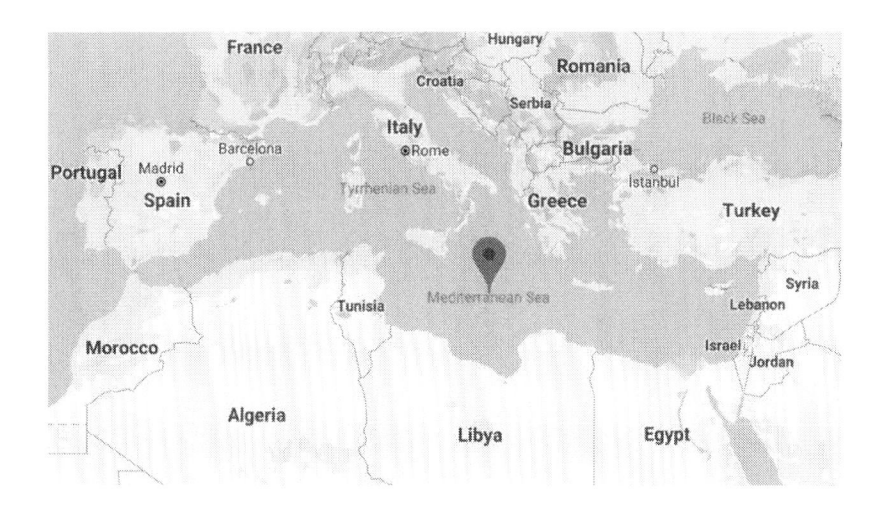

The map above shows us the Mediterranean Sea, and the countries that surround it. These countries don't really have much in common, and the same goes for their cuisines; this is actually a good thing. This diet is easy to follow as there will always be a dish to satisfy your craving. Craving something sweet and savoury? A fiery cuisine from morocco is sure to leave you satisfied. Craving something tangy and citrus? Maybe a Greek cuisine is what you're looking for.

Now if the cuisines of these countries are so far apart, why do we categorise their food into one single diet? The answer is simple: It's the healthy ingredients and use of heart-healthy oil. These ingredients are- vegetables, fruits, beans, lentils, whole grains, more seafood than meat and poultry, and heart-healthy olive oil. Different Mediterranean countries cook these ingredients in different ways, but the basics are the same with a focus on health.

The Mediterranean Diet Pyramid

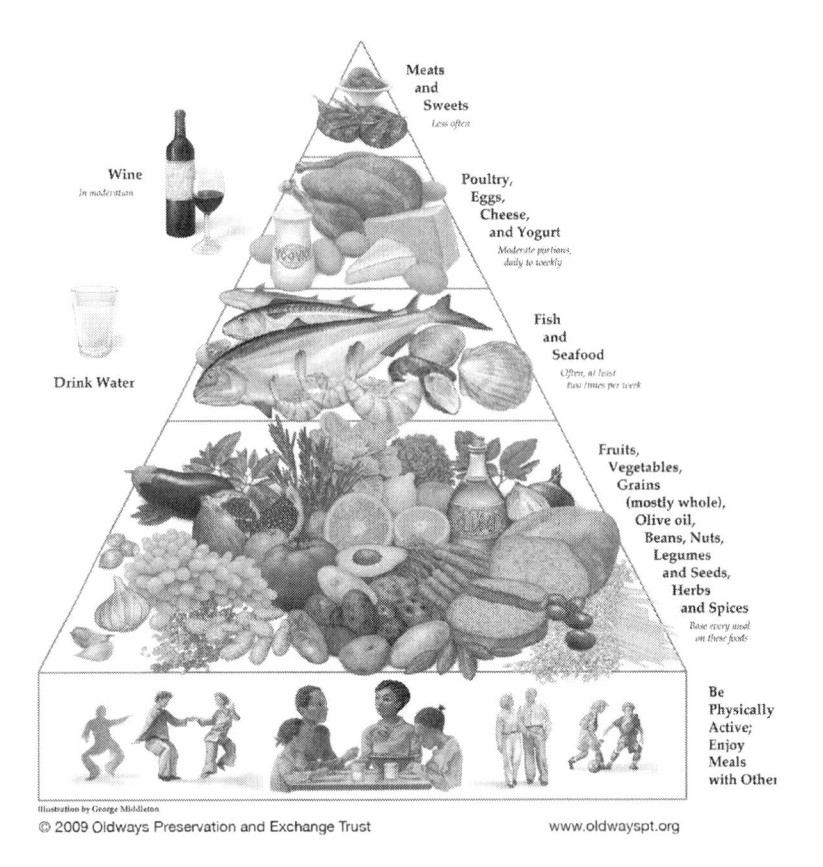

The above graphic illustration from www.oldwatspt.org clearly depicts what the Mediterranean diet, or rather the healthy Mediterranean way of life is based upon. In the year 1950, an American physiologist named Ankle Keys found that the people of Creda had among the lowest rates of coronary heart disease. After thorough research, the physiologist concluded that this was due to their traditional diet, which was loaded with vegetables, grains, and legumes, and included very low saturated fat. Based on this research, the pyramid you see above was formulated in the year 1990. All the recipes in this book have their foundation in the pyramid you see above. Which is to say, that most of the recipes you will find in this book are going to be those of the ingredients you see on the base of the pyramid, and fewer recipes of the ingredients that are placed on the higher levels of the pyramid.

Today, we know that vegetables and olive oil are related to low instances of heart diseases because they are rich in heart-healthy monosaturated fats. Since the Mediterranean diet is loaded with these, it is great for heart health, promotes healthy blood sugar levels, enhances cognitive abilities, and to a certain extent even helps prevent and manage diseases like cancer. The Mediterranean diet isn't low in fat, but today we know that fat doesn't make you fat. Sugar is the culprit. In fact, studies have found that high-fat diets like the popular ketogenic diet can promote fat loss by forcing your body to produce ketones to metabolize the fat, the very same ketones that can also metabolise body fat and hence promote weight loss.

The Mediterranean Flavours

A diet can be the most nutritious diet ever conceived, but it would be pointless if one cannot follow it for more than a day. We are all human, after all, and delicious food is one of the greatest pleasures we get to experience in our ephemeral lifetimes. With that in mind, it is important for any diet to provide the health benefits while tasting absolutely amazing. The Mediterranean diet does exactly that. Since the recipes are from such a wide spectrum of countries, the flavour never gets bland, and with a cookbook like this in your possession, you'll be living the Mediterranean way for years to come!

Although 21 countries have a coastline on the Mediterranean Sea, only a few of these countries truly represent the Mediterranean diet and way of life. Each country has its own flavour, and if you want to get into a little more detail about what the cuisines of a few of the most prominent countries taste like, refer to the table below.

Region	Most Common Ingredients	Overall Cuisine Flavor
Southern Italy	Anchovies, balsamic vinegar, basil, bay leaf, capers, garlic, mozzarella	Italian food is rich and savory, with strongly flavored ingredients. Look for tomato-

	cheese, olive oil, oregano, parsley, peppers, pine nuts, mushrooms, prosciutto, rosemary, sage, thyme, tomatoes	based sauces and even an occasional kick of spicy heat.
Greece	Basil, cucumbers, dill, fennel, feta cheese, garlic, honey, lemon, mint, olive oil, oregano, yogurt	Greek cuisines range from tangy with citrus accents to savory. Ingredients like feta cheese add a strong, bold flavor, while yogurt helps provide a creamy texture and soft flavor.
Morocco	Cinnamon, cumin, dried fruits, ginger, lemon, mint, paprika, parsley, pepper, saffron, turmeric	Moroccan cooking uses exotic flavors that include both sweet and savory, often in one dish. The food has strong flavors but isn't necessarily spicy.
Spain	Almonds, anchovies, cheeses (from goats, cows, and sheep), garlic, ham, honey, olive oil, onions, oregano, nuts, paprika, rosemary, saffron, thyme	Garlic and olive oil are a staple when it comes to Spanish dishes. Spanish dishes are often inspired by Arabic and Roman cuisine with emphasis on fresh seafood. Combinations of savory and sweet flavors, such as a seafood stew using sweet paprika are quite common.

Know the Ingredients

Today, we get our ingredients quite differently as compared to how the people living on the Mediterranean coast did 50 years ago. They couldn't just stroll into a grocery store and pick up whatever they wanted. They could only get their hands on what was farmed and fished locally. Today, however, the world is very different and much better connected. You can gain access to ingredients from across the planet with the flick of a finger (if you're shopping for groceries online). Having access to so many options may seem like a hurdle at first, but if you're truly determined to live the Mediterranean way, it has never been easier to do so. All you need to do is include more fresh ingredients into your food, and say no to junk and other processed foods.

Mediterranean Farm Produce

Most of the areas along the Mediterranean Sea are ideal for agriculture due to a moderate climate of wet winters and hot summers. Hence, Mediterranean areas have been growing their own food. Thanks to the climate, olives and fig trees grow well in most of these areas, and naturally have become a staple in the Mediterranean diet.

It is also important to note that relying on fresh produce also means eating seasonally. Not all crops grow all year round, so back in the day there was no option but to eat what was in season. Eating seasonally is highly beneficial as it incorporates a variety of foods into the diet. Today, however, it is easy to eat what you love all-year-round, and this is not a good practice if you do so. Living the Mediterranean way means eating a wide variety of ingredients to get the full spectrum of vitamins and minerals.

Below is a table showing a few of the most commonly farmed ingredients in this region: -

Category	Ingredient
Legumes	Chickpeas
	Lentils

Fruits	Peas
	Olives
	Mandarin oranges
	Figs
	Grapes
	Lemons
	Persimmons
	Pomegranates
Grains	Barley
	Corn
	Rice
	Wheat
Herbs	Rosemary
	Oregano
	Sage
	Parsley
	Basil
	Dill
	Thyme
	Mint
	Fennel
Nuts	Almonds
	Hazelnuts
	Pine nuts

Vegetables	Walnuts
	Asparagus
	Broccoli
	Cabbage
	Green beans
	Garlic
	Onions
	Eggplant
	Tomatoes
	Broccoli rabe
	Artichokes

Fishing the Mediterranean Sea

The Mediterranean Sea provided a bounty of seafood to the dwellers in that area, and naturally it became an indispensable part of the Mediterranean diet. Fish is rich in omega-3 fatty acids, and hence should be eaten a few times per week to reap all its health benefits. Due to their abundance, one could get sardines, anchovies, octopus, squid, and mackerel for quite cheap back in the day. A few slightly costlier options were mussels, trout, tuna, and clams. Extravagant meals included ingredients like lobster and red mullet.

Today, however, the marine life in the area has gone down significantly due to overfishing, and species vital to the marine ecosystem such as tuna are under threat.

The Mediterranean Way of Life

The healthy Mediterranean way of life is all about eating balanced foods rich in vitamins, minerals, antioxidants, and healthy fatty acids. However, the Mediterranean diet is just one aspect of it. The Mediterranean way of life calls for regular physical exercise, plenty of rest, healthy social interaction, and fun. Balancing all these aspects was the secret of good health of the Mediterranean folk back in the day. However, only the Mediterranean diet is the primary focus of this book, and we will spend most of our time talking about just that.

Eat Healthy Fats

The Mediterranean diet is by no means a low-fat diet, but the fat that is included in this diet is considered healthy for the body, and the heart in particular. Remember: not all fats are created equal. Certain kinds of fats are healthy, while others do more harm than good. Monosaturated fats and polyunsaturated omega-3 fatty acids, for example, are considered healthy. Omegs-6 polyunsaturated fatty acids and saturated fats are unhealthy, and these unhealthy fats are the ones primarily present in most of the common food worldwide. The United States, for example, absolutely loves saturated fats. According to a survey, saturated fats constitute 11% of the total calories of an average American, which is a very high number compared an average Mediterranean resident, who consumes less than 8% of his/her calories through saturated fat. So, if you wish to switch to the healthy Mediterranean way of life, the first thing to do is change the oils you consume. Eliminating fats like butter and lard in favour of healthier oils like olive oil would be the place to start.

Consume Dairy in Moderation

We all love cheese. Dairy products are delicious, nutritious, and great sources of calcium, and should be consumed in moderation if you're following the Mediterranean diet. It is usually a good idea to consume two to three servings of full-fat dairy products in a single day, where one serving can mean an 8-ounce glass of milk, or 8 ounces of yogurt, or an ounce of cheese.

Consume Tons of Plant-Based Foods
As we saw in the pyramid, fruits, vegetables, legumes, and whole grains form the basis of the Mediterranean diet. So, it is a good idea to eat five to ten servings of these in a single day, depending on your appetite. Basically, eat as much of these as you want, but don't overeat. Plant based foods are naturally low in calories, and high in fiber and nutrients. Fresh unprocessed plants are best, so always be on the lookout for the best sources of these around you!

Spice Things Up with Fresh Herbs and Spices
Fresh herbs and Spices are what make most of the recipes insanely delicious, while also providing health benefits. If you already use these in your daily cooking, more power to you! If not, we got you covered!

Consume Seafood Weekly
As we've talked before, one benefit of living close to the sea is the easy access to seafood. However, seafood holds a lower priority than plant-based foods in the Mediterranean diet, and should be consumed in moderation. If you're a vegetarian, consider taking fish oil supplements to get those omega-3 fatty acids into your system. Better yet, considering shunning your vegetarianism, and eating seafood to get the vital nourishment only seafood can provide.

Consume Meat Monthly
Red meat used to be a luxury for the Mediterranean people back in the day. Although not completely off-limits, you should try and reduce your red-meat intake as much as possible. If you absolutely love red meat, consider consuming it no more than two times per month. And even when you do eat it, make sure the serving size of the meat in the dish is small (two to three ounce serving). The main reason to limit meat intake is to limit the amount of unhealthy fats going into your system. As we talked before, saturated fats and omega-6 fatty acids are not good for health, but unfortunately, red meat contains significant quantities of these. As a beef lover myself, I eat a two-ounce serving of it per month, and when I do eat it, I make sure there are lots of vegetables on the side to satiate my hunger.

Drink Wine!

Love wine? Well, it is your lucky day. Having a glass of wine with dinner is a common practice in the Mediterranean regions. Red wine is especially good for the heart and it is a good idea to consume a glass of red wine twice a week. Excess of everything is bad, and wine is no exception so keep it in check. Also, if you're already suffering from health conditions, it is a good idea to check with your doctor before introducing wine to your daily diet.

Work Your Body

Now you don't have to hit the gym like a maniac to work your body. Walking to your destination instead of driving, taking the stairs instead of the lift, or kneading your own dough can all get the job done. So, be creative and work your body when you can. Better yet, play a sport or just hit the gym like a maniac. You don't have to, as I said at the start, but it will help... a lot.

Enjoy a Big Lunch

Lunch was usually the meal of the day when the Mediterranean residents sat with their families and took their time enjoying a big meal. This strengthens social bonds, and relaxes the mind during the most stressful time of the day, when you're just half done with your work, probably.

Have Fun with Friends and Family

Just spending a few minutes per day doing something fun with your loved ones is great for de-stressing. Today, we don't understand the importance of this, and people feel lonely, and in some cases, even depressed. Just doing this one thing has the power to solve a huge chunk of the problems our modern society faces.

Be Passionate

The Mediterranean people are passionate folk. Living on or close to sun-kissed coasts, their passion for life is naturally high. Being passionate about something in life can take you a long way towards health and wellness.

Benefits of the Mediterranean Diet

Now that we have talked about how you can follow the Mediterranean lifestyle; we should talk in detail about all the benefits you will get to reap if you are successful in doing so.

The Diet Fights Free Radicals

The Mediterranean diet is loaded with antioxidants, which help deter the process of oxidation in your body's cells. This reduces the number of free radicals or unstable molecules that cause harm to your cells, tissue, and DNA. In today's world, we have high exposure to harmful elements like vehicle exhaust, industrial waste, water contaminants, toxic foods, etc. These cause the free radicals in the body to escalate, which then increase the risk of chronic diseases of the heart, or even fatal diseases like cancer! Hence, it is absolutely vital to keep these free radicals in check as much as possible, and the best way of doing so naturally is to eat a diet rich in antioxidants, like the Mediterranean diet. The table below shoes a list of antioxidant-rich foods.

Antioxidant	*Foods*
Vitamin C	Asparagus
	Broccoli
	Cantaloupe
	Cauliflower
	Grapefruit
	Green and red bell peppers
	Guava
	Lemons

	Oranges
	Pineapple
	Strawberries
	Spinach, kale, and collard greens
	Tangerines
	Tomatoes
Vitamin E	Mustard greens, Swiss chard, spinach, and turnip and collard greens
	Almonds
	Peanuts
	Sunflower seeds
Beta carotene	Broccoli
	Cantaloupe
	Carrots
	Cilantro
	Kale, spinach, and turnip and collard greens
	Romaine lettuce

The Diet is Rich in Phytochemicals

We know that plants are rich in vitamins and minerals, but what few of us know is that they are also loaded with chemicals called phytochemicals. These are healthy chemicals contained in plants that provide numerous health benefits to the body, promote heart health, and help prevent certain types of cancers. Ever wondered why different fruits and vegetables exhibit different colours? The reason is the presence of different phytochemicals. Hence, it is possible to tell what kind of phytochemical a plant-based food contains simply by looking at its colour. Refer to the table below to gain some phytochemical knowledge.

Color	Health Benefits	Foods
Blue/purple	A lower risk of some cancers; improved memory; and healthy aging	Blueberries, eggplants, purple grapes, and plums
Green	A lower risk of some cancers; healthy vision; and strong bones and teeth	Broccoli, green peppers, honeydew melon, kiwi, salad greens, and spinach
Red	A lower risk of heart disease and of some cancers, and improved memory function	Pink watermelon, red bell peppers, and strawberries
White	A lower risk of heart disease and of some cancers	Bananas, garlic, and onions
Yellow/orange	A lower risk of heart disease and of some cancers; healthy vision; and a stronger immune system	Carrots, oranges, yellow and orange bell peppers, and yellow watermelon

The Diet is Rich in Vitamin D

The human body gets vitamin D from food sources and from exposure to sunlight. The Mediterranean residents have access to both, and hence have good levels of vitamin D. Some attribute their good health to their high vitamin D levels, and for good reason. Scientific research has demonstrated the numerous health benefits of the vitamin, and a few of these are listed below:

- Guards against Osteoporosis
- Reduces the risk of certain cancers
- Reduces the risk of coronary artery disease
- Reduces vulnerability to common infections such as the common flu

More Healthy Fats in Your Diet

As discussed before, the Mediterranean diet is rich in the healthy monosaturated fats omega-3 polyunsaturated fats, and has lower amounts of unhealthy omega-5 polyunsaturated fats and saturated fats. This has multiple health benefits that include:

- A lower risk of heart disease
- Enhanced insulin function and blood sugar control
- Lower cholesterol levels
- Reduced inflammation in the body
- Body weight management
- Enhanced immune system function
- Management of behavioural issues

More Fiber in Your Diet

It is common knowledge that fiber is great for health. The best sources of fiber are fruits, vegetables, whole grains, and legumes. All of these ingredients are dominant in the Mediterranean diet, and hence by following the Mediterranean diet, you can easily achieve your daily fiber goals. Fiber has multiple benefits for the body, a few of which are listed below:

- Helps maintain a healthy gastrointestinal tract by reducing constipation
- Decreases total cholesterol and bad cholesterol levels, hence promoting heart health
- Reduces the rate at which sugar is absorbed into the blood stream, hence helping maintain healthy blood sugar levels

- Since the body can't break down fiber for energy, it effectively has zero calories, but still fills up the stomach, hence reducing your calorie intake

More Functional Foods in Your Diet

Some foods provide specific health benefits other than basic nutritional benefits. These foods are called functional foods, and they are quite common in the Mediterranean diet. The table below shows the best functional foods to always have in your pantry, along with the benefits they provide.

Food	Benefits
Extra-virgin olive oil	Extra-virgin olive oil is loaded with monounsaturated fats and is an excellent source of phytochemicals, including polyphenolic compounds, squalene, and alpha-tocopherol. Health benefits include cardiovascular health, cancer prevention/protection, and immune boosting.
Lemons (zest and juice)	Citrus bioflavonoids benefit both cholesterol and triglycerides. Lemon is also dense source of vitamin C and exhibits anti-inflammatory properties.
Tomatoes and tomato products	Lycopene in tomato products promotes prostate health. Tomato is also a good source of vitamins A and C and carotenoids.
Grapes and grape products (such as red wine)	Phytochemicals in grapes, including polyphenols and resveratrol, promote heart health and brain protection.

Nuts	Nuts are loaded with monounsaturated fats and vitamin E; they also exhibit anti-inflammatory benefits and cardiovascular protection.
Yogurt	Yogurt is a fermented food providing healthy bacteria and healthy fats to your body.
Garlic	Garlic contains allicin, a phytochemical to help manage blood pressure.
Fresh herbs (parsley, basil, oregano, rosemary, and so on)	Herbs loaded with antioxidants and vitamins; plus, they contain heart-protective phytosterols. Some herbs are frequently used medicinally.
Olives	Olives are fermented foods providing healthy bacteria to the gut, along with heart-healthy omega-3 fatty acids.
Fatty fish	Fish are rich in omega-3 fatty acids and help reduce triglycerides and inflammation.
Leafy greens	Greens contain phytochemicals such as carotenoids, sulforaphanes, apigenin, and lutein/zeaxanthin. They're cancer protective, immune boosting, vision protective, and heart healthy.
Eggs	Eggs are loaded with vitamin D, lecithin, choline, and lutein/zeaxanthin. Benefits include vision health, brain health, hormone regulation, and bone health.

The Diet Includes Plenty of Pro-Biotic Foods

The human body is home to trillions of health-promoting microbes. These are commonly called "gut bacteria". Research has shown that a good balance of healthy bacteria in your system enhances your immune system, promotes digestion, and even helps with weight loss. The Mediterranean diet includes enough of these pro-biotic foods to make sure a healthy balance of these microbes is always maintained. A few of these pro-biotic foods are- cheese, wine yogurt, sourdough bread, and brined foods such as olives, artichokes, peppers, and capers.

The Diet is Anti-Diabetes

The Mediterranean diet is highly recommended for people with type-2 diabetes because the food in this diet is low on the **Glycaemic Index.** This index is a measure of how fast the carbohydrates in the food break down. If a food scores high on the index, that means that the food breaks down quickly, and causes a sudden spike in blood sugar. Foods low on this index break down slowly and steadily, providing a steady supply of energy to the body, which is healthy.

The Diet is Anti-Aging

The Mediterranean diet can help you feel younger, live longer, and look your best! Here's how the diet accomplishes this:

- **Anti-Disease:** The NIH-AARP Diet and Health Study published in the *Archives of Internal Medicine* in 2007 discovered that people who closely followed a Mediterranean-style diet were 12 to 20 percent less probable to die from cancer and all causes.
- **Anti-Wrinkle:** A study published in the *Journal of the American College of Nutrition* in 2001 discovered that people who followed a diet high in fruits, vegetables, nuts, legumes, and fish exhibited fewer wrinkles on their skin. More research is required on the subject, but you might as well try it out in the meantime.
- **Smoother skin:** The diet is loaded with vitamin C-rich foods, such as oranges, strawberries, and broccoli. These foods lead to higher production of collagen, the skin's support structure.

- **Anti-Inflammation:** Inflammation is an enemy of your heart health, joints, and skin. The Mediterranean diet is loaded with anti-inflammatory foods such as cold-water fish, walnuts, flaxseeds, and fresh herbs, which can help keep you feeling your best.
- **Anti-Alzheimer's:** A 2006 study at Columbia University Medical Canter discovered that participants who followed a Mediterranean-style diet had a 40 percent lower risk of Alzheimer's disease than those who didn't.
- **Forever Young Brain:** Brain structure changes as you age and can cause problems such as memory loss and dementia. According to a 2015 study published in *Neurology*, those who followed a Mediterranean diet, and consumed higher amounts of fish and lower amounts of meat, had less brain atrophy (loss of cells), providing better brain function as they grew older.

The Diet is Anti-Fat

The Mediterranean diet is great if you're looking to lose some weight. But it is even better if you follow the Mediterranean lifestyle while following the diet too. The overall composition of the diet when coupled with physical activity can work wonders!

Planning Your Meals

If you're a beginner and have not yet made the switch to the Mediterranean diet, you will need to identify what changes you need to make to your current diet to make it match closely with the Mediterranean diet. In time, the Mediterranean diet will come to you naturally, but to start off, you will need to plan in advance. You will need to plan your portion sizes, and how often you eat certain foods. The changes are small, but will benefit you in the long run. In this chapter, we will discuss these changes, and basic meal planning.

Importance of Meal Planning

Meal planning is all about creating a road map for what you're going to eat, when you will prepare the food, and what ingredients you will need to buy. It might sound simple, but will save you from a lot of headache, and make your transition to the Mediterranean diet much smoother. Meal planning is vital because:

- It enables you to be efficient with your time
- It enables you to plan what ingredients you will buy and when, so that when you cook them, they are at their freshest
- You don't have to worry about what to cook multiple times per day. You take care of it in one sitting.
- It saves money by reducing food wastage. You cook everything you buy while it is still fresh.

Meal Planning Techniques

Meal planning is a flexible process, and every person has their unique way of going for it. You will eventually discover how you like to plan your meals, but it would be useful to look at a few templates of the common ways of doing it.

- If you like to be moderately thorough and detailed, you can sit down and write what you will eat for breakfast, lunch, and dinner for each day of the week. If you like to munch on snacks from time to time, make sure you write those down too. Make sure the recipes you choose for that week are in season, and you can procure fresh ingredients for the written recipes.
- If you like to get all the thinking for the whole month done in a single sitting, you can prepare meal plans for multiple weeks, along with shopping lists that specify what you will buy, and when, in such a way that the ingredients are at their freshest at the time of cooking. This will take a while, but a good place to start if you have the time. Just make

- sure you don't plan for too long, and make a new plan with every season so you can get the good seasonal stuff.
- Once you get slightly well acquainted with the diet, you will start to have the Mediterranean staples in your pantry at all times, and you don't need to plan all three meals per day, or even your shopping list. You will have your favourite recipes that you will automatically shuffle as per your convenience. You will start to make larger batches so you can eat leftovers later if you're not in the mood to cook again. You might need to plan your big dinners once in a while, but that is about it. In a nutshell, Mediterranean cooking will come to you naturally and will require minimal planning.

Sample Summer Meal Plan

Making a meal plan is simple. Just pick a day, and now you have to pick a breakfast, a lunch, and a dinner recipe for that day. Look through the ingredients of each recipe to identify which recipes are in season, and then just pick one. For example, if you're deciding what to eat during a week in summer, you can make a table for each way in the week as follows:

	Monday
Breakfast	Any Breakfast recipe form this book you can prepare on a busy Monday morning during summer. Whip up an oatmeal, or boil a few eggs.
Snack	Any snack recipe from this book that will provide you the energy you need to get through to lunch. If you have leftovers from Sunday, grab those instead.
Lunch	Any big main course recipe from the book that will give you the energy to get through the rest of your workday.
Snack	Any snack recipe from the book to get you to dinner time. If you have leftovers from your previous meals, grab those instead.

| Dinner | Any big main course from this book. |

Now all you need to do is repeat the process for the rest of the days, and make sure there are at least two seafood recipes in the whole week, and as few meat recipes as possible. Slide a meat recipe in there once every four weeks if you absolutely have to, and even then, keep quantity of the meat small. It really is that simple. I hope you get the idea, and will be able to plan meals at your leisure now.

Buying the Ingredients

If you're used to heading to the market nearest to your home and picking up everything you need from there, you might need to change your habits a little; but only a little. You will still be getting most of your stuff at grocery stores, but you would do well to explore a little, and maybe you will find a few stores that sell fresher products. Below are a few guidelines you will need to follow when shopping for ingredients for the Mediterranean diet:

Shop Local if Possible: Big grocery stores usually source their items from the cheapest possible option they can find, and the cheapest option isn't necessarily the closest one. The farther they source their food from, the longer the food stays in transit, and the less fresh it is. Luckily, regardless of where you live, if you just set out to explore your nearby markets, you will definitely find speciality stores that source or produce their stuff locally. Good luck digging up these hidden gems in your locality! You could also run a google search for such stores, as most of these small stores are now starting to put their locations on google maps.

Local Farmer's Markets are your Friends: I'm not sure about you, but I personally love strolling through a farmer's market, picking out fresh seasonal produce. If you haven't tried it, what are you waiting for? Use the internet to find the nearest farmer's market and get shopping! Visit https://www.localharvest.org/ to find a nearby market if you're in the USA.

Get Into CSA: Community Supported Agriculture is a great way to grab some fresh seasonal produce. All you need to do is pay an upfront fee to a local farm, and in return they will send a box full of fresh produce every week!

More Stores to Look For: Do yourself a favour and look around till you find the best seafood seller, butcher, baker, Mediterranean market, green market, Italian market, or any other place you can get fresh ingredients for your diet.

Setting up Your Pantry

If you're serious about following the Mediterranean diet, you will need to set up your pantry accordingly. The Mediterranean diet has quite a few staple ingredients, and these are used often in the recipes in this book. Let us take a look at a few of these staples that you absolutely have to add to your pantry:

Canned and Dried Beans: Legumes are a staple in the Mediterranean diet, and vital source of protein. They are important ingredients in all kinds of Mediterranean recipes, and hence you will do well to have these on hand at all times. I personally prefer canned beans, but dried beans get the job done too.

Rice and Grains: Rice and grains are also staple ingredients of the Mediterranean diet, and will be used in a large percentage of the recipes in this book. Whole grains are the best. A few of the common grains you will want to keep on hand are: barley, farro, wheat berries, freekeh, and bulgur.

Pasta and Couscous: Pasta is an ingredient in quite a few Mediterranean dishes, and hence should be a staple in your pantry. Whole-wheat pasta is best. Mediterranean dishes also commonly use pearl couscous, which has a slightly bigger grains than regular couscous.

Olives and Olive Oil: Olives and Olive oil are two of the most important ingredients of the Mediterranean diet. When you head to your local market to buy olive oil, make sure you buy quality extra-virgin olive oil. Not all Extra-Virgin Olive Oils (EVOO) are created equal and the brand you choose definitely matters. I've done my fair share of testing in my lifetime, and if you're an American, the California Olive Ranch Everyday Extra Virgin Olive Oil is your best bet. It is quite popular and easily available on amazon.com if you can't find it in a nearby store. This oil is delicious and contains heart-healthy fats as discussed before. Never place olive oil on your kitchen counter, since strong sunlight will cause oxidation of the chlorophyll in the oil, producing stale, harsh flavours. Keeping your olive oil next to the stove is also a bad idea as heat greatly reduces shelf life. It is best to store EVOO in a dark pantry or cupboard; do not store olive oil in the fridge, as it can turn cloudy, thick, and viscous and can take a few hours to revert to normal. You can keep unopened oil for about a year; but once opened, it lasts only about ninety days—so don't buy too much in one go. And if possible, check the harvest date to ensure the freshest bottle possible. If you wish to store the oil in your own container or bottle, make sure it is not clear glass or plastic to reduce the amount of light entering the container/bottle.

When buying olives, it is best to buy unpitted ones, and then pit them later yourself. If, however, you're in a hurry, pre-pitted olives will do the job. To pit olives, start by placing the olives on a flat surface. After that, hold the blade of a knife flat on top of one of the olives. Now, lightly press down on the blade of the knife until the pit pops out. If the pit doesn't pop out all the way, pull it the rest of the way out using your fingers.

Fresh Herbs: Fresh herbs are vital flavouring ingredients in the Mediterranean diet. You will commonly see fresh herbs like mint, oregano, basil, dill, etc. used in the recipes in this book, and hence it is a good idea to keep your pantry stocked with these at all times. These ingredients are also commonly used to garnish the final dish. However, fresh herbs expire quite fast, and need to be stored correctly to make them keep for longer. Lightly wash and then dry your herbs thoroughly by rolling them in paper towels before storing them. These herbs should be placed in airtight bags such as a zipper-lock bag, and these bags should then be placed in the crisper drawer of your fridge.

Dried Herbs: Dried herbs are also a common ingredient in the recipes that follow, and you will do well to make a few of these a staple in your pantry. Rosemary and thyme are the most common dry herbs you should add to your pantry. A few of the recipes will also call for dried mint so make sure you have it before you start preparing a dish that calls for it. Dried herbs keep for longer than fresh ones. Once opened, dried herbs can last for six months to a year, depending on the type of herb. This information is usually provided on the packing. It is quite easy to convert fresh herbs to dry herbs by simply using the microwave. Just microwave them until they appear completely dehydrated. This proves usually takes about one to three minutes. Once dry, allow them to come to room temperature and then store them in a sealed container.

Spices, Spice Blends, and Pastes: Mediterranean dishes use common spices like cinnamon, saffron, paprika, etc. Most of these should be in your pantry already. You will find a few of the recipes in this book that use spices you don't have, and maybe haven't even heard of before, such as sumac, Aleppo pepper, parsley, etc. A few of the recipes in this book will also call for common spice blends and pastes such as:

- North African Ras El Hanout
- Harissa
- Za'atar

If you can't find these in a nearby store, just buy them online on amazon, or you could prepare these blends on your own. Make sure you store your spices away from heat and light to extend their shelf life.

Cheese, Cured Meats, and Nuts: Feta and Goat cheese are used in a few Mediterranean dishes in this book. Pancetta and Chorizo cured meats and nuts such as almonds and pine are also good to have on hand. When storing cheese, make sure to store it in your fridge after first coating it with a layer or parchment paper, and then with aluminium foil. It is best to store nuts in the freezer, and toast them before using in a recipe.

Yogurt: Although not a heavily used ingredient, a small amount of yogurt is used in quite a few recipes in this book and is hence nice to have on hand. Whole-milk yogurt is obviously best if you're going for the richest possible flavour.

Tahini: Used as a garnish, topping, or a base for sauces, Tahini is made using ground sesame seeds, and is good to have on hand as it is used in quite a few Mediterranean recipes. You can buy this from a nearby store, or online. You can also make your own.

Pomegranate molasses: This is basically dense pomegranate juice. It is used in quite a few Mediterranean recipes, and hence is good to have in your pantry. You can buy this from a nearby store, or online. You can also make your own.

Preserved lemons: Another important ingredient for quite a few Mediterranean dishes that you can buy, or make on your own. These last for several weeks, and are used to add a tangy flavour to the recipes.

Dukkah: It is an Egyptian condiment which is a mix of nuts, seeds, and spices. Make sure you have this with you if you plan to prepare a recipe that calls for it. You can buy this or prepare your own.

Mediterranean Spice Blends and Pastes

Most of these are easily available online, and probably even in a store near you. However, if you truly want full control over how your recipes turn out, you would do well to make these at home.

Dukkah

Yield: 2 cups

Ⓥ This is a Vegetarian Recipe Ⓥ

Ingredients:

- ⅓ cup black sesame seeds, toasted
- ½ cup shelled pistachios, toasted
- 1 (15-ounce) can chickpeas, rinsed
- 1 tablespoon cumin seeds, toasted
- 1 teaspoon extra-virgin olive oil
- 1¼ teaspoons 1½ teaspoons pepper
- 2 teaspoons fennel seeds, toasted
- 2½ tablespoons coriander seeds, toasted
- salt

Directions:

1. Place the oven rack in the centre of the oven and pre-heat your oven to 400 degrees. Pat chickpeas dry using paper towels and toss with oil. Lay out chickpeas into one layer in rimmed baking sheet and roast until browned and crisp, 40 to 45 minutes, stirring every 5 to 10 minutes; allow to cool fully.
2. Process chickpeas using a food processor until coarsely ground, about 10 seconds; move to medium bowl. Pulse pistachios and sesame seeds in now-empty food processor until coarsely ground, about 15 pulses; move to a container with chickpeas. Process coriander, cumin, and fennel seeds in again-empty food processor until finely ground, 2 to 3 minutes; move to a container with chickpeas. Put in pepper and salt and beat until mixture is thoroughly mixed. (Dukkah will keep safely in a fridge for maximum 1 month.)

Green Zhoug

Yield: Approximately ½ cup

This recipe can be made quickly

Ⓥ *This is a Vegetarian Recipe* Ⓥ

Ingredients:

- ¼ teaspoon ground cardamom
- ¼ teaspoon ground cumin
- ¼ teaspoon salt
- ½ cup fresh parsley leaves
- ½ teaspoon ground coriander
- ¾ cup fresh cilantro leaves
- 2 garlic cloves2 green Thai chiles, stemmed and chopped
- 6 tablespoons extra-virgin olive oil
- Pinch ground cloves
- , minced

Directions:

1. Microwave oil, coriander, cumin, cardamom, salt, and cloves in covered bowl until aromatic, approximately half a minute; allow to cool to room temperature.
2. Pulse oil-spice mixture, cilantro, parsley, chiles, and garlic using a food processor until coarse paste forms, about 15 pulses, scraping down sides of the container as required. (Green Zhoug will keep safely in a fridge for maximum 4 days.)

Harissa

Yield: Approximately ½ cup

✒ This recipe can be made quickly ✒

Ⓥ This is a Vegetarian Recipe Ⓥ

Ingredients:

- ½ teaspoon ¾ teaspoon caraway seeds
- 1 tablespoon ground coriander
- 1 tablespoon ground dried Aleppo pepper
- 1 teaspoon ground cumin
- 2 tablespoons paprika
- 6 garlic cloves, minced
- 6 tablespoons extra-virgin olive oil
- salt

Directions:

1. Mix all ingredients in a container and microwave until bubbling and very aromatic, approximately one minute, stirring halfway through microwaving.
2. Allow to cool to room temperature. (Harissa will keep safely in a fridge for maximum 4 days.)

Herbes de Provence

Yield: Approximately ½ cup

This recipe can be made quickly

Ⓥ This is a Vegetarian Recipe Ⓥ

Ingredients:

- 2 tablespoons dried marjoram
- 2 tablespoons dried rosemary
- 2 tablespoons dried thyme
- 2 teaspoons fennel seeds, toasted

Directions:

Mix all ingredients in a container. (Herbes de Provence can be stored at room temperature in airtight container for maximum 1 year.)

Ras el Hanout

Yield: Approximately ½ cup

This recipe can be made quickly

Ⓥ This is a Vegetarian Recipe Ⓥ

Ingredients:

- ¼ teaspoon black peppercorns
- ½ teaspoon allspice berries
- 16 cardamom pods
- 2 teaspoons 2 teaspoons anise seeds
- 2 teaspoons ground dried Aleppo pepper
- 2 teaspoons ground nutmeg
- 4 teaspoons coriander seeds
- 4 teaspoons cumin seeds

- 4 teaspoons ground ginger
- ground cinnamon

Directions:

1. Toast cardamom, coriander, cumin, anise, allspice, and peppercorns in small frying pan on moderate heat until aromatic, shaking frying pan occasionally to stop scorching, approximately two minutes. Allow it to cool to room temperature.
2. Move toasted spices, ginger, nutmeg, Aleppo, and cinnamon to spice grinder and process to fine powder. (Ras el hanout can be stored at room temperature in airtight container for maximum 1 year.)

Za'atar

Yield: Approximately ½ cup

This recipe can be made quickly

(V) This is a Vegetarian Recipe (V)

Ingredients:

- ½ cup dried thyme, ground
- 1½ tablespoons 2 tablespoons sesame seeds, toasted
- ground sumac

Directions:

Mix all ingredients in a container. (Za'atar can be stored at room temperature in airtight container for maximum 1 year.)

Pomegranate Molasses

Yield: ⅔ cup

This recipe can be made quickly

Ⓥ This is a Vegetarian Recipe Ⓥ

Ingredients:

- 1 tablespoon sugar
- 2 tablespoons water
- 2 teaspoons 4 cups unsweetened pomegranate juice
- If you over reduce the syrup in step 2, you can slowly beat in warm water as required to measure ⅔ cup.
- lemon juice

Directions:

1. Mix water and sugar in moderate-sized saucepan until sugar is completely moistened. Bring to boil on moderate to high heat and cook until sugar begins to turn golden, 2 to 3 minutes, gently swirling saucepan as required to ensure even cooking. Carry on cooking until sugar begins to smoke and is colour of peanut butter, approximately one minute. Remove from the heat, let caramel sit until mahogany brown, 45 to 60 seconds. Cautiously swirl in 2 tablespoons pomegranate juice until incorporated; mixture will bubble and steam. Slowly beat in remaining pomegranate juice and lemon juice, scraping up any caramel.
2. Bring mixture to boil on high heat and cook, stirring intermittently, until tight, slow-popping bubbles cover surface and syrup measures ⅔ cup, 30 to 35 minutes. Allow it to cool slightly, then move to container and continue to cool to room temperature. (Pomegranate molasses will keep safely in a fridge in airtight container for maximum 1 month.)

Preserved Lemons

Yield: 4 preserved lemons

Preserved Lemons are used in quite a few of the recipes that follow. You can buy these in a store, but it is best to make your own.

Ⓥ This is a Vegetarian Recipe Ⓥ

- 12 lemons, preferably Meyer
- ½ cup Diamond Crystal Kosher Salt or 6 tablespoons Morton Kosher Salt

Directions:

1. Wash and dry 4 lemons, then cut along the length into quarters, stopping 1 inch from bottom so lemons stay undamaged at base. Juice remaining lemons to yield 1½ cups juice; reserve extra juice to use as required.
2. Working over bowl, gently stretch 1 cut lemon open and pour 2 tablespoons salt into center. Gently rub cut surfaces of lemon together, then place in 1-quart jar. Replicate the process with the rest of the cut lemons and salt. Put in any accumulated salt and juice in a container to jar.
3. Pour 1½ cups lemon juice into jar and press gently to submerge lemons. (Put in more lemon juice to jar if needed to cover lemons fully.) Cover jar tightly with lid and shake. Refrigerate lemons, shaking jar once per day for first 4 days to redistribute salt and juice. Let lemons cure in refrigerator until glossy and softened, 6 to 8 weeks. (Preserved lemons will keep safely in a fridge for minimum 6 months.)
4. To use, cut off desired amount of preserved lemon. If desired, use knife to remove pulp and white pith from rind before using.

Quick Method:

1. It takes at least 6 weeks to make your own preserved lemons; however, if needed you can make a quick substitute: Mix four 2-inch strips lemon zest, minced, 1 teaspoon lemon juice, ½ teaspoon water, ¼ teaspoon sugar, and ¼ teaspoon salt. Microwave mixture at 50 percent power until liquid evaporates, about 1½ minutes, stirring and mashing lemon with back of spoon every 30 seconds. Makes about 1 tablespoon.

Gently stretch open quartered lemon, pour salt into center, and rub cut surfaces together; place in 1-quart jar. Pour lemon juice into jar and press gently to immerse lemons.

Snacks and Appetizers

Snacks and appetizers are great to munch on while you get to your next big meal. They also serve as a great first course if you're serving a multiple course meal. The Mediterranean diet offers numerous delicious and nutritious antipasti, tapas, meze, and other small plates to choose from. So, without much ado, let us dive into the recipes!

Baba Ghanoush

Yield: Approximately 2 cups

Ⓥ This is a Vegetarian Recipe Ⓥ

Baba ghanoush is a delicious and nutritious meze staple popular in Israel, Lebanon, Palestine, and many other countries!

Ingredients:

- 1 small garlic clove, minced
- 2 eggplants (1 pound each), pricked all over with fork
- 2 tablespoons extra-virgin olive oil, plus extra for serving
- 2 tablespoons tahini
- 2 teaspoons chopped fresh parsley
- 4 teaspoons lemon juice
- Salt and pepper to taste

Directions:

1. Place the oven rack in the centre of the oven and pre-heat your oven to 500 degrees. Place eggplants on a baking sheet coated with aluminium foil and roast, flipping the eggplants every fifteen minutes, until consistently soft when pressed using tongs, forty minutes to one hour. Allow eggplants to cool for 5 minutes over a baking sheet.
2. Place a colander on top of a container. Slice the top and bottom off each eggplant and slit eggplants along the length. Using

spoon, scoop hot pulp into colander (you should have about 2 cups pulp); discard skins. Allow the pulp to drain for about three minutes.
3. Move drained eggplant to your food processor. Put in tahini, oil, lemon juice, garlic, ¾ teaspoon salt, and ¼ teaspoon pepper. Pulse the mixture until a rough puree is achieved, approximately 8 pulses. Drizzle with salt and pepper to taste.
4. Move to serving bowl, cover firmly using plastic wrap, put inside your fridge until chilled, about 1 hour. (Dip will keep safely in a fridge for up to 24 hours; bring to room temperature before you serve.) Drizzle with salt and pepper to taste, sprinkle with extra oil to taste, and drizzle with parsley before you serve.

Brown Feta

Yield: 8 to 12 Servings

✐ This recipe can be made quickly ✐

Ⓥ This is a Vegetarian Recipe Ⓥ

This vegetarian appetizer is for all the Feta lovers out there. Quick and easy to prepare, this recipe tastes great with parsley and olive oil.

Ingredients:

- 2 (8-ounce) blocks feta cheese, sliced into ½-inch-thick slabs
- ¼ teaspoon red pepper flakes
- ¼ teaspoon pepper
- 2 tablespoons extra-virgin olive oil
- 2 teaspoons minced fresh parsley

Directions:

1. Place oven rack 4 inches from broiler element and heat broiler. Pat feta dry using paper towels and lay out on broiler-safe gratin dish.

2. Drizzle with red pepper flakes and pepper. Broil until edges of cheese start to look golden, three to eight minutes. Sprinkle with oil, drizzle with parsley, and serve instantly.

Bruschetta with Artichoke Hearts and Parmesan

Yield: 8 to 10 Servings

This recipe can be made quickly

Ⓥ This is a Vegetarian Recipe Ⓥ

Ingredients:

- 1 cup jarred whole baby artichoke hearts packed in water, rinsed and patted dry
- 1 garlic clove, minced
- 1 recipe Toasted Bread for Bruschetta
- 2 ounces Parmesan cheese, 1 ounce grated fine, 1 ounce shaved
- 2 tablespoons chopped fresh basil
- 2 tablespoons extra-virgin olive oil, plus extra for serving
- 2 teaspoons lemon juice
- Salt and pepper

Directions:

1. Pulse artichoke hearts, oil, basil, lemon juice, garlic, ¼ teaspoon salt, and ¼ teaspoon pepper using a food processor until coarsely pureed, about 6 pulses, scraping down sides of the container as required. Put in grated Parmesan and pulse to combine, about 2 pulses.
2. Lay out artichoke mixture uniformly toasts and top with shaved Parmesan. Season with pepper to taste, and sprinkle with extra oil to taste. Serve.

Bruschetta with Arugula Pesto and Goat Cheese

Yield: 8 to 10 Servings

This recipe can be made quickly

Ⓥ This is a Vegetarian Recipe Ⓥ

Ingredients:

- ¼ cup extra-virgin olive oil, plus extra for serving
- ¼ cup pine nuts, toasted
- 1 recipe Toasted Bread for Bruschetta
- 1 tablespoon minced shallot
- 1 teaspoon grated lemon zest plus 1 teaspoon juice
- 2 ounces goat cheese, crumbled
- 5 ounces (5 cups) baby arugula
- Salt and pepper

Directions:

1. Pulse arugula, oil, pine nuts, shallot, lemon zest and juice, ½ teaspoon salt, and ¼ teaspoon pepper using a food processor until mostly smooth, approximately 8 pulses, scraping down sides of the container as required.
2. Lay out arugula mixture uniformly toasts, top with goat cheese, and sprinkle with extra oil to taste. Serve.

Bruschetta with Black Olive Pesto, Ricotta, and Basil

Yield: 8 to 10 Servings

This recipe can be made quickly

Ⓥ *This is a Vegetarian Recipe* Ⓥ

Ingredients:

- ¾ cup pitted kalamata olives
- 1 garlic clove, minced
- 1 recipe Toasted Bread for Bruschetta
- 1 small shallot, minced
- 10 ounces whole-milk ricotta cheese
- 1½ teaspoons lemon juice
- 2 tablespoons extra-virgin olive oil, plus extra for serving
- 2 tablespoons shredded fresh basil
- Salt and pepper

Directions:

1. Pulse olives, shallot, oil, lemon juice, and garlic using a food processor until coarsely chopped, approximately ten pulses, scraping down sides of the container as required. Season ricotta with salt and pepper to taste.
2. Lay out ricotta mixture uniformly toasts, top with olive mixture, and sprinkle with extra oil to taste. Drizzle with basil before you serve.

Bruschetta with Ricotta, Tomatoes, and Basil

Yield: 8 to 10 Servings

This recipe can be made quickly

Ⓥ *This is a Vegetarian Recipe* Ⓥ

Ingredients:

- 1 pound cherry tomatoes, quartered
- 1 recipe Toasted Bread for Bruschetta
- 1 tablespoon extra-virgin olive oil, plus extra for serving
- 10 ounces whole-milk ricotta cheese
- 5 tablespoons shredded fresh basil
- Salt and pepper

Directions:

1. Toss tomatoes with 1 teaspoon salt using a colander and allow to drain for about fifteen minutes. Move drained tomatoes to a container, toss with oil and ¼ cup basil, and sprinkle with salt and pepper to taste. In a different container, combine ricotta with remaining 1 tablespoon basil and sprinkle with salt and pepper to taste.
2. Lay out ricotta mixture uniformly toasts, top with tomato mixture, and drizzle lightly with extra oil to taste. Serve.

Caponata

Yield: Approximately 3 cups

Ⓥ This is a Vegetarian Recipe Ⓥ

A delicious and nutritious snack for all eggplant lovers!

Ingredients:

- ¼ cup chopped fresh parsley
- ¼ cup pine nuts, toasted
- ¼ cup raisins
- ¼ cup red wine vinegar, plus extra for seasoning
- ½ teaspoon salt
- ¾ cup V8 juice
- 1 celery rib, chopped fine
- 1 large eggplant (1½ pounds), cut into ½-inch cubes
- 1 large tomato, cored, seeded, and chopped

- 1 red bell pepper, stemmed, seeded, and chopped fine
- 1 small onion, chopped fine (½ cup)
- 1½ teaspoons minced anchovy fillets (2 to 3 fillets)
- 2 tablespoons brown sugar
- 2 tablespoons extra-virgin olive oil
- 2 tablespoons minced black olives

Directions:

1. Toss eggplant with salt in a container. Thoroughly coat the full surface of big microwave-safe plate using double layer of coffee filters and lightly spray using vegetable oil spray. Lay out eggplant in a uniform layer on coffee filters. Microwave until eggplant is dry and shrivelled to one-third of its original size, about eight to fifteen minutes (Do not let it brown). Move eggplant instantly to paper towel–lined plate.
2. In the meantime, beat V8 juice, vinegar, sugar, parsley, and anchovies together in medium bowl. Mix in tomato, raisins, and olives.
3. Heat 1 tablespoon oil in 12-inch non-stick frying pan on moderate to high heat until it starts to shimmer. Put in eggplant and cook, stirring intermittently, until edges become browned, about four to eight minutes, adding 1 teaspoon more oil if pan seems to be dry; move to a container.
4. Put in remaining 2 teaspoons oil to now-empty frying pan and heat on moderate to high heat until it starts to shimmer. Put in celery, bell pepper, and onion and cook, stirring intermittently, till they become tender and edges are spotty brown, 6 to 8 minutes.
5. Decrease heat to moderate to low and mix in eggplant and V8 juice mixture. Bring to simmer and cook until V8 juice becomes thick and covers the vegetables, four to eight minutes. Move to serving bowl and allow to cool to room temperature. (Caponata will keep safely in a fridge for up to seven days; bring to room temperature before you serve.)
6. Drizzle with extra vinegar to taste and drizzle with pine nuts before you serve.

Classic Hummus

Yield: Approximately 2 cups

(V) This is a Vegetarian Recipe (V)

A popular recipe enjoyed throughout the eastern Mediterranean, Classic Hummus is an easy snack to prepare using simple ingredients!

Ingredients:

- ¼ cup water
- ¼ teaspoon ground cumin
- ½ teaspoon salt
- 1 (15-ounce) can chickpeas, rinsed
- 1 small garlic clove, minced
- 2 tablespoons extra-virgin olive oil, plus extra for serving
- 3 tablespoons lemon juice
- 6 tablespoons tahini
- Pinch cayenne pepper

Directions:

1. Mix water and lemon juice in a small-sized container. In a different container, beat tahini and oil together.
2. Process chickpeas, garlic, salt, cumin, and cayenne using a food processor until thoroughly ground, approximately fifteen seconds.
3. Scrape down sides of the container using a rubber spatula. While the machine runs, put in lemon juice mixture gradually. Scrape down sides of the container and carry on processing for about sixty seconds. While the machine runs, put in tahini mixture gradually and process until hummus is smooth and creamy, approximately fifteen seconds, scraping down sides of the container as required.

4. Move hummus to serving bowl, cover up using plastic wrap, and allow to sit at room temperature until flavours blend, approximately half an hour.
5. If you wish, you can refrigerate this dish for up to 5 days.
6. If needed, loosen hummus using 1 tablespoon warm water. Sprinkle with extra oil to taste before you serve.

Dolmathes

Yield: 24

(V) This is a Vegetarian Recipe (V)

A Greek delicacy, this recipe is basically stuffed grape leaves.

Ingredients:

- ¼ cup chopped fresh mint
- ⅓ cup chopped fresh dill
- ¾ cup short-grain white rice
- 1 (16-ounce) jar grape leaves
- 1 large onion, chopped fine
- 1½ tablespoons grated lemon zest plus 2 tablespoons juice
- 2 tablespoons extra-virgin olive oil, plus extra for serving
- Salt and pepper

Directions:

1. Reserve 24 intact grape leaves, approximately 6 inches in diameter; save for later rest of the leaves. Bring 6 cups water to boil in moderate-sized saucepan. Put in reserved grape leaves and cook for about sixty seconds. Gently drain leaves and move to a container of cold water to cool, about 5 minutes. Drain again, then move leaves to plate and cover loosely using plastic wrap.
2. Heat oil in now-empty saucepan over medium heat until it starts to shimmer. Put in onion and ½ teaspoon salt and cook till they become tender and lightly browned, 5 to 7 minutes. Put in

rice and cook, stirring frequently, until grain edges begin to turn translucent, approximately two minutes. Mix in ¾ cup water and bring to boil. Decrease heat to low, cover, and simmer gently until rice becomes soft but still firm in center and water has been absorbed, 10 to 12 minutes. Remove from the heat, let rice cool slightly, about 10 minutes. Mix in dill, mint, and lemon zest. (Blanched grape leaves and filling will keep safely in a fridge for up to 24 hours.)

3. Place 1 blanched leaf smooth side down on counter with stem facing you. Get rid of the stem from base of leaf by slicing along both sides of stem to form thin triangle. Pat leaf dry using paper towels. Overlap cut ends of leaf to stop any filling from leaking out. Place heaping tablespoon filling ¼ inch from bottom of leaf where ends overlap. Fold bottom over filling and fold in sides. Roll leaf tightly around filling to create tidy roll. Replicate the process with the rest of the blanched leaves and filling.

4. Line 12-inch frying pan with one layer of remaining leaves. Place rolled leaves seam side down in tight rows in prepared skillet. Mix 1¼ cups water and lemon juice, put in to skillet, and bring to simmer over medium heat. Cover, decrease the heat to moderate to low, and simmer until water is almost completely absorbed and leaves and rice are tender and cooked through, forty to sixty minutes.

5. Move stuffed grape leaves to serving platter and allow to cool to room temperature, approximately half an hour; discard leaves in skillet. Sprinkle with extra oil before you serve.

Easy Toasted Almonds

Yield: 2 cups

This recipe can be made quickly

Ⓥ This is a Vegetarian Recipe Ⓥ

Meze platters are a delicious part of the Mediterranean diet, and toasted nuts are a vital part of it.

Ingredients:

- ¼ teaspoon pepper
- 1 tablespoon extra-virgin olive oil
- 1 teaspoon salt
- 2 cups skin-on raw whole almonds

Directions:

1. Heat oil in 12-inch non-stick frying pan on moderate to high heat until it barely starts shimmering. Put in almonds, salt, and pepper and decrease the heat to moderate to low. Cook, stirring frequently, until almonds become aromatic and their colour becomes somewhat deep, approximately eight minutes.
2. Move almonds to plate coated using paper towels and allow to cool before you serve.
3. If you wish, you can store Almonds at room temperature for up to 5 days.

Fiery Red Whipped Feta

Yield: Approximately 2 cups

This recipe can be made quickly

(V) This is a Vegetarian Recipe (V)

The Greeks call this recipe "htipiti". This simple dish tastes great and is super quick and easy to make.

Ingredients:

- ¼ teaspoon pepper
- ⅓ cup extra-virgin olive oil, plus extra for serving
- ½ teaspoon cayenne pepper
- 1 cup jarred roasted red peppers, rinsed, patted dry, and chopped
- 1 tablespoon lemon juice

- 8 ounces feta cheese, crumbled (2 cups)

Directions:

1. Process feta, red peppers, oil, lemon juice, cayenne, and pepper using a food processor until smooth, approximately half a minute, scraping down sides of the container as required.
2. Move mixture to serving bowl, sprinkle with extra oil to taste, and serve. (Dip will keep safely in a fridge for up to 2 days; bring to room temperature before you serve.)

Flavourful Calamari with Oranges

Yield: 6 to 8 Servings

An aromatic snack from France!

Ingredients:

- ¼ cup extra-virgin olive oil
- ⅓ cup hazelnuts, toasted, skinned, and chopped
- 1 red bell pepper, stemmed, seeded, and cut into 2-inch-long matchsticks
- 1 shallot, sliced thin
- 1 teaspoon Dijon mustard
- 2 celery ribs, sliced thin on bias
- 2 garlic cloves, minced
- 2 oranges
- 2 pounds squid, bodies sliced crosswise into ¼-inch-thick rings, tentacles halved
- 2 tablespoons baking soda
- 2½ tablespoons harissa
- 3 tablespoons chopped fresh mint
- 3 tablespoons red wine vinegar
- Salt and pepper

Directions:

1. Dissolve baking soda and 1 tablespoon salt in 3 cups cold water in large container. Submerge squid in brine, cover, put inside your fridge for about fifteen minutes. Remove squid from brine and separate bodies from tentacles.
2. Bring 8 cups water to boil in a big saucepan on moderate to high heat. Fill big container with ice water. Put in 2 tablespoons salt and tentacles to boiling water and cook for 30 seconds. Put in bodies and cook until bodies are firm and opaque throughout, about 90 seconds. Drain squid, move to ice water, and allow to sit until chilled, about 5 minutes.
3. Beat oil, vinegar, harissa, garlic, mustard, 1½ teaspoons salt, and ½ teaspoon pepper together in a big container. Drain squid well and put in to a container with dressing.
4. Cut away peel and pith from oranges. Quarter oranges, then slice crosswise into ½-inch-thick pieces. Put in oranges, bell pepper, celery, and shallot to squid and toss to coat. Cover and put in the fridge for minimum sixty minutes or up to 24 hours. Mix in hazelnuts and mint and sprinkle with salt and pepper to taste before you serve.

Flavourful Green-Black Olives

Yield: 8 Servings

(V) This is a Vegetarian Recipe (V)

Why buy marinated olives from a store when you can create a much more delicious version of the snack right at home?

Ingredients:

- ½ teaspoon red pepper flakes
- ½ teaspoon salt
- ¾ cup extra-virgin olive oil
- 1 cup brine-cured black olives with pits
- 1 cup brine-cured green olives with pits
- 1 garlic clove, minced

- 1 shallot, minced
- 2 teaspoons grated lemon zest
- 2 teaspoons minced fresh oregano
- 2 teaspoons minced fresh thyme

Directions:

1. Wash olives comprehensively, then drain and pat dry using paper towels.
2. Toss olives with the rest of the ingredients in a container, cover, put inside your fridge for minimum 4 hours or for maximum 4 days. Allow to sit at room temperature for minimum half an hour before you serve.

Flavourful Saffron Caulipeas

Yield: 6 to 8 Servings

Ⓥ This is a Vegetarian Recipe Ⓥ

Marinated chickpeas and cauliflower taste absolutely amazing with saffron!

Ingredients:

- ⅛ teaspoon saffron threads, crumbled
- ⅓ cup extra-virgin olive oil
- ½ head cauliflower (1 pound), cored and cut into 1-inch florets
- ½ lemon, sliced thin
- 1 cup canned chickpeas, rinsed
- 1 small sprig fresh rosemary
- 1 tablespoon minced fresh parsley
- 1½ teaspoons smoked paprika
- 1½ teaspoons sugar
- 2 tablespoons sherry vinegar
- 5 garlic cloves, peeled and smashed
- Salt and pepper

Directions:

1. Bring 2 quarts water to boil in a big saucepan. Put in cauliflower and 1 tablespoon salt and cook until florets start to become tender, approximately three minutes. Drain florets and move to paper towel–lined baking sheet.
2. Mix ¼ cup hot water and saffron in a container; set aside. Heat oil and garlic in small saucepan over moderate to low heat until aromatic and starting to sizzle but not brown, four to eight minutes. Mix in sugar, paprika, and rosemary and cook until aromatic, approximately half a minute. Remove from the heat, mix in saffron mixture, vinegar, 1½ teaspoons salt, and ¼ teaspoon pepper.
3. Mix florets, saffron mixture, chickpeas, and lemon in a big container. Cover and place in the fridge, stirring intermittently, for minimum 4 hours or for maximum 3 days. To serve, discard rosemary sprig, move cauliflower and chickpeas to serving bowl using a slotted spoon, and drizzle with parsley.

Garmary White Bean Dip

Yield: Approximately 1¼ cups

✒ *This recipe can be made quickly* ✒

Ⓥ *This is a Vegetarian Recipe* Ⓥ

White beans are a staple ingredient in Mediterranean cuisines from Turkey to Tuscany. These beans are smooth and taste delicious!

Ingredients:

- ¼ cup extra-virgin olive oil
- 1 (15-ounce) can cannellini beans, rinsed
- 1 small garlic clove, minced
- 1 teaspoon minced fresh rosemary
- 2 tablespoons water

- 2 teaspoons lemon juice
- Pinch cayenne pepper
- Salt and pepper

Directions:

1. Process beans, 3 tablespoons oil, water, lemon juice, rosemary, garlic, ¼ teaspoon salt, ¼ teaspoon pepper, and cayenne using a food processor until smooth, approximately fifty seconds, scraping down sides of the container as required.
2. Move to serving bowl, cover up using plastic wrap, and allow to sit at room temperature until flavours blend, approximately half an hour.
3. (Dip will keep safely in a fridge for up to 24 hours; if needed, loosen dip using 1 tablespoon warm water before you serve.) Drizzle with salt and pepper to taste and drizzle with residual 1 tablespoon oil before you serve.

Giardiniera

Yield: four 1-pint jars

(V) This is a Vegetarian Recipe (V)

Love the taste of pickles? Try this Italian veggie delight.

Ingredients:

- ¼ cup sugar
- ½ head cauliflower (1 pound), cored and cut into ½-inch florets
- 1 cup chopped fresh dill
- 1 red bell pepper, stemmed, seeded, and cut into ½-inch-wide strips
- 2 serrano chiles, stemmed and sliced thin
- 2 tablespoons salt
- 2¼ cups water
- 2¾ cups white wine vinegar

- 3 carrots, peeled and sliced ¼ inch thick on bias
- 3 celery ribs, cut crosswise into ½-inch pieces
- 4 garlic cloves, sliced thin

Directions:

1. Mix cauliflower, carrots, celery, bell pepper, serranos, and garlic in a big container, then move to four 1-pint jars with tight-fitting lids.
2. Bundle dill in cheesecloth and tie using a kitchen twine to secure. Bring dill sachet, vinegar, water, sugar, and salt to boil in a big saucepan on moderate to high heat. Turn off the heat and allow to steep for about ten minutes. Discard dill sachet.
3. Return brine to brief boil, then pour uniformly over vegetables. Allow it to cool to room temperature, then cover put inside your fridge until vegetables taste pickled, minimum 7 days or maximum 1 month.

Infused Artichokes

Yield: 6 to 8 Servings

(V) This is a Vegetarian Recipe (V)

Marinated Artichokes taste absolutely amazing and can be thrown on pretty much everything.

Ingredients:

- ¼ teaspoon red pepper flakes
- 2 lemons
- 2 sprigs fresh thyme
- 2 tablespoons minced fresh mint
- 2½ cups extra-virgin olive oil
- 3 pounds baby artichokes (2 to 4 ounces each)
- 8 garlic cloves, peeled, 6 cloves smashed, 2 cloves minced
- Salt and pepper

Directions:

1. Take a vegetable peeler and use it to remove three 2-inch strips zest from 1 lemon. Grate ½ teaspoon zest from second lemon and set aside. Halve and juice lemons to yield ¼ cup juice, saving the spent lemon halves for later.
2. Mix oil and lemon zest strips in a big saucepan. Working with 1 artichoke at a time, cut top quarter off each artichoke, eliminate the outer leaves, and slice off any dark parts. Peel and trim stem, then cut artichoke in half along the length (quarter artichoke if large). Rub each artichoke half with previously saved spent lemon half and put in saucepan.
3. Put in smashed garlic, pepper flakes, thyme sprigs, 1 teaspoon salt, and ¼ teaspoon pepper to saucepan and quickly bring to simmer on high heat. Decrease heat to moderate to low and simmer, stirring intermittently to submerge all artichokes, until artichokes can be pierced with fork but are still firm, about 5 minutes. Remove from heat, cover, and allow to sit until artichokes are fork-tender and fully cooked, approximately twenty minutes.
4. Gently mix in ½ teaspoon reserved grated lemon zest, ¼ cup reserved lemon juice, and minced garlic. Move artichokes and oil to serving bowl and allow to cool to room temperature. Drizzle with salt to taste and drizzle with mint. Serve. (Artichokes and oil will keep safely in a fridge for up to 4 days.)

Labneh

Yield: Approximately 1 cup

Ⓥ This is a Vegetarian Recipe Ⓥ

Basically, this recipe is strained yogurt with its whey removed, making it a delicious, thick, rich, and tangy delicacy. It is highly popular in eastern Mediterranean regions.

Ingredients:

- 2 cups plain yogurt

Directions:

1. Cover fine-mesh strainer using 3 basket-style coffee filters or double layer of cheesecloth. Set strainer over big measuring vessel with plenty of room on the bottom.
2. Spoon yogurt into strainer, cover firmly using plastic wrap, put inside your fridge until yogurt has discharged approximately one cup liquid and has creamy, cream cheese–like texture, minimum 10 hours or for maximum 2 days.
3. Move drained yogurt to a clean bowl; discard liquid. Serve. (Yogurt will keep safely in a fridge for up to 2 days.)

Lavash Crackers

Yield: 10 to 12 Servings

Ⓥ *This is a Vegetarian Recipe* Ⓥ

This crispy eastern Mediterranean snack will taste great with a dip of your choice!

Ingredients:

- ⅓ cup extra-virgin olive oil, plus extra for brushing
- ¾ cup (3¾ ounces) all-purpose flour
- ¾ cup (4⅛ ounces) whole-wheat flour
- ¾ teaspoon salt
- 1 cup warm water
- 1 large egg, lightly beaten
- 1 teaspoon coarsely ground pepper
- 1½ cups (8⅝ ounces) semolina flour
- 2 tablespoons sesame seeds
- 2 teaspoons sea salt or kosher salt

Directions:

1. Use a stand mixer with a dough hook attachment to combine semolina flour, whole-wheat flour, all-purpose flour, and salt together on low speed. Progressively put in water and oil and knead until dough is smooth and elastic, seven to nine minutes. Turn dough out onto slightly floured counter and knead using your hands to form smooth, round ball. Split the dough into 4 equivalent pieces, brush with oil, and cover up using plastic wrap. Allow to rest at room temperature for about one hour.
2. Place two oven racks in your oven one just above, and one just below the middle position and pre-heat your oven to 425 degrees. Slightly coat two 18 by 13-inch rimless (or inverted) baking sheets using vegetable oil spray.
3. Work with two pieces of dough at a time while keeping the rest covered in plastic. Press dough into small rectangles, then move to the readied sheets. Using rolling pin and hands, roll and stretch dough uniformly to edges of sheet. Using fork, make holes in doughs at 2-inch gaps. Brush doughs with beaten egg, then drizzle each with 1½ teaspoons sesame seeds, ½ teaspoon salt, and ¼ teaspoon pepper. Push lightly on seasonings to help them stick.
4. Bake crackers until a deep golden brown colour is achieved, fifteen to twenty minutes, switching and rotating sheets halfway through baking. Move crackers to wire rack and allow to cool fully. Allow the baking sheets to cool to room temperature before rolling out and baking the rest of the dough. Break cooled lavash into big crackers and serve. (Lavash can be stored safely at room temperature for up to 2 weeks.)

Muhammara

Yield: Approximately 2 cups

✎ *This recipe can be made quickly* ✎

Ⓥ *This is a Vegetarian Recipe* Ⓥ

A delicious Syrian delicacy that goes swimmingly with any vegetable dish.

Ingredients:

- ⅛ teaspoon cayenne pepper
- ¼ cup plain wheat crackers, crumbled
- ½ teaspoon ground cumin
- ¾ teaspoon salt
- 1 cup walnuts, toasted
- 1 tablespoon minced fresh parsley (optional)
- 1½ cups jarred roasted red peppers, rinsed and patted dry
- 2 tablespoons extra-virgin olive oil
- 3 tablespoons pomegranate molasses
- Lemon juice, as required

Directions:

1. Pulse all ingredients except parsley using a food processor until smooth, approximately ten pulses. Move to serving bowl, cover, put inside your fridge for about fifteen minutes. (Dip will keep safely in a fridge for up to 24 hours; bring to room temperature before you serve.)
2. Drizzle with lemon juice, salt, and cayenne to taste and drizzle with parsley, if using, before you serve.

Mussels Escabèche

Yield: 6 to 8 Servings

This aromatic briny snack is goof for any occasion!

Ingredients:

- ¼ cup sherry vinegar
- ⅓ cup extra-virgin olive oil
- ½ small red onion, sliced ¼ inch thick
- ⅔ cup water

- ⅔ cup white wine
- ¾ teaspoon smoked paprika
- 2 bay leaves
- 2 pounds mussels, scrubbed and debearded
- 2 sprigs fresh thyme
- 2 tablespoons minced fresh parsley
- 4 garlic cloves, sliced thin
- Salt and pepper

Directions:

1. Bring wine and water to boil in Dutch oven on high heat. Put in mussels, cover, and cook, stirring intermittently, until mussels open, 3 to 6 minutes. Strain mussels and discard cooking liquid and any mussels that have not opened. Let mussels cool slightly, then remove mussels from shells and place in a big container; discard shells.
2. Heat oil in now-empty Dutch oven over medium heat until it starts to shimmer. Put in onion, garlic, bay leaves, thyme, 1 tablespoon parsley, and paprika. Cook, stirring frequently, until garlic is aromatic and onion is slightly wilted, about 1 minute.
3. Remove from the heat, mix in vinegar, ¼ teaspoon salt, and ⅛ teaspoon pepper. Pour mixture over mussels and allow to sit for about fifteen minutes. (Mussels will keep safely in a fridge for up to 2 days; bring to room temperature before you serve.) Drizzle with salt and pepper to taste and drizzle with remaining 1 tablespoon parsley before you serve.

Olive Oil–Sea Salt Pita Chips

Yield: 8 Servings

✎ *This recipe can be made quickly* ✎

Ⓥ *This is a Vegetarian Recipe* Ⓥ

Ingredients:

- ½ cup extra-virgin olive oil
- 1 teaspoon sea salt or kosher salt
- 4 (8-inch) pita breads

Directions:

1. Place two oven racks in your oven one just above, and one just below the middle position and pre-heat your oven to 350 degrees. Using kitchen shears, slice around perimeter of each pita and divide into 2 thin rounds.
2. Work with the rounds one at a time, and brush rough side heavily with oil and season with salt. Stack rounds one over the other, rough side up, as you go. Take a chef's knife and slice pita stack into 8 wedges. Lay out wedges, rough side up and in one layer, on 2 rimmed baking sheets.
3. Bake until wedges start to look golden brown and crisp, about fifteen minutes, rotating and switching sheets halfway through baking. Allow it to cool before you serve. (Pita chips can be stored safely at room temperature for up to 3 days.)

Packed Sardines

Yield: 8 Servings

Sardines make a scrumptious seafood snack.

Ingredients:

- ¼ cup golden raisins, chopped fine
- ¼ cup pine nuts, toasted and chopped fine
- ⅓ cup capers, rinsed and minced
- ⅓ cup panko bread crumbs
- 2 garlic cloves, minced
- 2 tablespoons minced fresh parsley
- 2 teaspoons grated orange zest plus wedges for serving
- 3 tablespoons extra-virgin olive oil

- 8 fresh sardines (2 to 3 ounces each), scaled, gutted, head and tail on
- Salt and pepper

Directions:

1. Place oven rack to lower-middle position and pre-heat your oven to 450 degrees. Coat rimmed baking sheet using aluminium foil. Mix capers, raisins, pine nuts, 1 tablespoon oil, parsley, orange zest, garlic, ¼ teaspoon salt, and ¼ teaspoon pepper in a container. Put in panko and slowly mix until blended.
2. Use a paring knife to slit belly of fish open from gill to tail, leaving spine undamaged. Gently rinse fish under cold running water and pat dry using paper towels. Rub skin of sardines evenly with remaining 2 tablespoons oil and sprinkle with salt and pepper.
3. Place sardines on readied sheet, spaced 1 inch apart. Stuff cavities of each sardine with 2 tablespoons filling and push on filling to help it stick; softly press fish closed.
4. Bake until fish flakes apart when softly poked using paring knife and filling is golden brown, about fifteen minutes. Serve with orange wedges.

Provençal Anchovy Dip

Yield: Approximately 1½ cups

A flavourful dip to go with vegetables!

Ingredients:

- ¼ cup extra-virgin olive oil, plus extra for serving
- ¼ cup water
- ¾ cup whole blanched almonds
- 1 garlic clove, minced

- 1 tablespoon minced fresh chives
- 1 teaspoon Dijon mustard
- 2 tablespoons lemon juice, plus extra for serving
- 2 tablespoons raisins
- 20 anchovy fillets (1½ ounces), rinsed, patted dry, and minced
- Salt and pepper

Directions:

1. Bring 4 cups water to boil in moderate-sized saucepan on moderate to high heat. Put in almonds and cook till they become tender, approximately twenty minutes. Drain and wash thoroughly.
2. Process drained almonds, anchovies, water, raisins, lemon juice, garlic, mustard, ¼ teaspoon pepper, and ⅛ teaspoon salt using a food processor until a somewhat smooth paste is achieved, approximately two minutes, scraping down sides of the container as required. While your food processor runs slowly put in oil and process to smooth puree, approximately two minutes.
3. Move mixture to a container, mix in 2 teaspoons chives, and sprinkle with salt and extra lemon juice to taste. (Dip will keep safely in a fridge for up to 2 days; bring to room temperature before you serve.) Drizzle with the rest of the chives and extra oil to taste before you serve.

Rich Turkish Nut Dip

Yield: Approximately 1 cup

✒ This recipe can be made quickly ✒

Ⓥ This is a Vegetarian Recipe Ⓥ

A delicious and nutritious ultra-smooth dip from Turkey!

Ingredients:

- ¼ cup extra-virgin olive oil
- ¾ cup water, plus extra as required
- 1 cup blanched almonds, blanched hazelnuts, pine nuts, or walnuts, toasted
- 1 slice hearty white sandwich bread, crusts removed, torn into 1-inch pieces
- 1 small garlic clove, minced
- 2 tablespoons lemon juice, plus extra as required
- Pinch cayenne pepper
- Salt and pepper

Directions:

1. Using a fork, mash bread and water together in a container till it turns into a paste. Process bread mixture, nuts, oil, lemon juice, garlic, ½ teaspoon salt, ⅛ teaspoon pepper, and cayenne using a blender until smooth, approximately two minutes. Put in extra water as required until sauce is slightly thicker than consistency of heavy cream.
2. Drizzle with salt, pepper, and extra lemon juice to taste. Serve at room temperature. (Sauce will keep safely in a fridge for up to 2 days; bring to room temperature before you serve.)

Searing Garlic Shrimp

Yield: 8 Servings

A Mediterranean classic, shrimp and garlic go hand in hand.

Ingredients:

- ¼ teaspoon salt
- ½ cup extra-virgin olive oil
- 1 (2-inch) piece mild dried chile, approximately broken, with seeds
- 1 bay leaf

- 1 pound medium-large shrimp (31 to 40 per pound), peeled, deveined, and tails removed
- 1 tablespoon minced fresh parsley
- 1½ teaspoons sherry vinegar
- 14 garlic cloves, peeled, 2 cloves minced, 12 cloves left whole

Directions:

1. Toss shrimp with minced garlic, 2 tablespoons oil, and salt in a container and allow to marinate at room temperature for minimum half an hour or maximum 1 hour.
2. In the meantime, use the flat side of a chef's knife to smash 4 garlic cloves. Heat smashed garlic and remaining 6 tablespoons oil in 12-inch frying pan over moderate to low heat, stirring intermittently, until garlic is light golden brown, four to eight minutes; allow the oil to cool to room temperature. Using slotted spoon, take out and discard smashed garlic.
3. Finely cut remaining 8 garlic cloves. Return frying pan with cooled oil to low heat and put in sliced garlic, bay leaf, and chile. Cook, stirring intermittently, until garlic becomes soft but not browned, four to eight minutes. If garlic does not begin to sizzle after 3 minutes, raise the heat to moderate to low.
4. Increase heat to moderate to low and put in shrimp with marinade. Cook, without stirring, until oil starts to bubble mildly, approximately two minutes. Using tongs, flip shrimp and carry on cooking until almost cooked through, approximately two minutes. Increase heat to high and put in vinegar and parsley. Cook, stirring continuously, until shrimp are cooked through and oil is bubbling heavily, 15 to 20 seconds. Take out and throw away the bay leaf. Serve instantly.

Skordalia

Yield: Approximately 2 cups

Ⓥ This is a Vegetarian Recipe Ⓥ

A thick garlic dip from Greece that tastes sensational with seafood and vegetables!

Ingredients:

- ¼ cup extra-virgin olive oil
- ¼ cup plain Greek yogurt
- 1 (10- to 12-ounce) russet potato, peeled and cut into 1-inch chunks
- 2 slices hearty white sandwich bread, crusts removed, torn into 1-inch pieces
- 3 garlic cloves, minced to paste
- 3 tablespoons lemon juice
- 6 tablespoons warm water, plus extra as required
- Salt and pepper

Directions:

1. Place potato in small saucepan and put in water to cover by 1 inch. Bring water to boil, then decrease heat to simmer and cook until potato becomes soft and paring knife can be inserted into potato easily, fifteen to twenty minutes. Drain potato using a colander, tossing to eliminate all surplus water.
2. In the meantime, combine garlic and lemon juice in a container and allow to sit for about ten minutes. In separate medium bowl, mash bread, ¼ cup warm water, and ½ teaspoon salt till it turns into a paste with fork.
3. Move potato to ricer (food mill fitted with small disk) and process into a container with bread mixture. Mix in lemon-garlic mixture, oil, yogurt, and remaining 2 tablespoons warm water until thoroughly mixed. (Sauce will keep safely in a fridge for up to 3 days; bring to room temperature before you serve.) Drizzle with salt and pepper to taste and adjust consistency with extra warm water as required before you serve.

Soft and Crispy Halloumi

Yield: 6 to 8 Servings

This recipe can be made quickly

This is a Vegetarian Recipe

Soft on the inside, and crispy on the outside, this recipe makes for a great first course.

Ingredients:

- 1 (8-ounce) block halloumi cheese, sliced into ½-inch-thick slabs
- 1 tablespoon all-purpose flour
- 2 tablespoons cornmeal
- 2 tablespoons extra-virgin olive oil
- Lemon wedges

Directions:

1. Mix cornmeal and flour in shallow dish. Working with 1 piece of cheese at a time, coat both wide sides with cornmeal mixture, pressing to help coating stick; move to plate.
2. Heat oil in 12-inch non-stick frying pan over medium heat until it starts to shimmer. Arrange halloumi in one layer in frying pan and cook until golden brown on both sides, 2 to 4 minutes each side. Move to platter and serve with lemon wedges.

Stuffed Dates Wrap

Yield: 6 to 8 Servings

This recipe can be made quickly

This one snack has a wide spectrum of flavours! What are the flavours? Only one way to find out!

Ingredients:

- ½ cup minced fresh parsley
- ½ teaspoon grated orange zest
- ⅔ cup walnuts, toasted and chopped fine
- 12 large pitted dates, halved along the length
- 12 thin slices prosciutto, halved along the length
- 2 tablespoons extra-virgin olive oil
- Salt and pepper

Directions:

1. Mix walnuts, parsley, oil, and orange zest in a container and sprinkle with salt and pepper to taste. Mound 1 large teaspoon filling into centre of each date half.
2. Wrap prosciutto tightly around dates. Serve. (Dates will keep safely in a fridge for up to 8 hours; bring to room temperature before you serve.)

Toasted Bread for Bruschetta

Yield: 8 to 10 Servings

This recipe can be made quickly

Ⓥ *This is a Vegetarian Recipe* Ⓥ

Ingredients:

- 1 (10 by 5-inch) loaf country bread with thick crust, ends discarded, sliced crosswise into ¾-inch-thick pieces
- 1 garlic clove, peeled
- Extra-virgin olive oil
- Salt

Directions:

1. Toast the bread immediately before assembling the bruschetta.
2. Place oven rack 4 inches from broiler element and heat broiler. Place bread on a baking sheet coated with an aluminium foil.

3. Broil until bread becomes deeply golden and toasted on both sides, 1 to 2 minutes each side. Lightly rub 1 side of each toast with garlic. Brush with oil and sprinkle with salt to taste.

Tzatziki

Yield: Approximately 2 cups

Ⓥ This is a Vegetarian Recipe Ⓥ

Tzatziki is a classic Greek sauce made out of strained yogurt and cucumber, and can be enjoyed as a dip for raw vegetables, or dolloped over grilled meat of your choice.

Ingredients:

- 1 (12-ounce) cucumber, peeled, halved along the length, seeded, and shredded
- 1 cup whole-milk Greek yogurt
- 1 small garlic clove, minced
- 2 tablespoons extra-virgin olive oil
- 2 tablespoons minced fresh mint and/or dill
- Salt and pepper

Directions:

1. Toss cucumber with ½ teaspoon salt using a colander and allow to drain for about fifteen minutes.
2. Beat yogurt, oil, mint, and garlic together in a container, then combine in the drained cucumber. Cover and put in the fridge until chilled, minimum sixty minutes or up to 2 days. Drizzle with salt and pepper to taste before you serve.

Soups

Soups go well before a big meal. Go ahead and try these delicious and nutritious soups!

Artichoke-Mushroom Soup

Yield: **4 to 6 Servings**

Artichokes, mushrooms, and root vegetables taste great together in s soup!

Ingredients:

- ¼ cup dry white wine
- ¼ cup heavy cream
- 1 leek, white and light green parts only, halved along the length, sliced ¼ inch thick, and washed thoroughly
- 1 teaspoon minced fresh thyme or ¼ teaspoon dried
- 1 teaspoon white wine vinegar, plus extra for seasoning
- 12 ounces white mushrooms, trimmed and sliced thin
- 2 anchovy fillets, rinsed, patted dry, and minced
- 2 bay leaves
- 2 tablespoons minced fresh tarragon
- 3 cups chicken broth
- 3 cups jarred whole baby artichokes packed in water, quartered, rinsed, and patted dry
- 3 cups vegetable broth
- 3 tablespoons all-purpose flour
- 3 tablespoons extra-virgin olive oil
- 4 garlic cloves, minced
- 6 ounces parsnips, peeled and cut into ½-inch pieces
- Salt and pepper

Directions:

1. Heat 1 tablespoon oil in Dutch oven on moderate heat until it starts to shimmer. Put in artichokes and cook until browned, eight to ten minutes. Move to slicing board, allow to cool slightly, then chop coarse.
2. Heat 1 tablespoon oil in now-empty pot on moderate heat until it starts to shimmer. Put in mushrooms, cover, and cook until they have released their liquid, approximately five minutes. Uncover and carry on cooking until mushrooms are dry, approximately five minutes.
3. Mix in leek and residual 1 tablespoon oil and cook until leek is softened and mushrooms become browned, eight to ten minutes. Mix in garlic, anchovies, and thyme and cook until aromatic, approximately half a minute. Mix in flour and cook for about sixty seconds. Mix in wine, scraping up any browned bits, and cook until nearly evaporated, about 1 minute.
4. Slowly beat in chicken broth and vegetable broth, smoothing out any lumps. Mix in artichokes, parsnips, and bay leaves and bring to simmer. Decrease heat to low, cover, and simmer gently until parsnips are tender, fifteen to twenty minutes. Remove from the heat, discard bay leaves. Mix in cream, tarragon, and vinegar. Drizzle with salt, pepper, and extra vinegar to taste. Serve.

Classic Chicken Broth

Yield: Approximately 8 cups

Chicken broth is a timeless classic, almost all over the planet.

Ingredients:

- 1 onion, chopped
- 14 cups water
- 2 bay leaves
- 2 teaspoons salt
- 4 pounds chicken backs and wings

Directions:

1. Heat chicken and water in big stockpot or Dutch oven on moderate to high heat until boiling, skimming off any scum that comes to surface. Decrease heat to low and simmer slowly for three hours.
2. Put in onion, bay leaves, and salt and continue to simmer for another 2 hours.
3. Strain broth through fine-mesh strainer into a big container, pressing on solids to extract as much liquid as possible. Allow broth to settle for approximately five minutes, then skim off fat. (Cooled broth will keep safely in a fridge for maximum 4 days or frozen for maximum 1 month.)

Classic Croutons

Yield: Approximately 3 cups

This recipe can be made quickly

Ⓥ *This is a Vegetarian Recipe* Ⓥ

Got some stale bread lying around you want to get rid of? This recipe will get the job done.

Ingredients:

- 3 tablespoons extra-virgin olive oil
- 6 slices hearty white sandwich bread, crusts removed, cut into ½-inch cubes (3 cups)
- Salt and pepper

Directions:

1. Place the oven rack in the centre of the oven and pre-heat your oven to 350 degrees. Toss bread with oil, sprinkle with salt and pepper, and spread in rimmed baking sheet. Bake until a golden

brown colour is achieved and it becomes crunchy, 20 minutes to half an hour, stirring halfway through baking.
2. Allow it to cool and serve. (Croutons can be stored safely at room temperature for up to 3 days.)

Classic Gazpacho

Yield: 8 to 10 Servings

Ⓥ This is a Vegetarian Recipe Ⓥ

A refreshing cold chilli tomato soup popular in southern Spain!

Ingredients:

- ⅓ cup sherry vinegar
- ½ small sweet onion or 2 large shallots, chopped fine
- 1 teaspoon hot sauce (optional)
- 1½ pounds tomatoes, cored and cut into ¼-inch pieces
- 2 garlic cloves, minced
- 2 red bell peppers, stemmed, seeded, and cut into ¼-inch pieces
- 2 small cucumbers (1 peeled, both sliced along the length, seeded, and cut into ¼-inch pieces)
- 5 cups tomato juice
- 8 ice cubes
- Extra-virgin olive oil
- Salt and pepper

Directions:

1. Mix tomatoes, bell peppers, cucumbers, onion, vinegar, garlic, and 2 teaspoons salt in a big container (at least 4-quart) and season with pepper to taste. Allow to stand until vegetables barely start to discharge their juices, approximately five minutes. Mix in tomato juice, ice cubes, and hot sauce, if using. Cover and put in the fridge to blend flavours, minimum 4 hours or for maximum 2 days.

2. Scoop out and throw away any ice cubes that remain, and sprinkle soup with salt and pepper to taste. Pour into your soup bowls, drizzle with oil, and serve.

Cold Cucumber-Yogurt Soup

Yield: 6 Servings

(V) This is a Vegetarian Recipe (V)

A fresh-tasting chilled soup popular in Turkey and Greece.

Ingredients:

- ¼ teaspoon sugar
- 1 tablespoon lemon juice
- 1½ tablespoons minced fresh dill
- 1½ tablespoons minced fresh mint
- 2 cups plain Greek yogurt
- 2 cups water
- 4 scallions, green parts only, chopped coarse
- 5 pounds English cucumbers, peeled and seeded (1 cucumber cut into ½-inch pieces, remaining cucumbers cut into 2-inch pieces)
- Extra-virgin olive oil
- Salt and pepper

Directions:

1. Toss 2-inch pieces of cucumber with scallions. Working in 2 batches, process cucumber-scallion mixture using a blender with water until smoothened thoroughly, approximately two minutes; move to big container. Beat in yogurt, lemon juice, 1½ teaspoons salt, sugar, and pinch pepper. Cover and put in the fridge to combine the flavours, minimum sixty minutes or maximum 12 hours.

2. Mix in dill and mint and sprinkle with salt and pepper to taste. Serve, topped with remaining ½-inch pieces of cucumber and drizzled with oil.

Fiery Moroccan Chicken Lentil Soup

Yield: 8 Servings

Ingredients:

- ¼ cup harissa, plus extra for serving
- ¼ teaspoon cayenne pepper
- ¼ teaspoon ground cinnamon
- ⅓ cup minced fresh cilantro
- ½ teaspoon paprika
- ¾ cup green or brown lentils, picked over and rinsed
- 1 (15-ounce) can chickpeas, rinsed
- 1 onion, chopped fine
- 1 tablespoon all-purpose flour
- 1 tablespoon extra-virgin olive oil
- 1 teaspoon grated fresh ginger
- 1 teaspoon ground cumin
- 10 cups chicken broth
- 1½ pounds bone-in split chicken breasts, trimmed
- 4 plum tomatoes, cored and cut into ¾-inch pieces
- Pinch saffron threads, crumbled
- Salt and pepper

Directions:

1. Pat chicken dry using paper towels and sprinkle with salt and pepper. Heat oil in Dutch oven on moderate to high heat until just smoking. Brown chicken lightly, approximately three minutes each side; move to plate.
2. Put in onion to fat left in pot and cook on moderate heat till they become tender, approximately five minutes. Mix in ginger, cumin, paprika, cinnamon, cayenne, ¼ teaspoon pepper, and

saffron and cook until aromatic, approximately half a minute. Mix in flour and cook for about sixty seconds. Slowly beat in broth, scraping up any browned bits and smoothing out any lumps, and bring to boil.
3. Mix in lentils and chickpeas, then nestle chicken into pot and bring to simmer. Cover, decrease the heat to low, and simmer gently until chicken registers 160 degrees, fifteen to twenty minutes.
4. Move chicken to slicing board, allow to cool slightly, then shred into bite-size pieces using 2 forks, discarding skin and bones. In the meantime, continue to simmer lentils, covered, for 25 to 30 minutes.
5. Mix in shredded chicken and cook until heated through, approximately two minutes. Mix in tomatoes, cilantro, and harissa and sprinkle with salt and pepper to taste. Serve, passing extra harissa separately.

French Lentil Soup

Yield: 4 to 6 Servings

Ingredients:

- ½ cup dry white wine
- 1 (14.5-ounce) can diced tomatoes, drained
- 1 bay leaf
- 1 cup lentilles du Puy, picked over and rinsed
- 1 large onion, chopped fine
- 1 teaspoon minced fresh thyme or ¼ teaspoon dried
- 1½ cups water
- 1½ teaspoons balsamic vinegar
- 2 carrots, peeled and chopped
- 3 garlic cloves, minced
- 3 slices bacon, cut into ¼-inch pieces
- 3 tablespoons minced fresh parsley
- 4½ cups chicken broth, plus extra as required

- Salt and pepper

Directions:

1. Cook bacon in Dutch oven on moderate to high heat, stirring frequently, until crisp, approximately five minutes. Mix in onion and carrots and cook until vegetables start to become tender, approximately two minutes. Mix in garlic and thyme and cook until aromatic, approximately half a minute. Mix in tomatoes and bay leaf and cook until aromatic, approximately half a minute. Mix in lentils and ¼ teaspoon salt. Cover, decrease the heat to moderate to low, and cook until vegetables are softened and lentils have darkened, eight to ten minutes.
2. Increase heat to high, mix in wine, and bring to simmer. Mix in broth and water and bring to boil. Partially cover pot, decrease the heat to low, and simmer gently until lentils are tender but still hold their shape, 30 to 35 minutes.
3. Discard bay leaf. Process 3 cups soup using a blender until smooth, approximately half a minute, then return to pot. Heat soup gently over low heat until hot (do not boil) and adjust consistency with extra hot broth as required. Mix in vinegar and parsley and sprinkle with salt and pepper to taste. Serve.

Greek White Bean Soup

Yield: 6 Servings

Ⓥ This is a Vegetarian Recipe Ⓥ

Ingredients:

- 1 onion, chopped
- 1 pound (2½ cups) dried cannellini beans, picked over and rinsed
- 1 teaspoon ground dried Aleppo pepper
- 2 tablespoons chopped fresh parsley
- 2 tablespoons extra-virgin olive oil, plus extra for serving

- 2½ teaspoons minced fresh oregano or ¾ teaspoon dried
- 3 tablespoons lemon juice
- 4 celery ribs, cut into ½-inch pieces
- 6 cups chicken or vegetable broth, plus extra as required
- Salt and pepper

Directions:

1. Dissolve 3 tablespoons salt in 4 quarts cold water in large container. Put in beans and soak at room temperature for minimum 8 hours or for maximum 24 hours. Drain and wash thoroughly.
2. Heat oil in Dutch oven on moderate heat until it starts to shimmer. Put in onion, ½ teaspoon salt, and ½ teaspoon pepper and cook till they become tender and lightly browned, 5 to 7 minutes. Mix in oregano and cook until aromatic, approximately half a minute. Mix in broth, celery, and soaked beans and bring to boil. Decrease heat to low, cover, and simmer until beans are tender, 45 to 60 minutes.
3. Process 2 cups soup using a blender until smooth, approximately half a minute, then return to pot. Heat soup gently over low heat until hot (do not boil) and adjust consistency with extra hot broth as required. Mix in lemon juice, Aleppo, and parsley and sprinkle with salt and pepper to taste. Serve, drizzling individual portions with extra oil.

Green Pea Soup

Yield: 6 Servings

Ingredients:

QUICK PEA BROTH

- 1 carrot, chopped
- 1 garlic clove, lightly crushed
- 1 small onion, chopped

- 1 teaspoon salt
- 1¾ cups chicken broth
- 2 bay leaves
- 6 cups water
- 8 ounces snow peas, chopped

SOUP

- ½ cup dry white wine
- 1 cup Arborio rice
- 1 garlic clove, minced
- 1 onion, chopped fine
- 1½ ounces Parmesan cheese, grated (¾ cup)
- 2 ounces pancetta, chopped fine
- 2 tablespoons extra-virgin olive oil
- 2 teaspoons lemon juice
- 20 ounces frozen peas
- 4 teaspoons minced fresh parsley
- Salt and pepper

Directions:

1. FOR THE QUICK PEA BROTH Mix all ingredients in Dutch oven and bring to boil on moderate to high heat. Decrease heat to moderate to low, partially cover, and simmer for 30 minutes. Strain broth through fine-mesh strainer into moderate-sized saucepan, pressing on solids with wooden spoon to extract as much liquid as possible. Cover and keep warm over low heat until ready to use.
2. FOR THE SOUP Heat oil in now-empty pot on moderate heat until it starts to shimmer. Put in onion and pancetta and cook, stirring intermittently, until onion is softened and lightly browned, 5 to 7 minutes. Mix in garlic and cook until aromatic, approximately half a minute. Put in rice and cook, stirring often, until grain edges begin to turn translucent, approximately three minutes.
3. Put in wine and cook, stirring continuously, until fully absorbed, about 1 minute. Mix in warm broth and bring to boil. Decrease

heat to moderate to low, cover, and simmer, stirring intermittently, until rice is just cooked, about fifteen minutes. Mix in peas and cook until heated through, approximately two minutes. Remove from the heat, mix in Parmesan, parsley, and lemon juice and sprinkle with salt and pepper to taste. Serve instantly.

Italian Pasta e Fagioli

Yield: 8 to 10 Servings

Ingredients:

- ¼ cup minced fresh parsley
- ¼ teaspoon red pepper flakes
- ½ teaspoon fennel seeds
- 1 (28-ounce) can diced tomatoes
- 1 celery rib, minced
- 1 cup orzo
- 1 fennel bulb, stalks discarded, bulb halved, cored, and chopped fine
- 1 onion, chopped fine
- 1 Parmesan cheese rind, plus grated Parmesan for serving
- 1 tablespoon extra-virgin olive oil, plus extra for serving
- 1 tablespoon minced fresh oregano or 1 teaspoon dried
- 2 (15-ounce) cans cannellini beans, rinsed
- 2 teaspoons grated orange zest
- 2½ cups water
- 3 anchovy fillets, rinsed and minced
- 3 ounces pancetta, chopped fine
- 3½ cups chicken broth
- 4 garlic cloves, minced
- Salt and pepper

Directions:

1. Heat oil in Dutch oven on moderate to high heat until it starts to shimmer. Put in pancetta and cook, stirring intermittently, until starting to brown, 3 to 5 minutes. Mix in onion, fennel, and celery and cook until vegetables are softened, 5 to 7 minutes. Mix in garlic, anchovies, oregano, orange zest, fennel seeds, and pepper flakes and cook until aromatic, about 1 minute.
2. Mix in tomatoes and their juice, scraping up any browned bits. Mix in Parmesan rind and beans, bring to simmer, and cook until flavours blend, about 10 minutes.
3. Mix in broth, water, and 1 teaspoon salt. Increase heat to high and bring to boil. Mix in pasta and cook until al dente, about 10 minutes. Remove from the heat, discard Parmesan rind. Mix in parsley and sprinkle with salt and pepper to taste. Serve, drizzling individual portions with extra oil and sprinkling with grated Parmesan.

Libyan Lamb-Mint Sharba

Yield: 6 to 8 Servings

Ingredients:

- ¼ teaspoon ground cumin
- ½ teaspoon ground cinnamon
- 1 (15-ounce) can chickpeas, rinsed
- 1 cup orzo
- 1 onion, chopped fine
- 1 pound lamb shoulder chops (blade or round bone), 1 to 1½ inches thick, trimmed and halved
- 1 tablespoon extra-virgin olive oil
- 1 teaspoon ground turmeric
- 1 teaspoon paprika
- 10 cups chicken broth
- 1½ teaspoons dried mint, crumbled
- 2 tablespoons tomato paste
- 4 plum tomatoes, cored and cut into ¼-inch pieces

- Salt and pepper

Directions:

1. Place oven rack to lower-middle position and pre-heat your oven to 325 degrees. Pat lamb dry using paper towels and sprinkle with salt and pepper. Heat oil in Dutch oven on moderate to high heat until just smoking. Brown lamb, about 4 minutes each side; move to plate. Pour off all but 2 tablespoons fat from pot.
2. Put in onion to fat left in pot and cook on moderate heat till they become tender, approximately five minutes. Mix in tomatoes and cook till they become tender and juice has evaporated, approximately two minutes. Mix in tomato paste, 1 teaspoon mint, turmeric, paprika, 1 teaspoon salt, cinnamon, cumin, and ¼ teaspoon pepper and cook until aromatic, about 1 minute. Mix in broth, scraping up any browned bits, and bring to boil.
3. Mix in chickpeas, then nestle lamb into pot along with any accumulated juices. Cover, place pot in oven, and cook until fork slips easily in and out of lamb, about 1 hour.
4. Move lamb to slicing board, allow to cool slightly, then shred into bite-size pieces using 2 forks, discarding excess fat and bones. In the meantime, stir orzo into soup, bring to simmer on moderate heat, and cook until tender, 10 to 12 minutes.
5. Mix in shredded lamb and cook until heated through, approximately two minutes. Remove from the heat, mix in remaining ½ teaspoon mint and allow to sit until aromatic, about 1 minute. Serve.

Moroccan Chickpea Soup

Yield: 4 to 6 Servings

(V) This is a Vegetarian Recipe (V)

Ingredients:

- ¼ cup minced fresh parsley or mint
- ¼ teaspoon ground cumin
- ¼ teaspoon ground ginger
- ¼ teaspoon saffron threads, crumbled
- ½ teaspoon hot paprika
- 1 (14.5-ounce) can diced tomatoes
- 1 onion, chopped fine
- 1 pound red potatoes, unpeeled, cut into ½-inch pieces
- 1 teaspoon sugar
- 1 zucchini, cut into ½-inch pieces
- 2 (15-ounce) cans chickpeas, rinsed
- 3 tablespoons extra-virgin olive oil
- 3½ cups chicken or vegetable broth
- 4 garlic cloves, minced
- Lemon wedges
- Salt and pepper

Directions:

1. Heat oil in Dutch oven on moderate to high heat until it starts to shimmer. Put in onion, sugar, and ½ teaspoon salt and cook until onion is softened, approximately five minutes. Mix in garlic, paprika, saffron, ginger, and cumin and cook until aromatic, approximately half a minute. Mix in chickpeas, potatoes, tomatoes and their juice, zucchini, and broth. Bring to simmer and cook, stirring intermittently, until potatoes are tender, 20 to 30 minutes.
2. Using wooden spoon, mash some of potatoes against side of pot to thicken soup. Remove from the heat, mix in parsley and sprinkle with salt and pepper to taste. Serve with lemon wedges.

Moroccan Spicy Fava Bean Soup

Yield: **4 to 6 Servings**

Ⓥ This is a Vegetarian Recipe Ⓥ

Ingredients:

- ¼ cup lemon juice (2 lemons)
- 1 onion, chopped
- 1 pound (3 cups) dried split fava beans, picked over and rinsed
- 2 cups water
- 2 teaspoons cumin, plus extra for serving
- 2 teaspoons paprika, plus extra for serving
- 3 tablespoons extra-virgin olive oil, plus extra for serving
- 5 garlic cloves, minced
- 6 cups chicken or vegetable broth, plus extra as required
- Salt and pepper

Directions:

1. Heat oil in Dutch oven on moderate heat until it starts to shimmer. Put in onion, ¾ teaspoon salt, and ¼ teaspoon pepper and cook till they become tender and lightly browned, 5 to 7 minutes. Mix in garlic, paprika, and cumin and cook until aromatic, approximately half a minute.
2. Mix in beans, broth, and water and bring to boil. Cover, decrease the heat to low, and simmer gently, stirring intermittently, until beans are soft and broken down, 1½ to 2 hours.
3. Remove from the heat, beat soup heavily until broken down to coarse puree, approximately half a minute. Adjust consistency with extra hot broth as required. Mix in lemon juice and sprinkle with salt and pepper to taste. Serve, drizzling individual portions with extra oil and sprinkling with extra paprika and cumin.

Provençal Vegetable Soup

Yield: 6 Servings

Ⓥ *This is a Vegetarian Recipe* Ⓥ

This is a timeless French soup made with seasonal vegetables, creamy white beans, and aromatic herbs.

Ingredients:

PISTOU

- ⅓ cup extra-virgin olive oil
- ½ cup fresh basil leaves
- 1 garlic clove, minced
- 1 ounce Parmesan cheese, grated (½ cup)

SOUP

- ½ cup orecchiette
- 1 (15-ounce) can cannellini or navy beans, rinsed
- 1 carrot, peeled and sliced ¼ inch thick
- 1 celery rib, cut into ½-inch pieces
- 1 large tomato, cored, seeded, and chopped
- 1 leek, white and light green parts only, halved along the length, sliced ½ inch thick, and washed thoroughly
- 1 small zucchini, halved along the length, seeded, and cut into ¼-inch pieces
- 1 tablespoon extra-virgin olive oil
- 2 garlic cloves, minced
- 3 cups vegetable broth
- 3 cups water
- 8 ounces haricots verts, trimmed and cut into ½-inch lengths
- Salt and pepper

Directions:

1. **For the Pistou**: Process all ingredients using a food processor until smooth, approximately fifteen seconds, scraping down sides of the container as required. (Pistou will keep safely in a fridge for maximum 4 hours.)

2. **For the Soup**: Heat oil in Dutch oven on moderate heat until it starts to shimmer. Put in leek, celery, carrot, and ½ teaspoon salt and cook until vegetables are softened, eight to ten minutes. Mix in garlic and cook until aromatic, approximately half a minute. Mix in broth and water and bring to simmer.
3. Mix in pasta and simmer until slightly softened, approximately five minutes. Mix in haricots verts and simmer until bright green but still crunchy, approximately three minutes. Mix in cannellini beans, zucchini, and tomato and simmer until pasta and vegetables are tender, approximately three minutes. Drizzle with salt and pepper to taste. Serve, topping individual portions with pistou.

Provene Fish Soup

Yield: 6 to 8 Servings

Ingredients:

- ⅛ teaspoon red pepper flakes
- 1 cup dry white wine or dry vermouth
- 1 fennel bulb, 2 tablespoons fronds minced, stalks discarded, bulb halved, cored, and cut into ½-inch pieces
- 1 onion, chopped
- 1 tablespoon extra-virgin olive oil, plus extra for serving
- 1 tablespoon grated orange zest
- 1 teaspoon paprika
- 2 (8-ounce) bottles clam juice
- 2 bay leaves
- 2 celery ribs, halved along the length and cut into ½-inch pieces
- 2 pounds skinless hake fillets, 1 to 1½ inches thick, sliced crosswise into 6 equivalent pieces
- 2 tablespoons minced fresh parsley
- 4 cups water
- 4 garlic cloves, minced
- 6 ounces pancetta, chopped fine

- Pinch saffron threads, crumbled
- Salt and pepper

Directions:

1. Heat oil in Dutch oven on moderate heat until it starts to shimmer. Put in pancetta and cook, stirring intermittently, until starting to brown, 3 to 5 minutes. Mix in fennel pieces, onion, celery, and 1½ teaspoons salt and cook until vegetables are softened and lightly browned, 12 to 14 minutes. Mix in garlic, paprika, pepper flakes, and saffron and cook until aromatic, approximately half a minute.
2. Mix in wine, scraping up any browned bits. Mix in water, clam juice, and bay leaves. Bring to simmer and cook until flavours blend, fifteen to twenty minutes.
3. Remove from the heat, discard bay leaves. Nestle hake into cooking liquid, cover, and allow to sit until fish flakes apart when softly poked using paring knife and registers 140 degrees, eight to ten minutes. Gently mix in parsley, fennel fronds, and orange zest and break fish into large pieces. Drizzle with salt and pepper to taste. Serve, drizzling individual portions with extra oil.

Red Pepper Roast Soup with Sides

Yield: 6 Servings

Ⓥ This is a Vegetarian Recipe Ⓥ

Roasted red peppers bring a rich smoky flavour to the soup.

Ingredients:

- ½ cup half-and-half
- ½ cup whole-milk yogurt
- ½ teaspoon ground cumin
- ½ teaspoon smoked paprika
- 1 bay leaf

- 1 red onion, chopped
- 1 tablespoon all-purpose flour
- 1 tablespoon extra-virgin olive oil
- 1 teaspoon lime juice
- 2 garlic cloves, minced
- 2 tablespoons dry sherry
- 2 tablespoons tomato paste
- 3 tablespoons minced fresh cilantro
- 4 cups chicken or vegetable broth, plus extra as required
- 8 red bell peppers, cored and flattened
- Salt and pepper

Directions:

1. Beat yogurt, 1 tablespoon cilantro, and lime juice together in a container. Drizzle with salt and pepper to taste. Cover and put in the fridge until needed.
2. Place oven rack 3 inches from broiler element and heat broiler. Lay out half of peppers skin side up on a baking sheet coated with an aluminium foil. Broil until skin is charred and puffed but flesh is still firm, eight to ten minutes, rotating sheet halfway through broiling. Move broiled peppers to a container, cover up using plastic wrap or foil, and let steam until skins peel off easily, 10 to fifteen minutes. Replicate the process with the rest of the peppers. Peel broiled peppers, discarding skins, and chop coarse.
3. Cook oil and garlic together in Dutch oven over low heat, stirring continuously, until garlic is foamy, sticky, and straw-coloured, six to eight minutes. Mix in onion and ¼ teaspoon salt, increase heat to medium, and cook till they become tender, approximately five minutes.
4. Mix in cumin and paprika and cook until aromatic, approximately half a minute. Mix in tomato paste and flour and cook for about sixty seconds. Slowly beat in broth, scraping up any browned bits and smoothing out any lumps. Mix in bay leaf and chopped peppers, bring to simmer, and cook until peppers are very tender, 5 to 7 minutes.

5. Discard bay leaf. Working in batches, process soup using a blender until smooth, approximately two minutes. Return soup to clean pot and mix in half-and-half and sherry. Heat soup gently over low heat until hot (do not boil) and adjust consistency with extra hot broth as required. Mix in remaining 2 tablespoons cilantro and sprinkle with salt and pepper to taste. Serve, drizzling individual portions with yogurt mixture.

Shellfish Soup

Yield: 6 to 8 Servings

Ingredients:

- ⅛ teaspoon red pepper flakes
- ⅓ cup minced fresh parsley
- ½ teaspoon ground turmeric
- 1 cup dry white wine or dry vermouth
- 1 teaspoon grated fresh ginger
- 1 teaspoon ground coriander
- 1½ pounds leeks, white and light green parts only, halved along the length, sliced thin, and washed thoroughly
- 12 ounces large sea scallops, tendons removed
- 12 ounces large shrimp (26 to 30 per pound), peeled and deveined, shells reserved
- 12 ounces squid, bodies sliced crosswise into ½-inch-thick rings, tentacles halved
- 2 (8-ounce) bottles clam juice
- 2 garlic cloves, minced
- 2 tablespoons extra-virgin olive oil, plus extra for serving
- 3 tablespoons tomato paste
- 4 cups water
- 4 ounces pancetta, chopped fine
- Salt and pepper

Directions:

1. Heat 1 tablespoon oil in Dutch oven on moderate heat until it starts to shimmer. Put in shrimp shells and cook, stirring often, until starting to turn spotty brown and pot starts to brown, 2 to 4 minutes. Put in wine and simmer, stirring intermittently, for 2 minutes. Mix in water, bring to simmer, and cook for 4 minutes. Strain mixture through fine-mesh strainer into a container, pressing on solids to extract as much liquid as possible; discard solids.
2. Heat residual 1 tablespoon oil in now-empty pot on moderate heat until it starts to shimmer. Put in leeks and pancetta and cook until leeks are softened and lightly browned, approximately eight minutes. Mix in tomato paste, garlic, 1 teaspoon salt, ginger, coriander, turmeric, and pepper flakes and cook until aromatic, about 1 minute. Mix in wine mixture and clam juice, scraping up any browned bits. Bring to simmer and cook until flavours blend, fifteen to twenty minutes.
3. Decrease heat to gentle simmer, put in sea scallops, and cook for 2 minutes. Mix in shrimp and cook until just opaque throughout, approximately two minutes. Remove from the heat, mix in squid, cover, and allow to sit until just opaque and tender, 1 to 2 minutes. Mix in parsley and sprinkle with salt and pepper to taste. Serve, drizzling individual portions with extra oil.

Sicilian Chickpea-Escarole Soup

Yield: 6 to 8 Servings

Ⓥ This is a Vegetarian Recipe Ⓥ

Ingredients:

- ¼ teaspoon red pepper flakes
- 1 (3-inch) strip orange zest
- 1 head escarole (1 pound), trimmed and cut into 1-inch pieces

- 1 large tomato, cored and chopped
- 1 Parmesan cheese rind, plus grated Parmesan for serving
- 1 pound (2¾ cups) dried chickpeas, picked over and rinsed
- 1 small onion, chopped
- 2 bay leaves
- 2 fennel bulbs, stalks discarded, bulbs halved, cored, and chopped fine
- 2 tablespoons extra-virgin olive oil, plus extra for serving
- 2 teaspoons minced fresh oregano or ½ teaspoon dried
- 5 cups chicken or vegetable broth
- 5 garlic cloves, minced
- Salt and pepper

Directions:

1. Dissolve 3 tablespoons salt in 4 quarts cold water in large container. Put in chickpeas and soak at room temperature for minimum 8 hours or for maximum 24 hours. Drain and wash thoroughly.
2. Heat oil in Dutch oven on moderate heat until it starts to shimmer. Put in fennel, onion, and 1 teaspoon salt and cook until vegetables are softened, 7 to 10 minutes. Mix in garlic, oregano, and pepper flakes and cook until aromatic, approximately half a minute.
3. Mix in 7 cups water, broth, soaked chickpeas, Parmesan rind, bay leaves, and orange zest and bring to boil. Reduce to gentle simmer and cook until chickpeas are tender, 1¼ to 1¾ hours.
4. Mix in escarole and tomato and cook until escarole is wilted, 5 to 10 minutes. Remove from the heat, discard bay leaves and Parmesan rind (scraping off any cheese that has melted and adding it back to pot). Drizzle with salt and pepper to taste. Serve, drizzling individual portions with extra oil and sprinkling with grated Parmesan.

Spanish Lentil-Chorizo Soup

Yield: 6 to 8 Servings

Ingredients:

- ⅛ teaspoon ground cloves
- 1 large onion
- 1 pound (2¼ cups) lentils, picked over and rinsed
- 1 tablespoon all-purpose flour
- 1½ pounds Spanish-style chorizo sausage, pricked with fork several times
- 2 bay leaves
- 2 tablespoons sweet smoked paprika
- 3 carrots, peeled and cut into ¼-inch pieces
- 3 garlic cloves, minced
- 3 tablespoons minced fresh parsley
- 3 tablespoons sherry vinegar, plus extra for seasoning
- 5 tablespoons extra-virgin olive oil
- Salt and pepper

Directions:

1. Place lentils and 2 teaspoons salt in heatproof container. Cover with 4 cups boiling water and let soak for 30 minutes. Drain well.
2. In the meantime, finely chop three-quarters of onion (you should have about 1 cup) and grate remaining quarter (you should have about 3 tablespoons). Heat 2 tablespoons oil in Dutch oven on moderate heat until it starts to shimmer. Put in chorizo and cook until browned on all sides, six to eight minutes. Move chorizo to large plate. Decrease heat to low and put in chopped onion, carrots, 1 tablespoon parsley, and 1 teaspoon salt. Cover and cook, stirring intermittently, until vegetables are very soft but not brown, 25 to 30 minutes. If vegetables begin to brown, put in 1 tablespoon water to pot.
3. Put in lentils and vinegar to vegetables, increase heat to medium-high, and cook, stirring often, until vinegar starts to

evaporate, three to five minutes. Put in 7 cups water, chorizo, bay leaves, and cloves; bring to simmer. Decrease heat to low; cover; and cook until lentils are tender, approximately half an hour.

4. Heat remaining 3 tablespoons oil in small saucepan on moderate heat until it starts to shimmer. Put in paprika, grated onion, garlic, and ½ teaspoon pepper; cook, stirring continuously, until aromatic, 2 minutes. Put in flour and cook, stirring continuously, 1 minute longer. Remove chorizo and bay leaves from lentils. Stir paprika mixture into lentils and carry on cooking until flavours have blended and soup has thickened, 10 to fifteen minutes. When chorizo is cool enough to handle, cut in half along the length, then cut each half into ¼-inch-thick slices. Return chorizo to soup along with remaining 2 tablespoons parsley and heat through, about 1 minute. Drizzle with salt, pepper, and up to 2 teaspoons vinegar to taste and serve. (Soup can be made up to 3 days in advance.)

Spanish Meatball-Saffron Soup

Yield: **6 to 8 Servings**

Ingredients:

MEATBALLS

- ⅓ cup whole milk
- ½ teaspoon pepper
- ½ teaspoon salt
- 1 ounce Manchego cheese, grated (½ cup)
- 1 shallot, minced
- 2 slices hearty white sandwich bread, torn into quarters
- 2 tablespoons extra-virgin olive oil
- 3 tablespoons minced fresh parsley
- 8 ounces 80 percent lean ground beef
- 8 ounces ground pork

SOUP

- ⅛ teaspoon red pepper flakes
- ¼ teaspoon saffron threads, crumbled
- 1 cup dry white wine
- 1 onion, chopped fine
- 1 recipe Picada
- 1 red bell pepper, stemmed, seeded, and cut into ¾-inch pieces
- 1 tablespoon extra-virgin olive oil
- 1 teaspoon paprika
- 2 garlic cloves, minced
- 2 tablespoons minced fresh parsley
- 8 cups chicken broth
- Salt and pepper

Directions:

1. FOR THE MEATBALLS Using fork, mash bread and milk together till it turns into a paste in a big container. Mix in ground pork, Manchego, parsley, shallot, oil, salt, and pepper until combined. Put in ground beef and knead with your hands until combined. Pinch off and roll 2-teaspoon-size pieces of mixture into balls and lay out on rimmed baking sheet (you should have 30 to 35 meatballs). Cover using plastic wrap put inside your fridge until firm, minimum 30 minutes.
2. FOR THE SOUP Heat oil in large Dutch oven on moderate to high heat until it starts to shimmer. Put in onion and bell pepper and cook till they become tender and lightly browned, eight to ten minutes. Mix in garlic, paprika, saffron, and pepper flakes and cook until aromatic, approximately half a minute. Mix in wine, scraping up any browned bits, and cook until almost completely evaporated, about 1 minute.
3. Mix in broth and bring to simmer. Gently put in meatballs and simmer until cooked through, 10 to 12 minutes. Remove from the heat, mix in picada and parsley and sprinkle with salt and pepper to taste. Serve.

Spicy Moroccan Lamb Lentil Soup

Yield: 6 to 8 Servings

Ingredients:

- ¼ cup harissa, plus extra for serving
- ¼ teaspoon cayenne pepper
- ¼ teaspoon ground cinnamon
- ⅓ cup minced fresh cilantro
- ½ teaspoon paprika
- ¾ cup green or brown lentils, picked over and rinsed
- 1 (15-ounce) can chickpeas, rinsed
- 1 onion, chopped fine
- 1 pound lamb shoulder chops (blade or round bone), 1 to 1½ inches thick, trimmed and halved
- 1 tablespoon all-purpose flour
- 1 tablespoon extra-virgin olive oil
- 1 teaspoon grated fresh ginger
- 1 teaspoon ground cumin
- 10 cups chicken broth
- 4 plum tomatoes, cored and cut into ¾-inch pieces
- Pinch saffron threads, crumbled
- Salt and pepper

Directions:

1. Place oven rack to lower-middle position and pre-heat your oven to 325 degrees. Pat lamb dry using paper towels and sprinkle with salt and pepper. Heat oil in Dutch oven on moderate to high heat until just smoking. Brown lamb, about 4 minutes each side; move to plate. Pour off all but 2 tablespoons fat from pot.
2. Put in onion to fat left in pot and cook on moderate heat till they become tender, approximately five minutes. Mix in ginger, cumin, paprika, cinnamon, cayenne, ¼ teaspoon pepper, and saffron and cook until aromatic, approximately half a minute. Mix in flour and cook for about sixty seconds. Slowly beat in

broth, scraping up any browned bits and smoothing out any lumps, and bring to boil.
3. Nestle lamb into pot along with any accumulated juices, bring to simmer, and cook for about ten minutes. Mix in lentils and chickpeas, cover, and place pot in oven. Cook until fork slips easily in and out of lamb and lentils are tender, fifty to sixty minutes.
4. Move lamb to slicing board, allow to cool slightly, then shred into bite-size pieces using 2 forks, discarding excess fat and bones. Stir shredded lamb into soup and allow to sit until heated through, approximately two minutes. Mix in tomatoes, cilantro, and harissa and sprinkle with salt and pepper to taste. Serve, passing extra harissa separately.

Spicy Red Lentil Soup

Yield: 4 to 6 Servings

Ⓥ This is a Vegetarian Recipe Ⓥ

Ingredients:

- ⅛ teaspoon ground cinnamon
- ¼ cup chopped fresh cilantro
- ¼ cup extra-virgin olive oil
- ¼ teaspoon ground ginger
- ½ teaspoon ground cumin
- ¾ teaspoon ground coriander
- 1 garlic clove, minced
- 1 large onion, chopped fine
- 1 tablespoon tomato paste
- 1 teaspoon paprika
- 10½ ounces (1½ cups) red lentils, picked over and rinsed
- 1½ teaspoons dried mint, crumbled
- 2 cups water
- 2 tablespoons lemon juice, plus extra for seasoning

- 4 cups chicken or vegetable broth, plus extra as required
- Pinch cayenne pepper
- Salt and pepper

Directions:

1. Heat 2 tablespoons oil in a big saucepan on moderate heat until it starts to shimmer. Put in onion and 1 teaspoon salt and cook, stirring intermittently, till they become tender, approximately five minutes. Mix in coriander, cumin, ginger, cinnamon, ¼ teaspoon pepper, and cayenne and cook until aromatic, approximately two minutes. Mix in tomato paste and garlic and cook for about sixty seconds.
2. Mix in broth, water, and lentils and bring to vigorous simmer. Cook, stirring intermittently, until lentils are soft and about half are broken down, about fifteen minutes.
3. Beat soup heavily until broken down to coarse puree, approximately half a minute. Adjust consistency with extra hot broth as required. Mix in lemon juice and sprinkle with salt and extra lemon juice to taste. Cover and keep warm.
4. Heat remaining 2 tablespoons oil in small frying pan on moderate heat until it starts to shimmer. Remove from the heat, mix in mint and paprika. Serve soup, drizzling individual portions with 1 teaspoon spiced oil and sprinkling with cilantro.

Tomato Soup with Eggplant Roast

Yield: 4 to 6 Servings

Ⓥ This is a Vegetarian Recipe Ⓥ

Eastern Mediterranean countries love to couple tomatoes with eggplant!

Ingredients:

- ¼ cup raisins
- ½ teaspoon ground cumin

- 1 (14.5-ounce) can diced tomatoes, drained
- 1 bay leaf
- 1 onion, chopped
- 1½ teaspoons ras el hanout
- 2 garlic cloves, minced
- 2 pounds eggplant, cut into ½-inch pieces
- 2 tablespoons minced fresh cilantro
- 2 tablespoons slivered almonds, toasted
- 2 teaspoons lemon juice
- 4 cups chicken or vegetable broth, plus extra as required
- 6 tablespoons extra-virgin olive oil, plus extra for serving
- Salt and pepper

Directions:

1. Place oven rack 4 inches from broiler element and heat broiler. Toss eggplant with 5 tablespoons oil, then spread in aluminium foil–lined rimmed baking sheet. Broil eggplant for about ten minutes. Stir eggplant and continue to broil until mahogany brown, 5 to 7 minutes. Measure out and reserve 2 cups eggplant.
2. Heat residual 1 tablespoon oil in a big saucepan on moderate heat until it starts to shimmer. Put in onion, ¾ teaspoon salt, and ¼ teaspoon pepper and cook till they become tender and lightly browned, 5 to 7 minutes. Mix in garlic, ras el hanout, and cumin and cook until aromatic, approximately half a minute. Mix in broth, tomatoes, raisins, bay leaf, and remaining eggplant and bring to simmer. Decrease heat to low, cover, and simmer gently until eggplant is softened, approximately twenty minutes.
3. Discard bay leaf. Working in batches, process soup using a blender until smooth, approximately two minutes. Return soup to clean saucepan and mix in reserved eggplant. Heat soup gently over low heat until hot (do not boil) and adjust consistency with extra hot broth as required. Mix in lemon juice and sprinkle with salt and pepper to taste. Serve, sprinkling

individual portions with almonds and cilantro and drizzling with extra oil.

Traditional Greek Avgolemono

Yield: 6 to 8 Servings

Ingredients:

- ½ cup long-grain white rice
- 1 bay leaf
- 1 scallion, sliced thin, or 3 tablespoons chopped fresh mint
- 1½ teaspoons salt
- 12 (4-inch) strips lemon zest plus ¼ cup juice (2 lemons)
- 2 large eggs plus 2 large yolks, room temperature
- 4 green cardamom pods, crushed, or 2 whole cloves
- 8 cups chicken broth

Directions:

1. Bring broth to boil in moderate-sized saucepan on high heat. Mix in rice, lemon zest, cardamom pods, bay leaf, and salt. Reduce to simmer and cook until rice becomes soft and broth is aromatic, 16 to 20 minutes.
2. Gently beat whole eggs, egg yolks, and lemon juice together in medium bowl until combined. Discard bay leaf, cardamom, and zest strips. Decrease heat to low. Whisking continuously, slowly ladle about 2 cups hot broth into egg mixture and beat until combined. Pour egg mixture back into saucepan and cook, stirring continuously, until soup is slightly thickened and wisps of steam appear, approximately five minutes (do not simmer or boil). Sprinkle individual portions with scallion and serve instantly.

Turkish Tomato Grain Soup

Yield: 6 to 8 Servings

(V) This is a Vegetarian Recipe (V)

A Turkish tomato soup empowered by flavourful grains!

Ingredients:

- ⅛ teaspoon red pepper flakes
- ⅓ cup chopped fresh mint
- ½ cup dry white wine
- ½ teaspoon smoked paprika
- ¾ cup medium-grind bulgur, rinsed
- 1 (28-ounce) can diced fire-roasted tomatoes
- 1 onion, chopped
- 1 tablespoon tomato paste
- 1 teaspoon dried mint, crumbled
- 2 cups water
- 2 red bell peppers, stemmed, seeded, and chopped
- 2 tablespoons extra-virgin olive oil
- 3 garlic cloves, minced
- 4 cups chicken or vegetable broth
- Salt and pepper

Directions:

1. Heat oil in Dutch oven on moderate heat until it starts to shimmer. Put in onion, bell peppers, ¾ teaspoon salt, and ¼ teaspoon pepper and cook till they become tender and lightly browned, six to eight minutes. Mix in garlic, dried mint, smoked paprika, and pepper flakes and cook until aromatic, approximately half a minute. Mix in tomato paste and cook for about sixty seconds.
2. Mix in wine, scraping up any browned bits, and simmer until reduced by half, about 1 minute. Put in tomatoes and their juice

and cook, stirring intermittently, until tomatoes soften and begin to break apart, about 10 minutes.
3. Mix in broth, water, and bulgur and bring to simmer. Decrease heat to low, cover, and simmer gently until bulgur is tender, approximately twenty minutes. Drizzle with salt and pepper to taste. Serve, sprinkling individual portions with fresh mint.

Vegetable Broth Base

Yield: Approximately 1¾ cups base, or about 1¾ gallons broth

✓ This recipe can be made quickly ✓

Ⓥ This is a Vegetarian Recipe Ⓥ

A quick, easy, and flavourful vegetable broth.

Ingredients:

- ½ cup (½ ounce) fresh parsley leaves and thin stems
- ½ small celery root, peeled and cut into ½-inch pieces (¾ cup)
- 1 pound leeks, white and light green parts only, chopped and washed (2½ cups)
- 1½ tablespoons tomato paste
- 2 carrots, peeled and cut into ½-inch pieces (⅔ cup)
- 3 tablespoons dried minced onion
- 3 tablespoons kosher salt

Directions:

1. Process leeks, carrots, celery root, parsley, dried minced onion, and salt using a food processor, pausing to scrape down sides of the container often, until paste is as fine as possible, three to five minutes. Put in tomato paste and process for 2 minutes, scraping down sides of the container every 30 seconds. Move mixture to airtight container and tap tightly on counter to eliminate air bubbles. Press small piece of parchment paper

flush against surface of mixture and cover firmly. Freeze for maximum 6 months.
2. For each cup you wish to serve, stir 1 tablespoon fresh or frozen broth base into 1 cup boiling water. If particle-free broth is desired, allow broth to steep for about five minutes, then strain through fine-mesh strainer.

White Gazpacho

Yield: 6 to 8 Servings

(V) This is a Vegetarian Recipe (V)

A rich and elegant soup for when you want to impress!

Ingredients:

- ⅛ teaspoon almond extract
- ½ cup plus 2 teaspoons extra-virgin olive oil, plus extra for serving
- 1 garlic clove, peeled and smashed
- 2½ cups (8¾ ounces) plus ⅓ cup sliced blanched almonds
- 3 tablespoons sherry vinegar
- 4 cups water
- 6 ounces seedless green grapes, sliced thin (1 cup)
- 6 slices hearty white sandwich bread, crusts removed
- Pinch cayenne pepper
- Salt and pepper

Directions:

1. Mix bread and water in a container and let soak for about five minutes. Process 2½ cups almonds using a blender until finely ground, approximately half a minute, scraping down sides of blender jar as required. Using your hands, remove bread from water, squeeze it lightly, and move to blender with almonds. Measure out 3 cups soaking water and set aside; move remaining soaking water to blender. Put in garlic, vinegar, ½

teaspoon salt, and cayenne to blender and process until mixture has consistency of cake batter, 30 to 45 seconds. With blender running, put in ½ cup oil in thin, steady stream, approximately half a minute. Put in reserved soaking water and process for about sixty seconds.
2. Season soup with salt and pepper to taste, then strain through fine-mesh strainer into a container, pressing on solids to extract as much liquid as possible; discard solids.
3. Move 1 tablespoon soup to different container and mix in almond extract. Return 1 teaspoon extract-soup mixture to soup; discard remaining mixture. Cover and put in the fridge to combine the flavours, minimum 4 hours or for maximum 24 hours.
4. Heat remaining 2 teaspoons oil in 8-inch frying pan on moderate to high heat until it starts to shimmer. Put in remaining ⅓ cup almonds and cook, stirring continuously, until golden brown, three to five minutes. Immediately move almonds to a container, mix in ¼ teaspoon salt, and allow to cool slightly.
5. Ladle soup into shallow bowls. Mound grapes in center of each bowl, drizzle with almonds, and drizzle with extra oil. Serve instantly.

Salad and Salad Dressings

Salad Dressings

The dressing is the life of the salad.

Balsamic-Mustard Vinaigrette

Yield: ¼ cup

✒ *This recipe can be made quickly* ✒

Ⓥ *This is a Vegetarian Recipe* Ⓥ

This is best for dressing assertive greens.

Ingredients:

- ⅛ teaspoon salt
- ½ teaspoon mayonnaise
- ½ teaspoon minced fresh thyme
- 1 tablespoon balsamic vinegar
- 1½ teaspoons minced shallot
- 2 teaspoons Dijon mustard
- 3 tablespoons extra-virgin olive oil
- Pinch pepper

Directions:

1. Beat vinegar, mustard, shallot, mayonnaise, thyme, salt, and pepper together in a container until smooth.
2. Whisking continuously, slowly drizzle in oil until completely blended. (Vinaigrette will keep safely in a fridge for maximum 2 weeks.)

Classic Vinaigrette

Yield: ¼ cup

✎ *This recipe can be made quickly* ✎

Ⓥ *This is a Vegetarian Recipe* Ⓥ

This dressing works well with all types of greens.

Ingredients:

- ⅛ teaspoon salt
- ½ teaspoon Dijon mustard
- ½ teaspoon mayonnaise
- 1 tablespoon wine vinegar
- 1½ teaspoons minced shallot
- 3 tablespoons extra-virgin olive oil
- Pinch pepper

Directions:

1. Beat vinegar, shallot, mayonnaise, mustard, salt, and pepper together in a container until smooth.
2. Whisking continuously, slowly drizzle in oil until completely blended. (Vinaigrette will keep safely in a fridge for maximum 2 weeks.)

Herb Vinaigrette

Yield: ¼ cup

✎ *This recipe can be made quickly* ✎

Ⓥ *This is a Vegetarian Recipe* Ⓥ

Serve this vinaigrette immediately.

Ingredients:

- ⅛ teaspoon salt
- ½ teaspoon Dijon mustard
- ½ teaspoon mayonnaise
- ½ teaspoon minced fresh thyme, tarragon, marjoram, or oregano
- 1 tablespoon minced fresh parsley or chives
- 1 tablespoon wine vinegar
- 1½ teaspoons minced shallot
- 3 tablespoons extra-virgin olive oil
- Pinch pepper

Directions:

1. Beat vinegar, parsley, shallot, thyme, mayonnaise, mustard, salt, and pepper together in a container until smooth.
2. Whisking continuously, slowly drizzle in oil until completely blended.

Lemon Vinaigrette

Yield: ¼ cup

This recipe can be made quickly

(V) *This is a Vegetarian Recipe* (V)

This is best for dressing mild greens.

Ingredients:

- ⅛ teaspoon salt
- ¼ teaspoon grated lemon zest plus
- ½ teaspoon Dijon mustard
- ½ teaspoon mayonnaise
- 1 tablespoon juice
- 3 tablespoons extra-virgin olive oil
- Pinch pepper

- Pinch sugar

Directions:

1. Beat lemon zest and juice, mayonnaise, mustard, salt, pepper, and sugar together in a container until smooth.
2. Whisking continuously, slowly drizzle in oil until completely blended. (Vinaigrette will keep safely in a fridge for maximum 2 weeks.)

Tahini-Lemon Dressing

Yield: Approximately ½ cup

This recipe can be made quickly

Ⓥ This is a Vegetarian Recipe Ⓥ

Ingredients:

- ⅛ teaspoon pepper
- ¼ cup extra-virgin olive oil
- ½ teaspoon salt
- 1 garlic clove, minced
- 1 tablespoon water
- 2 tablespoons tahini
- 2½ tablespoons lemon juice

Directions:

1. Beat lemon juice, tahini, water, garlic, salt, and pepper together in a container until smooth.
2. Whisking continuously, slowly drizzle in oil until completely blended. (Dressing will keep safely in a fridge for maximum seven days.)

Walnut Vinaigrette

Yield: ¼ cup

✒ This recipe can be made quickly ✒

Ⓥ *This is a Vegetarian Recipe* Ⓥ

Ingredients:

- ⅛ teaspoon salt
- ½ teaspoon Dijon mustard
- ½ teaspoon mayonnaise
- 1 tablespoon wine vinegar
- 1½ tablespoons extra-virgin olive oil
- 1½ tablespoons roasted walnut oil
- 1½ teaspoons minced shallot
- Pinch pepper

Directions:

1. Beat vinegar, shallot, mayonnaise, mustard, salt, and pepper together in a container until smooth.
2. Whisking continuously, slowly drizzle in oils until completely blended. (Vinaigrette will keep safely in a fridge for maximum 2 weeks.)

Green Salads

Salads are a vital component of the Mediterranean diet. Enjoy these with a dressing of your choice!

Arugula Fennel Parmesan Salad

Yield: 4 to 6 Servings

This recipe can be made quickly

Ⓥ *This is a Vegetarian Recipe* Ⓥ

Ingredients:

- ¼ cup extra-virgin olive oil
- 1 large fennel bulb, stalks discarded, bulb halved, cored, and sliced thin
- 1 ounce Parmesan cheese, shaved
- 1 small garlic clove, minced
- 1 small shallot, minced
- 1 teaspoon Dijon mustard
- 1 teaspoon minced fresh thyme
- 1½ tablespoons lemon juice
- 6 ounces (6 cups) baby arugula
- Salt and pepper

Directions:

1. Gently toss arugula and fennel together in a big container. Beat lemon juice, shallot, mustard, thyme, garlic, ⅛ teaspoon salt, and pinch pepper together in a small-sized container.
2. Whisking continuously, slowly drizzle in oil. Sprinkle dressing over salad and gently toss to coat. Sprinkle with salt and pepper to taste. Serve, topping individual portions with Parmesan.

Arugula Mix Salad

Yield: 6 Servings

This recipe can be made quickly

Ingredients:

- ¼ cup extra-virgin olive oil
- ½ cup dried figs, stemmed and chopped
- ½ cup walnuts, toasted and chopped

- 1 small shallot, minced
- 1 tablespoon raspberry jam
- 2 ounces Parmesan cheese, shaved
- 2 ounces thinly sliced prosciutto, cut into ¼-inch-wide ribbons
- 3 tablespoons balsamic vinegar
- 8 ounces (8 cups) baby arugula
- Salt and pepper

Directions:

1. Heat 1 tablespoon oil in 10-inch non-stick frying pan on moderate heat. Put in prosciutto and cook, stirring frequently, until crisp, approximately seven minutes. Use a slotted spoon to move prosciutto to paper towel–lined plate; set aside.
2. Beat vinegar, jam, shallot, ¼ teaspoon salt, and ⅛ teaspoon pepper together in a big container. Mix in figs, cover, and microwave until steaming, about 1 minute. Whisking continuously, slowly drizzle in remaining 3 tablespoons oil. Allow to sit until figs are softened and vinaigrette has cooled to room temperature, about fifteen minutes.
3. Just before you serve, beat vinaigrette to re-emulsify. Put in arugula and gently toss to coat. Sprinkle with salt and pepper to taste. Serve, topping individual portions with prosciutto, walnuts, and Parmesan.

Arugula Sweet Salad

Yield: 6 Servings

✔ This recipe can be made quickly ✔

Ⓥ This is a Vegetarian Recipe Ⓥ

Honey can be substituted for the apricot jam.

Ingredients:

- ¼ small red onion, sliced thin

- ⅓ cup sliced almonds, toasted
- ½ cup dried apricots, chopped
- 1 ripe but firm pear, halved, cored, and sliced ¼ inch thick
- 1 small shallot, minced
- 1 tablespoon apricot jam
- 3 ounces goat cheese, crumbled (¾ cup)
- 3 tablespoons extra-virgin olive oil
- 3 tablespoons white wine vinegar
- 8 ounces (8 cups) baby arugula
- Salt and pepper

Directions:

1. Beat vinegar, jam, shallot, ¼ teaspoon salt, and ⅛ teaspoon pepper together in a big container. Put in apricots, cover, and microwave until steaming, about 1 minute. Whisking continuously, slowly drizzle in oil. Mix in onion and allow to sit until figs are softened and vinaigrette has cooled to room temperature, about fifteen minutes.
2. Just before you serve, beat vinaigrette to re-emulsify. Put in arugula and pear and gently toss to coat. Sprinkle with salt and pepper to taste. Serve, topping individual portions with almonds and goat cheese.

Asparagus Arugula Cannellini Salad

Yield: 4 to 6 Servings

This recipe can be made quickly

(V) This is a Vegetarian Recipe (V)

Ingredients:

- ½ red onion, sliced thin
- 1 (15-ounce) can cannellini beans, rinsed
- 1 pound asparagus, trimmed and cut on bias into 1-inch lengths

- 2 tablespoons plus 2 teaspoons balsamic vinegar
- 5 tablespoons extra-virgin olive oil
- 6 ounces (6 cups) baby arugula
- Salt and pepper

Directions:

1. Heat 2 tablespoons oil in 12-inch non-stick frying pan on high heat until just smoking. Put in onion and cook until lightly browned, about 1 minute. Put in asparagus, ¼ teaspoon salt, and ¼ teaspoon pepper and cook, stirring intermittently, until asparagus is browned and crisp-tender, about 4 minutes. Move to a container, mix in beans, and allow to cool slightly.
2. Beat vinegar, ¼ teaspoon salt, and ⅛ teaspoon pepper together in a small-sized container. Whisking continuously, slowly drizzle in remaining 3 tablespoons oil. Gently toss arugula with 2 tablespoons dressing until coated. Sprinkle with salt and pepper to taste. Divide arugula among plates. Toss asparagus mixture with remaining dressing, arrange over arugula, and serve.

Asparagus-Red Pepper-Spinach-Goat Cheese Salad

Yield: 4 to 6 Servings

✒ This recipe can be made quickly ✒

Ⓥ This is a Vegetarian Recipe Ⓥ

Ingredients:

- 1 garlic clove, minced
- 1 pound asparagus, trimmed and cut on bias into 1-inch lengths
- 1 red bell pepper, stemmed, seeded, and cut into 2-inch-long matchsticks
- 1 shallot, halved and sliced thin
- 1 tablespoon plus 1 teaspoon sherry vinegar

- 2 ounces goat cheese, crumbled (½ cup)
- 5 tablespoons extra-virgin olive oil
- 6 ounces (6 cups) baby spinach
- Salt and pepper

Directions:

1. Heat 1 tablespoon oil in 12-inch non-stick frying pan on high heat until just smoking. Put in bell pepper and cook until lightly browned, approximately two minutes. Put in asparagus, ¼ teaspoon salt, and ⅛ teaspoon pepper and cook, stirring intermittently, until asparagus is browned and almost tender, approximately two minutes. Mix in shallot and cook till they become tender and asparagus is crisp-tender, about 1 minute. Move to a container and allow to cool slightly.
2. Beat vinegar, garlic, ¼ teaspoon salt, and ⅛ teaspoon pepper together in a small-sized container. Whisking continuously, slowly drizzle in remaining ¼ cup oil. Gently toss spinach with 2 tablespoons dressing until coated. Sprinkle with salt and pepper to taste. Divide spinach among plates. Toss asparagus mixture with remaining dressing and arrange over spinach. Sprinkle with goat cheese and serve.

Bitter Greens Olive Feta Salad

Yield: 4 to 6 Servings

This recipe can be made quickly

Ⓥ *This is a Vegetarian Recipe* Ⓥ

Ingredients:

- ⅓ cup chopped fresh dill
- ⅓ cup pepperoncini, seeded and cut into ¼-inch-thick strips
- ½ cup pitted kalamata olives, halved
- 1 garlic clove, minced

- 1 head escarole (1 pound), trimmed and cut into 1-inch pieces
- 1 small head frisée (4 ounces), trimmed and torn into 1-inch pieces
- 2 ounces feta cheese, crumbled (½ cup)
- 2 tablespoons lemon juice
- 3 tablespoons extra-virgin olive oil
- Salt and pepper

Directions:

1. Gently toss escarole, frisée, olives, feta, and pepperoncini together in a big container. Beat dill, lemon juice, garlic, ¼ teaspoon salt, and ⅛ teaspoon pepper together in a small-sized container.
2. Whisking continuously, slowly drizzle in oil. Sprinkle dressing over salad and gently toss to coat. Serve.

Fiery Tuna-Olive Salad

Yield: 4 to 6 Servings

This recipe can be made quickly

Ingredients:

- ½ cup pimento-stuffed green olives, chopped
- 1 (15-ounce) can cannellini beans, rinsed
- 1 garlic clove, minced
- 1 tablespoon chopped fresh parsley
- 12 ounces cherry tomatoes, halved
- 2 (12-ounce) tuna steaks, 1 to 1¼ inches thick
- 3 tablespoons lemon juice
- 5 ounces (5 cups) baby arugula
- 6 tablespoons extra-virgin olive oil
- Salt and pepper

Directions:

1. Beat olives, lemon juice, parsley, and garlic together in a big container. Whisking continuously, slowly drizzle in 5 tablespoons oil. Sprinkle with salt and pepper to taste.
2. Pat tuna dry using paper towels and sprinkle with salt and pepper. Heat residual 1 tablespoon oil in 12-inch non-stick frying pan on moderate to high heat until just smoking. Cook tuna until thoroughly browned and translucent red at center when checked with tip of paring knife and registers 110 degrees (for rare), approximately two minutes each side. Move to slicing board and slice into ½-inch-thick slices.
3. Beat dressing to re-emulsify, then drizzle 1 tablespoon dressing over tuna. Put in arugula, tomatoes, and beans to a container with remaining dressing and gently toss to combine. Sprinkle with salt and pepper to taste. Divide salad among plates and top with tuna. Serve.

Fundamental Green Salad

Yield: 4 Servings

This recipe can be made quickly

Ⓥ *This is a Vegetarian Recipe* Ⓥ

Ingredients:

- ½ garlic clove, peeled
- 8 ounces (8 cups) lettuce, torn into bite-size pieces if needed
- Extra-virgin olive oil
- Salt and pepper
- Vinegar

Directions:

1. Take a salad bowl and coat its inside with garlic. Put in lettuce. Cautiously sprinkle lettuce with a little oil. Slowly toss the

contents of the bowl. Carry on drizzling with oil and toss gently until greens are mildly coated and barely starting to shine.
2. Drizzle with small amounts of vinegar, salt, and pepper to taste and toss gently to coat. Serve.

Green Artichoke Olive Salad

Yield: **4 to 6 Servings**

◢ This recipe can be made quickly ◣

Ⓥ This is a Vegetarian Recipe Ⓥ

Ingredients:

- ⅓ cup fresh parsley leaves
- ⅓ cup pitted kalamata olives, halved
- 1 cup jarred whole baby artichoke hearts packed in water, quartered, rinsed, and patted dry
- 1 ounce Asiago cheese, shaved
- 1 romaine lettuce heart (6 ounces), cut into 1-inch pieces
- 1 small garlic clove, minced
- 2 tablespoons white wine vinegar or white balsamic vinegar
- 3 ounces (3 cups) baby arugula
- 3 tablespoons extra-virgin olive oil
- Salt and pepper

Directions:

1. Gently toss romaine, arugula, artichoke hearts, parsley, and olives together in a big container. Beat vinegar, garlic, ¼ teaspoon salt, and pinch pepper together in a small-sized container.
2. Whisking continuously, slowly drizzle in oil. Sprinkle vinaigrette over salad and gently toss to coat. Sprinkle with salt and pepper to taste. Serve, topping individual portions with Asiago.

Green Marcona Manchego Salad

Yield: **4 to 6 Servings**

This recipe can be made quickly

(V) This is a Vegetarian Recipe (V)

Ingredients:

- ¼ cup extra-virgin olive oil
- ⅓ cup Marcona almonds, chopped coarse
- 1 shallot, minced
- 1 teaspoon Dijon mustard
- 2 ounces Manchego cheese, shaved
- 5 teaspoons sherry vinegar
- 6 ounces (6 cups) mesclun greens
- Salt and pepper

Directions:

1. Place mesclun in a big container. Beat vinegar, shallot, mustard, ¼ teaspoon salt, and ¼ teaspoon pepper together in a small-sized container. Whisking continuously, slowly drizzle in oil.
2. Sprinkle vinaigrette over mesclun and gently toss to coat. Sprinkle with salt and pepper to taste. Serve, topping individual portions with almonds and Manchego.

Kale-Sweet Potato Salad

Yield: **6 to 8 Servings**

(V) This is a Vegetarian Recipe (V)

Ingredients:

SALAD

- ⅓ cup pecans, toasted and chopped
- ½ head radicchio (5 ounces), cored and sliced thin
- 1½ pounds sweet potatoes, peeled, cut into ½-inch pieces
- 12 ounces Tuscan kale, stemmed and sliced crosswise into ½-inch-wide strips (7 cups)
- 2 teaspoons extra-virgin olive oil
- Salt and pepper
- Shaved Parmesan cheese

VINAIGRETTE

- ¼ cup extra-virgin olive oil
- 1 small shallot, minced
- 1 tablespoon cider vinegar
- 1 tablespoon honey
- 1½ tablespoons pomegranate molasses
- 2 tablespoons water
- Salt and pepper

Directions:

1. **For the Salad:** Place the oven rack in the centre of the oven and pre-heat your oven to 400 degrees. Toss sweet potatoes with oil and sprinkle with salt and pepper. Arrange potatoes in one layer in rimmed baking sheet and roast until browned, 25 to 30 minutes, flipping potatoes halfway through roasting. Move to plate and allow to cool for 20 minutes. In the meantime, heavily squeeze and massage kale with hands until leaves are uniformly darkened and slightly wilted, about 1 minute.
2. **For the Vinaigrette**: Beat water, pomegranate molasses, shallot, honey, vinegar, ¼ teaspoon salt, and ¼ teaspoon pepper together in a big container. Whisking continuously, slowly drizzle in oil.
3. Put in potatoes, kale, and radicchio to vinaigrette and gently toss to coat. Sprinkle with salt and pepper to taste. Move to serving platter and drizzle with pecans and shaved Parmesan to taste. Serve.

Mâche-Cucumber-Mint Salad

Yield: 6 to 8 Servings

This recipe can be made quickly

Ⓥ This is a Vegetarian Recipe Ⓥ

Ingredients:

- ¼ cup extra-virgin olive oil
- ⅓ cup pine nuts, toasted
- ½ cup chopped fresh mint
- 1 cucumber, sliced thin
- 1 garlic clove, minced
- 1 tablespoon capers, rinsed and minced
- 1 tablespoon lemon juice
- 1 tablespoon minced fresh parsley
- 1 teaspoon minced fresh thyme
- 12 ounces (12 cups) mâche
- Salt and pepper

Directions:

1. Gently toss mâche, cucumber, mint, and pine nuts together in a big container. Beat lemon juice, parsley, capers, thyme, garlic, ¼ teaspoon salt, and ¼ teaspoon pepper together in a small-sized container.
2. Whisking continuously, slowly drizzle in oil. Sprinkle dressing over salad and gently toss to coat. Sprinkle with salt and pepper to taste. Serve.

Salade Niçoise

Yield: 6 Servings

Ingredients:

DRESSING

- ¼ cup lemon juice (2 lemons)
- ¼ teaspoon pepper
- ½ cup extra-virgin olive oil
- ½ teaspoon salt
- 1 shallot, minced
- 1 teaspoon Dijon mustard
- 2 tablespoons minced fresh basil
- 2 teaspoons minced fresh oregano
- 2 teaspoons minced fresh thyme

SALAD

- ¼ cup pitted niçoise olives
- 1 small red onion, sliced thin
- 10–12 anchovy fillets, rinsed (optional)
- 1¼ pounds small red potatoes, unpeeled, quartered
- 2 (5-ounce) cans solid white tuna in water, drained and flaked
- 2 heads Boston lettuce or Bibb lettuce (1 pound), torn into bite-size pieces
- 2 tablespoons capers, rinsed (optional)
- 2 tablespoons dry vermouth
- 3 hard-cooked large eggs, peeled and quartered
- 3 small tomatoes, cored and cut into ½-inch-thick wedges
- 8 ounces green beans, trimmed and halved
- Salt and pepper

Directions:

1. **FOR THE DRESSING**: Beat lemon juice, shallot, basil, thyme, oregano, mustard, salt, and pepper together in a small-sized container. Whisking continuously, slowly drizzle in oil.
2. **FOR THE SALAD**: Place potatoes in a big saucepan, put in water to cover by 1 inch, and bring to boil on high heat. Put in 1 tablespoon salt, reduce to simmer, and cook until potatoes are soft and paring knife can be slipped in and out of potatoes with

little resistance, 5 to 8 minutes. With slotted spoon, gently move potatoes to a container (do not discard water). Toss warm potatoes with ¼ cup vinaigrette and vermouth. Sprinkle with salt and pepper to taste; set aside.
3. As potatoes cook, mildly toss lettuce with ¼ cup vinaigrette in a container until coated. Arrange bed of lettuce on very large, flat serving platter. Place tuna in now-empty bowl and break up using a fork. Put in ¼ cup vinaigrette and stir to combine. Mound tuna in center of lettuce. In now-empty bowl, toss tomatoes and red onion with 2 tablespoons vinaigrette and sprinkle with salt and pepper to taste. Arrange tomato-onion mixture in mound at edge of lettuce bed. Arrange rest of the potatoes in separate mound at edge of lettuce bed.
4. Return water to boil and put in 1 tablespoon salt and green beans. Cook until crisp-tender, 3 to 5 minutes. In the meantime, fill big container halfway with ice and water. Drain green beans, move to ice water, and allow to sit until just cool, approximately half a minute. Move beans to triple layer of paper towels and dry well. In now-empty bowl, toss green beans with remaining 2 tablespoons vinaigrette and sprinkle with salt and pepper to taste. Arrange in separate mound at edge of lettuce bed.
5. Place eggs, olives, and anchovies, if using, in separate mounds at edge of lettuce bed. Sprinkle the whole salad with capers, if using. Serve.

Spinach-Feta-Pistachio Salad

Yield: 6 Servings

✔ *This recipe can be made quickly* ✔

Ⓥ *This is a Vegetarian Recipe* Ⓥ

Ingredients:

- 1 (2-inch) strip lemon zest plus 1½ tablespoons juice
- 1 shallot, minced

- 10 ounces curly-leaf spinach, stemmed and torn into bite-size pieces
- 1½ ounces feta cheese, crumbled (⅓ cup)
- 2 teaspoons sugar
- 3 tablespoons chopped toasted pistachios
- 3 tablespoons extra-virgin olive oil
- 6 radishes, trimmed and sliced thin
- Salt and pepper

Directions:

1. Place feta on plate and freeze until mildly stiff, about fifteen minutes.
2. Cook oil, lemon zest, shallot, and sugar in Dutch oven over moderate to low heat until shallot is softened, approximately five minutes. Remove from the heat, discard zest and mix in lemon juice. Put in spinach, cover, and let steam off heat until it just begins to wilt, approximately half a minute.
3. Move spinach mixture and liquid left in pot to big container. Put in radishes, pistachios, and chilled feta and toss to combine. Sprinkle with salt and pepper to taste. Serve.

Tangy Salad

Yield: 4 to 6 Servings

This recipe can be made quickly

Ⓥ *This is a Vegetarian Recipe* Ⓥ

Ingredients:

- ½ cup smoked almonds, chopped coarse
- ⅔ cup chopped pitted dates
- 1 small head radicchio (6 ounces), cored and sliced thin
- 1 small shallot, minced
- 1 teaspoon Dijon mustard

- 1 teaspoon sugar
- 2 red grapefruits
- 3 oranges
- 3 tablespoons extra-virgin olive oil
- Salt and pepper

Directions:

1. Cut away peel and pith from grapefruits and oranges. Cut each fruit in half from pole to pole, then slice crosswise ¼ inch thick. Move to a container, toss with sugar and ½ teaspoon salt, and allow to sit for about fifteen minutes.
2. Drain fruit in fine-mesh strainer set over bowl, reserving 2 tablespoons juice. Arrange fruit on serving platter and drizzle with oil. Beat reserved juice, shallot, and mustard together in medium bowl. Put in radicchio, ⅓ cup dates, and ¼ cup almonds and gently toss to coat. Sprinkle with salt and pepper to taste. Arrange radicchio mixture over fruit, leaving 1-inch border of fruit around edges. Sprinkle with remaining ⅓ cup dates and remaining ¼ cup almonds. Serve.

Tri-Balsamic Salad

Yield: 4 to 6 Servings

This recipe can be made quickly

Ⓥ *This is a Vegetarian Recipe* Ⓥ

Ingredients:

- 1 head Belgian endive (4 ounces), cut into 2-inch pieces
- 1 small head radicchio (6 ounces), cored and cut into 1-inch pieces
- 1 tablespoon balsamic vinegar
- 1 teaspoon red wine vinegar
- 3 ounces (3 cups) baby arugula

- 3 tablespoons extra-virgin olive oil
- Salt and pepper

Directions:

1. Gently toss radicchio, endive, and arugula together in a big container. Beat balsamic vinegar, red wine vinegar, ⅛ teaspoon salt, and pinch pepper together in a small-sized container.
2. Whisking continuously, slowly drizzle in oil. Drizzle vinaigrette over salad and gently toss to coat. Drizzle with salt and pepper to taste. Serve.

Vegetable Salads

Algerian Mix Salad

Yield: 4 to 6 Servings

This recipe can be made quickly

Ⓥ *This is a Vegetarian Recipe* Ⓥ

Ingredients:

- ¼ cup coarsely chopped fresh mint
- ¼ cup extra-virgin olive oil
- ½ cup pitted oil-cured black olives, quartered
- 2 fennel bulbs, stalks discarded, bulbs halved, cored, and sliced thin
- 2 tablespoons lemon juice
- 4 blood oranges
- Salt and pepper

Directions:

1. Cut away peel and pith from oranges. Quarter oranges, then slice crosswise into ¼-inch-thick pieces. Mix oranges, fennel, olives, and mint in a big container.
2. Beat lemon juice, ¼ teaspoon salt, and ⅛ teaspoon pepper together in a small-sized container. Whisking continuously, slowly drizzle in oil. Sprinkle dressing over salad and gently toss to coat. Sprinkle with salt and pepper to taste. Serve.

Asparagus Mix Salad

Yield: 4 to 6 Servings

This recipe can be made quickly

Ⓥ This is a Vegetarian Recipe Ⓥ

Ingredients:

PESTO

- ¼ cup fresh basil leaves
- ¼ cup grated Pecorino Romano cheese
- ½ cup extra-virgin olive oil
- 1 garlic clove, minced
- 1 teaspoon grated lemon zest plus 2 teaspoons juice
- 2 cups fresh mint leaves
- Salt and pepper

SALAD

- ¾ cup hazelnuts, toasted, skinned, and chopped
- 2 oranges
- 2 pounds asparagus, trimmed
- 4 ounces feta cheese, crumbled (1 cup)
- Salt and pepper

Directions:

1. **For the Pesto:** Process mint, basil, Pecorino, lemon zest and juice, garlic, and ¾ teaspoon salt using a food processor until finely chopped, approximately half a minute, scraping down sides of the container as required. Move to big container. Mix in oil and sprinkle with salt and pepper to taste.
2. **For the Salad:** Chop asparagus tips from stalks into ¾-inch-long pieces. Cut asparagus stalks ⅛ inch thick on bias into approximate 2-inch lengths. Cut away the peel and pith from oranges. Holding fruit over bowl, use paring knife to cut between membranes to release segments. Put in asparagus tips and stalks, orange segments, feta, and hazelnuts to pesto and toss to combine. Sprinkle with salt and pepper to taste. Serve.

Brussels Pecorino Pine Salad

Yield: 4 to 6 Servings

✎ This recipe can be made quickly ✎

Ⓥ This is a Vegetarian Recipe Ⓥ

Ingredients:

- ¼ cup extra-virgin olive oil
- ¼ cup pine nuts, toasted
- 1 garlic clove, minced
- 1 pound Brussels sprouts, trimmed, halved, and sliced very thin
- 1 small shallot, minced
- 1 tablespoon Dijon mustard
- 2 ounces Pecorino Romano cheese, shredded (⅔ cup)
- 2 tablespoons lemon juice
- Salt and pepper

Directions:

1. Beat lemon juice, mustard, shallot, garlic, and ½ teaspoon salt together in a big container. Whisking continuously, slowly

drizzle in oil. Put in Brussels sprouts, toss to coat, and allow to sit for minimum half an hour or maximum 2 hours.
2. Mix in Pecorino and pine nuts. Sprinkle with salt and pepper to taste. Serve.

Cauliflower Chermoula Salad

Yield: 4 to 6 Servings

Ⓥ This is a Vegetarian Recipe Ⓥ

Ingredients:

SALAD

- ½ cup raisins
- ½ red onion, sliced ¼ inch thick
- 1 cup shredded carrot
- 1 head cauliflower (2 pounds), cored and cut into 2-inch florets
- 2 tablespoons chopped fresh cilantro
- 2 tablespoons extra-virgin olive oil
- 2 tablespoons sliced almonds, toasted
- Salt and pepper

CHERMOULA

- ⅛ teaspoon cayenne pepper
- ¼ cup extra-virgin olive oil
- ¼ teaspoon salt
- ½ teaspoon ground cumin
- ½ teaspoon paprika
- ¾ cup fresh cilantro leaves
- 2 tablespoons lemon juice
- 4 garlic cloves, minced

Directions:

1. **For the Salad:** Place oven rack to lowest position and pre-heat your oven to 475 degrees. Toss cauliflower with oil and sprinkle with salt and pepper. Arrange cauliflower in one layer in parchment paper–lined rimmed baking sheet. Cover tightly with aluminium foil and roast till they become tender, 5 to 7 minutes. Remove foil and spread onion evenly in sheet. Roast until vegetables are tender, cauliflower becomes deeply golden brown, and onion slices are charred at edges, 10 to fifteen minutes, stirring halfway through roasting. Allow it to cool slightly, approximately five minutes.
2. **For the Chermoula:** Process all ingredients using a food processor until smooth, about 1 minute, scraping down sides of the container as required. Move to big container.
3. Gently toss cauliflower-onion mixture, carrot, raisins, and cilantro with chermoula until coated. Move to serving platter and drizzle with almonds. Serve warm or at room temperature.

Cherry Tomato Mix Salad

Yield: 4 to 6 Servings

Ⓥ This is a Vegetarian Recipe Ⓥ

Ingredients:

- ½ cup pitted kalamata olives, chopped
- ½ teaspoon sugar
- 1 shallot, minced
- 1 small cucumber, peeled, halved along the length, seeded, and cut into ½-inch pieces
- 1 tablespoon red wine vinegar
- 1½ pounds cherry tomatoes, quartered
- 2 garlic cloves, minced
- 2 tablespoons extra-virgin olive oil
- 2 teaspoons minced fresh oregano
- 3 tablespoons chopped fresh parsley

- 4 ounces feta cheese, crumbled (1 cup)
- Salt and pepper

Directions:

1. Toss tomatoes with sugar and ¼ teaspoon salt in a container and allow to sit for 30 minutes. Move tomatoes to salad spinner and spin until seeds and excess liquid have been removed, 45 to 60 seconds, stopping to redistribute tomatoes several times during spinning. Put in tomatoes, cucumber, olives, feta, and parsley to big container; set aside.
2. Strain ½ cup tomato liquid through fine-mesh strainer into liquid measuring cup; discard remaining liquid. Bring tomato liquid, shallot, vinegar, garlic, and oregano to simmer in small saucepan on moderate heat and cook until reduced to 3 tablespoons, six to eight minutes. Move to small-sized container and allow to cool to room temperature, approximately five minutes. Whisking continuously, slowly drizzle in oil. Sprinkle dressing over salad and gently toss to coat. Sprinkle with salt and pepper to taste. Serve.

Classic Greek Salad

Yield: 6 to 8 Servings

✒ This recipe can be made quickly ✒

Ⓥ This is a Vegetarian Recipe Ⓥ

Ingredients:

- ¼ cup chopped fresh mint
- ¼ cup chopped fresh parsley
- ½ cup pitted kalamata olives, quartered
- ½ red onion, sliced thin
- 1 cup jarred roasted red peppers, rinsed, patted dry, and cut into ½-inch strips

- 1 garlic clove, minced
- 1 teaspoon lemon juice
- 1½ tablespoons red wine vinegar
- 2 cucumbers, peeled, halved along the length, seeded, and sliced thin
- 2 teaspoons minced fresh oregano
- 5 ounces feta cheese, crumbled (1¼ cups)
- 6 large ripe tomatoes, cored, seeded, and cut into ½-inch-thick wedges
- 6 tablespoons extra-virgin olive oil
- Salt and pepper

Directions:

1. Beat oil, vinegar, oregano, lemon juice, garlic, ½ teaspoon salt, and ⅛ teaspoon pepper together in a big container. Put in cucumbers and onion, toss to coat, and allow to sit for 20 minutes.
2. Put in tomatoes, red peppers, olives, parsley, and mint to a container with cucumber-onion mixture and toss to combine. Sprinkle with salt and pepper to taste. Move salad to wide, shallow serving bowl or platter and drizzle with feta. Serve instantly.

Crunchy Mushroom Salad

Yield: 6 Servings

✒This recipe can be made quickly ✒

Ⓥ This is a Vegetarian Recipe Ⓥ

Ingredients:

- ¼ cup extra-virgin olive oil
- ½ cup fresh parsley leaves
- 1 shallot, halved and sliced thin

- 1½ tablespoons lemon juice
- 2 ounces Parmesan cheese, shaved
- 2 tablespoons chopped fresh tarragon
- 4 celery ribs, sliced thin, plus ½ cup celery leaves
- 8 ounces cremini mushrooms, trimmed and sliced thin
- Salt and pepper

Directions:

1. Beat oil, lemon juice, and ¼ teaspoon salt together in a big container. Put in mushrooms and shallot, toss to coat, and allow to sit for about ten minutes.
2. Put in sliced celery and leaves, Parmesan, parsley, and tarragon to mushroom-shallot mixture and toss to combine. Sprinkle with salt and pepper to taste. Serve.

Cucumber Sesame-Lemon Salad

Yield: 4 Servings

(V) This is a Vegetarian Recipe (V)

Ingredients:

- ⅛ teaspoon red pepper flakes, plus extra for seasoning
- ¼ cup rice vinegar
- 1 tablespoon lemon juice
- 1 tablespoon sesame seeds, toasted
- 2 tablespoons toasted sesame oil
- 2 teaspoons sugar
- 3 cucumbers, peeled, halved along the length, seeded, and sliced ¼ inch thick
- Salt and pepper

Directions:

1. Toss cucumbers with 1 tablespoon salt using a colander set over big container. Weight cucumbers with 1 gallon-size zipper-lock bag filled with water; drain for 1 to three hours. Wash and pat dry.
2. Beat vinegar, oil, lemon juice, sesame seeds, sugar, and pepper flakes together in a big container. Put in cucumbers and toss to coat. Sprinkle with salt and pepper to taste. Serve at room temperature or chilled.

Cut Up Salad

Yield: 4 Servings

ⓥ This is a Vegetarian Recipe ⓥ

Ingredients:

- ½ cup chopped fresh parsley
- ½ cup pitted kalamata olives, chopped
- ½ small red onion, chopped fine
- 1 (15-ounce) can chickpeas, rinsed
- 1 cucumber, peeled, halved along the length, seeded, and cut into ½-inch pieces
- 1 garlic clove, minced
- 1 romaine lettuce heart (6 ounces), cut into ½-inch pieces
- 10 ounces grape tomatoes, quartered
- 3 tablespoons extra-virgin olive oil
- 3 tablespoons red wine vinegar
- 4 ounces feta cheese, crumbled (1 cup)
- Salt and pepper

Directions:

1. Toss cucumber and tomatoes with 1 teaspoon salt and allow to drain using a colander for about fifteen minutes.
2. Beat vinegar and garlic together in a big container. Whisking continuously, slowly drizzle in oil. Put in cucumber-tomato

mixture, chickpeas, olives, onion, and parsley and toss to coat. Allow to sit for minimum 5 minutes or maximum 20 minutes.
3. Put in lettuce and feta and gently toss to combine. Sprinkle with salt and pepper to taste. Serve.

Fattoush

Yield: 4 to 6 Servings

Ⓥ *This is a Vegetarian Recipe* Ⓥ

Ingredients:

- ¼ teaspoon minced garlic
- ½ cup chopped fresh cilantro
- ½ cup chopped fresh mint
- 1 cup arugula, chopped coarse
- 1 English cucumber, peeled and sliced ⅛ inch thick
- 1 pound ripe tomatoes, cored and cut into ¾-inch pieces
- 2 (8-inch) pita breads
- 3 tablespoons lemon juice
- 4 scallions, sliced thin
- 4 teaspoons ground sumac, plus extra for sprinkling
- 7 tablespoons extra-virgin olive oil
- Salt and pepper

Directions:

1. Place the oven rack in the centre of the oven and pre-heat your oven to 375 degrees. Using kitchen shears, slice around perimeter of each pita and divide into 2 thin rounds. Cut each round in half. Place pitas smooth side down on wire rack set in rimmed baking sheet. Brush 3 tablespoons oil on surface of pitas. (Pitas do not need to be uniformly coated. Oil will spread during baking.) Sprinkle with salt and pepper. Bake until pitas are crisp and pale golden brown, 10 to 14 minutes. Allow it to cool to room temperature.

2. Beat lemon juice, sumac, garlic, and ¼ teaspoon salt together in a small-sized container and allow to sit for about ten minutes. Whisking continuously, slowly drizzle in remaining ¼ cup oil.
3. Break pitas into ½-inch pieces and place in a big container. Put in tomatoes, cucumber, arugula, cilantro, mint, and scallions. Sprinkle dressing over salad and gently toss to coat. Sprinkle with salt and pepper to taste. Serve, sprinkling individual portions with extra sumac.

French Potato Dijon Herb Salad

Yield: 4 to 6 Servings

Ⓥ This is a Vegetarian Recipe Ⓥ

Ingredients:

- ¼ cup extra-virgin olive oil
- ½ teaspoon pepper
- 1 garlic clove, peeled and threaded on skewer
- 1 small shallot, minced
- 1 tablespoon minced fresh chervil
- 1 tablespoon minced fresh chives
- 1 tablespoon minced fresh parsley
- 1 teaspoon minced fresh tarragon
- 1½ tablespoons white wine vinegar or Champagne vinegar
- 2 pounds small red potatoes, unpeeled, sliced ¼ inch thick
- 2 tablespoons salt
- 2 teaspoons Dijon mustard

Directions:

1. Place potatoes in a big saucepan, put in water to cover by 1 inch, and bring to boil on high heat. Put in salt, decrease the heat to simmer, and cook until potatoes are soft and paring knife can be slipped in and out of potatoes with little resistance, about 6 minutes.

2. While potatoes are cooking, lower skewered garlic into simmering water and blanch for 45 seconds. Run garlic under cold running water, then remove from skewer and mince.
3. Reserve ¼ cup cooking water, then drain potatoes and lay out on tight one layer in rimmed baking sheet. Beat oil, minced garlic, vinegar, mustard, pepper, and reserved potato cooking water together in a container, then drizzle over potatoes. Let potatoes sit until flavours blend, about 10 minutes. (Potatoes will keep safely in a fridge for maximum 8 hours; return to room temperature before you serve.)
4. Move potatoes to big container. Mix shallot and herbs in a small-sized container, then drizzle over potatoes and gently toss to coat using rubber spatula. Serve.

Green Bean Cilantro Salad

Yield: 6 to 8 Servings

✒ *This recipe can be made quickly* ✒

Ⓥ *This is a Vegetarian Recipe* Ⓥ

Ingredients:

- ¼ cup walnuts
- ½ cup extra-virgin olive oil
- 1 scallion, sliced thin
- 2 garlic cloves, unpeeled
- 2 pounds green beans, trimmed
- 2½ cups fresh cilantro leaves and stems, tough stem ends trimmed (about 2 bunches)
- 4 teaspoons lemon juice
- Salt and pepper

Directions:

1. Cook walnuts and garlic in 8-inch frying pan on moderate heat, stirring frequently, until toasted and aromatic, 5 to 7 minutes; move to a container. Let garlic cool slightly, then peel and approximately chop.
2. Process walnuts, garlic, cilantro, oil, lemon juice, scallion, ½ teaspoon salt, and ⅛ teaspoon pepper using a food processor until smooth, about 1 minute, scraping down sides of the container as required; move to big container.
3. Bring 4 quarts water to boil in large pot on high heat. In the meantime, fill big container halfway with ice and water. Put in 1 tablespoon salt and green beans to boiling water and cook until crisp-tender, 3 to 5 minutes. Drain green beans, move to ice water, and allow to sit until chilled, approximately two minutes. Move green beans to a container with cilantro sauce and gently toss until coated. Sprinkle with salt and pepper to taste. Serve. (Salad will keep safely in a fridge for maximum 4 hours.)

Halloumi-Veg Salad

Yield: 4 to 6 Servings

✏ This recipe can be made quickly ✏

Ⓥ This is a Vegetarian Recipe Ⓥ

Ingredients:

- ¼ cup extra-virgin olive oil
- ½ teaspoon grated lemon zest plus 3 tablespoons juice
- 1 (8-ounce) block halloumi cheese, sliced into ½-inch-thick slabs
- 1 garlic clove, minced
- 1 head radicchio (10 ounces), quartered
- 1 pound eggplant, sliced into ½-inch-thick rounds
- 1 tablespoon minced fresh thyme
- 1 zucchini, halved along the length
- 3 tablespoons honey
- Salt and pepper

Directions:

1. Beat honey, thyme, lemon zest and juice, garlic, ⅛ teaspoon salt, and ⅛ teaspoon pepper together in a big container; set aside. Brush eggplant, radicchio, zucchini, and halloumi with 2 tablespoons oil and sprinkle with salt and pepper.
2. **FOR A CHARCOAL GRILL:** Open bottom vent fully. Light large chimney starter half filled with charcoal briquettes (3 quarts). When top coals are partially covered with ash, pour uniformly over grill. Set cooking grate in place, cover, and open lid vent fully. Heat grill until hot, approximately five minutes.
3. **FOR A GAS GRILL:** Turn all burners to high, cover, and heat grill until hot, about fifteen minutes. Turn all burners to medium.
4. Clean cooking grate, then repetitively brush grate with thoroughly oiled paper towels until grate is black and glossy, 5 to 10 times. Place vegetables and cheese on grill. Cook (covered if using gas), flipping as required, until radicchio becomes tender and mildly charred, 3 to 5 minutes, and remaining vegetables and cheese are softened and mildly charred, about 10 minutes. Move vegetables and cheese to slicing board as they finish cooking, allow to cool slightly, then cut into 1-inch pieces.
5. Whisking continuously, slowly drizzle remaining 2 tablespoons oil into honey mixture. Put in vegetables and cheese and gently toss to coat. Sprinkle with salt and pepper to taste. Serve.

Italian Panzanella Mix Salad

Yield: 6 Servings

Ⓥ This is a Vegetarian Recipe Ⓥ

Ingredients:

- 1 (15-ounce) can cannellini beans, rinsed
- 1 small red onion, halved and sliced thin

- 1½ pounds ripe tomatoes, cored and chopped, seeds and juice reserved
- 12 ounces rustic Italian bread, cut into 1-inch pieces (4 cups)
- 2 ounces Parmesan cheese, shaved
- 2 tablespoons minced fresh oregano
- 3 ounces (3 cups) baby arugula
- 3 tablespoons chopped fresh basil
- 3 tablespoons red wine vinegar
- 5 tablespoons extra-virgin olive oil
- Salt and pepper

Directions:

1. Place the oven rack in the centre of the oven and pre-heat your oven to 350 degrees. Toss bread pieces with 1 tablespoon oil and sprinkle with salt and pepper. Arrange bread in one layer in rimmed baking sheet and bake, stirring intermittently, until light golden brown, fifteen to twenty minutes. Allow it to cool to room temperature.
2. Beat vinegar and ¼ teaspoon salt together in a big container. Whisking continuously, slowly drizzle in remaining ¼ cup oil. Put in tomatoes with their seeds and juice, beans, onion, 1½ tablespoons basil, and 1 tablespoon oregano, toss to coat, and allow to sit for 20 minutes.
3. Put in cooled croutons, arugula, remaining 1½ tablespoons basil, and remaining 1 tablespoon oregano and gently toss to combine. Sprinkle with salt and pepper to taste. Move salad to serving platter and drizzle with Parmesan. Serve.

Mackerel-Fennel-Apple Salad

Yield: 4 to 6 Servings

Ingredients:

- ¼ cup extra-virgin olive oil

- 1 fennel bulb, stalks discarded, bulb halved, cored, and sliced thin
- 1 small shallot, minced
- 1 tablespoon whole-grain mustard
- 2 Granny Smith apples, peeled, cored, and cut into 3-inch-long matchsticks
- 2 teaspoons minced fresh tarragon
- 3 tablespoons lemon juice
- 5 ounces (5 cups) watercress
- 6 ounces smoked mackerel, skin and pin bones removed, flaked
- Salt and pepper

Directions:

1. Beat lemon juice, mustard, shallot, 1 teaspoon tarragon, ½ teaspoon salt, and ¼ teaspoon pepper together in a big container. Whisking continuously, slowly drizzle in oil. Put in watercress, apples, and fennel and gently toss to coat. Sprinkle with salt and pepper to taste.
2. Divide salad among plates and top with flaked mackerel. Sprinkle any remaining dressing over mackerel and drizzle with remaining 1 teaspoon tarragon. Serve instantly.

Moroccan Carrot Salad

Yield: 4 to 6 Servings

This recipe can be made quickly

Ⓥ *This is a Vegetarian Recipe* Ⓥ

Ingredients:

- ⅛ teaspoon cayenne pepper
- ⅛ teaspoon ground cinnamon
- ¾ teaspoon ground cumin
- 1 pound carrots, peeled and shredded

- 1 tablespoon lemon juice
- 1 teaspoon honey
- 2 oranges
- 3 tablespoons extra-virgin olive oil
- 3 tablespoons minced fresh cilantro
- Salt and pepper

Directions:

1. Cut away peel and pith from oranges. Holding fruit over bowl, use paring knife to slice between membranes to release segments. Cut segments in half crosswise and allow to drain in fine-mesh strainer set over big container, reserving juice.
2. Beat lemon juice, honey, cumin, cayenne, cinnamon, and ½ teaspoon salt into reserved orange juice. Put in drained oranges and carrots and gently toss to coat. Allow to sit until liquid starts to pool in bottom of bowl, 3 to 5 minutes.
3. Drain salad in fine-mesh strainer and return to now-empty bowl. Mix in cilantro and oil and sprinkle with salt and pepper to taste. Serve.

Radish-Fava Salad

Yield: 4 to 6 Servings

This recipe can be made quickly

(V) This is a Vegetarian Recipe (V)

Ingredients:

- ¼ cup chopped fresh basil
- ¼ cup extra-virgin olive oil
- ¼ teaspoon ground coriander
- ¼ teaspoon pepper
- ½ teaspoon salt
- 10 radishes, trimmed, halved, and sliced thin

- 1½ ounces (1½ cups) pea shoots
- 2 garlic cloves, minced
- 3 pounds fava beans, shelled (3 cups)
- 3 tablespoons lemon juice

Directions:

1. Bring 4 quarts water to boil in large pot on high heat. In the meantime, fill big container halfway with ice and water. Put in fava beans to boiling water and cook for about sixty seconds. Drain fava beans, move to ice water, and allow to sit until chilled, approximately two minutes. Move fava beans to triple layer of paper towels and dry well. Use a paring knife to make small cut along edge of each bean through waxy sheath, then gently squeeze sheath to release bean; discard sheath.
2. Beat lemon juice, garlic, salt, pepper, and coriander together in a big container. Whisking continuously, slowly drizzle in oil. Put in fava beans, radishes, pea shoots, and basil and gently toss to coat. Serve instantly.

Roasted Beet-Carrot Salad with

Yield: 4 to 6 Servings

Ⓥ *This is a Vegetarian Recipe* Ⓥ

Ingredients:

- ½ cup shelled pistachios, toasted and chopped
- ½ teaspoon ground cumin
- 1 pound beets, trimmed
- 1 pound carrots, peeled and sliced on bias ¼ inch thick
- 1 small shallot, minced
- 1 tablespoon grated lemon zest plus 3 tablespoons juice
- 1 teaspoon honey
- 2 tablespoons minced fresh parsley
- 2½ tablespoons extra-virgin olive oil

- Salt and pepper

Directions:

1. Adjust oven racks to middle and lowest positions. Place rimmed baking sheet on lower rack and pre-heat your oven to 450 degrees.
2. Wrap each beet individually in aluminium foil and place in second rimmed baking sheet. Toss carrots with 1 tablespoon oil, ½ teaspoon salt, and ½ teaspoon pepper.
3. Quickly, arrange carrots in one layer in hot baking sheet and place baking sheet with beets on middle rack. Roast until carrots are soft and thoroughly browned on 1 side, 20 minutes to half an hour, and skewer can be inserted easily into the center of the beets with aluminium foil removed 35 to 45 minutes.
4. Cautiously open foil packets and allow beets to sit until cool enough to handle. Cautiously rub off beet skins using paper towel. Slice beets into ½-inch-thick wedges, and, if large, cut in half crosswise.
5. Beat lemon juice, shallot, honey, cumin, ¼ teaspoon salt, and ⅛ teaspoon pepper together in a big container. Whisking continuously, slowly drizzle in remaining 1½ tablespoons oil. Put in beets and carrots, toss to coat, and allow to cool to room temperature, approximately twenty minutes.
6. Put in pistachios, parsley, and lemon zest to a container with beets and carrots and toss to coat. Sprinkle with salt and pepper to taste. Serve.

Scorched Beet Almond Salad

Yield: 4 to 6 Servings

Ⓥ This is a Vegetarian Recipe Ⓥ

Ingredients:

- 2 blood oranges
- 2 ounces (2 cups) baby arugula
- 2 ounces ricotta salata cheese, shaved
- 2 pounds beets, trimmed
- 2 tablespoons extra-virgin olive oil
- 2 tablespoons sliced almonds, toasted
- 4 teaspoons sherry vinegar
- Salt and pepper

Directions:

1. Place the oven rack in the centre of the oven and pre-heat your oven to 400 degrees. Wrap each beet individually in aluminium foil and place in rimmed baking sheet. Roast beets until it is easy to skewer the centre of beets with foil removed, forty minutes to one hour.
2. Cautiously open foil packets and allow beets to sit until cool enough to handle. Cautiously rub off beet skins using a paper towel. Slice beets into ½-inch-thick wedges, and, if large, cut in half crosswise.
3. Beat vinegar, ¼ teaspoon salt, and ¼ teaspoon pepper together in a big container. Whisking continuously, slowly drizzle in oil. Put in beets, toss to coat, and allow to cool to room temperature, approximately twenty minutes.
4. Cut away peel and pith from oranges. Quarter oranges, then slice crosswise into ½-inch-thick pieces. Put in oranges and arugula to a container with beets and gently toss to coat. Sprinkle with salt and pepper to taste. Move to serving platter and drizzle with ricotta salata and almonds. Serve.

Sweet Nut Winter Squash Salad

Yield: 4 to 6 Servings

(V) This is a Vegetarian Recipe (V)

Ingredients:

- ¼ cup extra-virgin olive oil
- ⅓ cup roasted, unsalted pepitas
- ½ cup pomegranate seeds
- ¾ cup fresh parsley leaves
- 1 small shallot, minced
- 1 teaspoon za'atar
- 2 tablespoons honey
- 2 tablespoons lemon juice
- 3 pounds butternut squash, peeled, seeded, and cut into ½-inch pieces (8 cups)
- Salt and pepper

Directions:

1. Place oven rack to lowest position and pre-heat your oven to 450 degrees. Toss squash with 1 tablespoon oil and sprinkle with salt and pepper. Arrange squash in one layer in rimmed baking sheet and roast until thoroughly browned and tender, 30 to 35 minutes, stirring halfway through roasting. Sprinkle squash with za'atar and allow to cool for about fifteen minutes.
2. Beat shallot, lemon juice, honey, and ¼ teaspoon salt together in a big container. Whisking continuously, slowly drizzle in remaining 3 tablespoons oil. Put in squash, parsley, and pepitas and gently toss to coat. Arrange salad on serving platter and drizzle with pomegranate seeds. Serve.

Tomato Mix Salad

Yield: 6 Servings

✐ This recipe can be made quickly ✐

Ⓥ This is a Vegetarian Recipe Ⓥ

Ingredients:

- ¼ cup plain Greek yogurt

- 1 garlic clove, minced
- 1 scallion, sliced thin
- 1 tablespoon extra-virgin olive oil
- 1 tablespoon lemon juice
- 1 tablespoon minced fresh oregano
- 1 teaspoon ground cumin
- 2½ pounds ripe tomatoes, cored and cut into ½-inch-thick wedges
- 3 ounces feta cheese, crumbled (¾ cup)
- Salt and pepper

Directions:

1. Toss tomatoes with ½ teaspoon salt and allow to drain using a colander set over bowl for fifteen to twenty minutes.
2. Microwave oil, garlic, and cumin in a container until aromatic, approximately half a minute; allow to cool slightly. Move 1 tablespoon tomato liquid to big container; discard remaining liquid. Beat in yogurt, lemon juice, scallion, oregano, and oil mixture until combined. Put in tomatoes and feta and gently toss to coat. Sprinkle with salt and pepper to taste. Serve.

Tomato-Burrata Mix Salad

Yield: 4 to 6 Servings

Ⓥ *This is a Vegetarian Recipe* Ⓥ

Ingredients:

- ½ cup chopped fresh basil
- 1 garlic clove, minced
- 1 shallot, halved and sliced thin
- 1½ pounds ripe tomatoes, cored and cut into 1-inch pieces
- 1½ tablespoons white balsamic vinegar
- 3 ounces rustic Italian bread, cut into 1-inch pieces (1 cup)
- 6 tablespoons extra-virgin olive oil

- 8 ounces burrata cheese, room temperature
- 8 ounces ripe cherry tomatoes, halved
- Salt and pepper

Directions:

1. Toss tomatoes with ¼ teaspoon salt and allow to drain using a colander for 30 minutes.
2. Pulse bread using a food processor into large crumbs measuring between ⅛ and ¼ inch, approximately ten pulses. Mix crumbs, 2 tablespoons oil, pinch salt, and pinch pepper in 12-inch non-stick skillet. Cook on moderate heat, stirring frequently, until crumbs are crisp and golden, about 10 minutes. Clear center of skillet, put in garlic, and cook, mashing it into skillet, until aromatic, approximately half a minute. Stir garlic into crumbs. Move to plate and allow to cool slightly.
3. Beat shallot, vinegar, and ¼ teaspoon salt together in a big container. Whisking continuously, slowly drizzle in remaining ¼ cup oil. Put in tomatoes and basil and gently toss to combine. Sprinkle with salt and pepper to taste and arrange on serving platter. Cut buratta into 1-inch pieces, collecting creamy liquid. Sprinkle burrata over tomatoes and drizzle with creamy liquid. Sprinkle with bread crumbs and serve instantly.

Tomato-Tuna Mix Salad

Yield: 6 Servings

This recipe can be made quickly

Ingredients:

- ¼ cup capers, rinsed and minced
- ¼ cup extra-virgin olive oil
- ¼ cup finely chopped red onion
- ⅓ cup pitted kalamata olives, chopped coarse
- 1 (5-ounce) can solid white tuna in water, drained and flaked

- 1 tablespoon lemon juice
- 2 tablespoons chopped fresh parsley
- 2½ pounds ripe tomatoes, cored and cut into ½-inch-thick wedges
- Salt and pepper

Directions:

1. Toss tomatoes with ½ teaspoon salt and allow to drain using a colander set over bowl for fifteen to twenty minutes.
2. Move 1 tablespoon tomato liquid to big container; discard remaining liquid. Beat in oil, olives, capers, onion, parsley, and lemon juice until combined. Put in tomatoes and tuna and gently toss to coat. Sprinkle with salt and pepper to taste. Serve.

Yogurt-Mint Cucumber Salad

Yield: 4 Servings

(V) This is a Vegetarian Recipe (V)

Ingredients:

- ¼ cup minced fresh mint
- ½ teaspoon ground cumin
- 1 cup plain low-fat yogurt
- 1 garlic clove, minced
- 1 small red onion, sliced thin
- 2 tablespoons extra-virgin olive oil
- 3 cucumbers, peeled, halved along the length, seeded, and sliced ¼ inch thick
- Salt and pepper

Directions:

1. Toss cucumbers and onion with 1 tablespoon salt using a colander set over big container. Weight cucumber-onion

mixture with 1 gallon-size zipper-lock bag filled with water; drain for 1 to three hours. Wash and pat dry.
2. Beat yogurt, mint, oil, garlic, and cumin together in a big container. Put in cucumber-onion mixture and toss to coat. Sprinkle with salt and pepper to taste. Serve at room temperature or chilled within one hour.

Zucchini Parmesan Salad

Yield: 6 to 8 Servings

This recipe can be made quickly

This is a Vegetarian Recipe

Ingredients:

- ¼ cup lemon juice (2 lemons)
- ½ cup extra-virgin olive oil
- 1½ pounds small zucchini, trimmed and sliced along the length into ribbons
- 2 tablespoons minced fresh mint
- 6 ounces Parmesan cheese, shaved
- Salt and pepper

Directions:

1. Gently toss zucchini with salt and pepper to taste, then arrange beautifully on serving platter.
2. Sprinkle with oil and lemon juice, then drizzle with Parmesan and mint. Serve instantly.

Rice and Grain Recipes

Grains are a staple in the Mediterranean diet.

Aromatic Baked Brown Rice

Yield: 4 to 6 Servings

Ⓥ *This is a Vegetarian Recipe* Ⓥ

Ingredients:

- ½ cup minced fresh parsley
- ¾ cup jarred roasted red peppers, rinsed, patted dry, and chopped
- 1 cup chicken or vegetable broth
- 1½ cups long-grain brown rice, rinsed
- 2 onions, chopped fine
- 2¼ cups water
- 4 teaspoons extra-virgin olive oil
- Grated Parmesan cheese
- Lemon wedges
- Salt and pepper

Directions:

1. Place the oven rack in the centre of the oven and pre-heat your oven to 375 degrees. Heat oil in a Dutch oven on moderate heat until it starts to shimmer. Put in onions and 1 teaspoon salt and cook, stirring intermittently, till they become tender and well browned, 12 to 14 minutes.
2. Mix in water and broth and bring to boil. Mix in rice, cover, and move pot to oven. Bake until rice becomes soft and liquid is absorbed, 65 to 70 minutes.
3. Remove pot from oven. Sprinkle red peppers over rice, cover, and allow to sit for about five minutes. Put in parsley to rice and

fluff gently with fork to combine. Sprinkle with salt and pepper to taste. Serve with grated Parmesan and lemon wedges.

Aromatic Barley Pilaf

Yield: 4 to 6 Servings

Ⓥ This is a Vegetarian Recipe Ⓥ

Ingredients:

- ¼ cup minced fresh parsley
- 1 small onion, chopped fine
- 1½ cups pearl barley, rinsed
- 1½ teaspoons lemon juice
- 1½ teaspoons minced fresh thyme or ½ teaspoon dried
- 2 garlic cloves, minced
- 2 tablespoons minced fresh chives
- 2½ cups water
- 3 tablespoons extra-virgin olive oil
- Salt and pepper

Directions:

1. Heat oil in a big saucepan on moderate heat until it starts to shimmer. Put in onion and ½ teaspoon salt and cook till they become tender, approximately five minutes. Mix in barley, garlic, and thyme and cook, stirring often, until barley is lightly toasted and aromatic, approximately three minutes.
2. Mix in water and bring to simmer. Decrease heat to low, cover, and simmer until barley becomes soft and water is absorbed, 20 to 40 minutes.
3. Remove from the heat, lay clean dish towel underneath lid and let pilaf sit for about ten minutes. Put in parsley, chives, and lemon juice to pilaf and fluff gently with fork to combine. Sprinkle with salt and pepper to taste. Serve.

Basmati Rice Pilaf Mix

Yield: 4 to 6 Servings

Ⓥ *This is a Vegetarian Recipe* Ⓥ

Ingredients:

- ¼ cup currants
- ¼ cup sliced almonds, toasted
- ¼ teaspoon ground cinnamon
- ½ teaspoon ground turmeric
- 1 small onion, chopped fine
- 1 tablespoon extra-virgin olive oil
- 1½ cups basmati rice, rinsed
- 2 garlic cloves, minced
- 2¼ cups water
- Salt and pepper

Directions:

1. Heat oil in a big saucepan on moderate heat until it starts to shimmer. Put in onion and ¼ teaspoon salt and cook till they become tender, approximately five minutes. Put in rice, garlic, turmeric, and cinnamon and cook, stirring often, until grain edges begin to turn translucent, approximately three minutes.
2. Mix in water and bring to simmer. Decrease heat to low, cover, and simmer gently until rice becomes soft and water is absorbed, 16 to 18 minutes.
3. Remove from the heat, drizzle currants over pilaf. Cover, laying clean dish towel underneath lid, and let pilaf sit for about ten minutes. Put in almonds to pilaf and fluff gently with fork to combine. Sprinkle with salt and pepper to taste. Serve.

Brown Rice Salad with Asparagus, Goat Cheese, and Lemon

Yield: 4 to 6 Servings

Ⓥ This is a Vegetarian Recipe Ⓥ

Ingredients:

- ¼ cup minced fresh parsley
- ¼ cup slivered almonds, toasted
- 1 pound asparagus, trimmed and cut into 1-inch lengths
- 1 shallot, minced
- 1 teaspoon grated lemon zest plus 3 tablespoons juice
- 1½ cups long-grain brown rice
- 2 ounces goat cheese, crumbled (½ cup)
- 3½ tablespoons extra-virgin olive oil
- Salt and pepper

Directions:

1. Bring 4 quarts water to boil in a Dutch oven. Put in rice and 1½ teaspoons salt and cook, stirring intermittently, until rice is tender, about half an hour. Drain rice, spread onto rimmed baking sheet, and drizzle with 1 tablespoon lemon juice. Allow it to cool completely, about fifteen minutes.
2. Heat 1 tablespoon oil in 12-inch frying pan on high heat until just smoking. Put in asparagus, ¼ teaspoon salt, and ¼ teaspoon pepper and cook, stirring intermittently, until asparagus is browned and crisp-tender, about 4 minutes; move to plate and allow to cool slightly.
3. Beat remaining 2½ tablespoons oil, lemon zest and remaining 2 tablespoons juice, shallot, ½ teaspoon salt, and ½ teaspoon pepper together in a big container. Put in rice, asparagus, 2 tablespoons goat cheese, 3 tablespoons almonds, and 3 tablespoons parsley. Gently toss to combine and allow to sit for about ten minutes. Sprinkle with salt and pepper to taste. Move

to serving platter and drizzle with remaining 2 tablespoons goat cheese, remaining 1 tablespoon almonds, and remaining 1 tablespoon parsley. Serve.

Carrot-Almond-Bulgur Salad

Yield: 4 to 6 Servings

Ⓥ This is a Vegetarian Recipe Ⓥ

Ingredients:

- ⅛ teaspoon cayenne pepper
- ⅓ cup chopped fresh cilantro
- ⅓ cup chopped fresh mint
- ⅓ cup extra-virgin olive oil
- ½ cup sliced almonds, toasted
- ½ teaspoon ground cumin
- 1 cup water
- 1½ cups medium-grind bulgur, rinsed
- 3 scallions, sliced thin
- 4 carrots, peeled and shredded
- 6 tablespoons lemon juice (2 lemons)
- Salt and pepper

Directions:

1. Mix bulgur, water, ¼ cup lemon juice, and ¼ teaspoon salt in a container. Cover and allow to sit at room temperature until grains are softened and liquid is fully absorbed, about 1½ hours.
2. Beat remaining 2 tablespoons lemon juice, oil, cumin, cayenne, and ½ teaspoon salt together in a big container. Put in bulgur, carrots, scallions, almonds, mint, and cilantro and gently toss to combine. Sprinkle with salt and pepper to taste. Serve.

Chickpea-Spinach-Bulgur

Yield: 4 to 6 Servings

Ⓥ This is a Vegetarian Recipe Ⓥ

Ingredients:

- ¾ cup chicken or vegetable broth
- ¾ cup water
- 1 (15-ounce) can chickpeas, rinsed
- 1 cup medium-grind bulgur, rinsed
- 1 onion, chopped fine
- 1 tablespoon lemon juice
- 2 tablespoons za'atar
- 3 garlic cloves, minced
- 3 ounces (3 cups) baby spinach, chopped
- 3 tablespoons extra-virgin olive oil
- Salt and pepper

Directions:

1. Heat 2 tablespoons oil in a big saucepan on moderate heat until it starts to shimmer. Put in onion and ½ teaspoon salt and cook till they become tender, approximately five minutes. Mix in garlic and 1 tablespoon za'atar and cook until aromatic, approximately half a minute.
2. Mix in bulgur, chickpeas, broth, and water and bring to simmer. Decrease heat to low, cover, and simmer gently until bulgur is tender, 16 to 18 minutes.
3. Remove from the heat, lay clean dish towel underneath lid and let bulgur sit for about ten minutes. Put in spinach, lemon juice, remaining 1 tablespoon za'atar, and residual 1 tablespoon oil and fluff gently with fork to combine. Sprinkle with salt and pepper to taste. Serve.

Classic Baked Brown Rice

Yield: **4 Servings**

Ⓥ This is a Vegetarian Recipe Ⓥ

Ingredients:

- 1½ cups long-grain brown rice, rinsed
- 2 teaspoons extra-virgin olive oil
- 2⅓ cups boiling water
- Salt and pepper

Directions:

1. Place the oven rack in the centre of the oven and pre-heat your oven to 375 degrees. Mix boiling water, rice, oil, and ½ teaspoon salt in 8-inch square baking dish.
2. Cover dish tightly using double layer of aluminium foil. Bake until rice becomes soft and water is absorbed, about 1 hour. Remove dish from oven, uncover, and gently fluff rice with fork, scraping up any rice that has stuck to bottom. Cover dish with clean dish towel and let rice sit for about five minutes. Uncover and let rice sit for about five minutes longer.
3. Sprinkle with salt and pepper to taste. Serve.

Classic Italian Seafood Risotto

Yield: **4 to 6 Servings**

Ingredients:

- ⅛ teaspoon saffron threads, crumbled
- 1 (14.5-ounce) can diced tomatoes, drained
- 1 cup dry white wine
- 1 onion, chopped fine
- 1 tablespoon lemon juice
- 1 teaspoon minced fresh thyme or ¼ teaspoon dried

- 12 ounces large shrimp (26 to 30 per pound), peeled and deveined, shells reserved
- 12 ounces small bay scallops
- 2 bay leaves
- 2 cups Arborio rice
- 2 cups chicken broth
- 2 tablespoons minced fresh parsley
- 2½ cups water
- 4 (8-ounce) bottles clam juice
- 5 garlic cloves, minced
- 5 tablespoons extra-virgin olive oil
- Salt and pepper

Directions:

1. Bring shrimp shells, broth, water, clam juice, tomatoes, and bay leaves to boil in a big saucepan on moderate to high heat. Decrease the heat to a simmer and cook for 20 minutes. Strain mixture through fine-mesh strainer into big container, pressing on solids to extract as much liquid as possible; discard solids. Return broth to now-empty saucepan, cover, and keep warm on low heat.
2. Heat 2 tablespoons oil in a Dutch oven on moderate heat until it starts to shimmer. Put in onion and cook till they become tender, approximately five minutes. Put in rice, garlic, thyme, and saffron and cook, stirring often, until grain edges begin to turn translucent, approximately three minutes.
3. Put in wine and cook, stirring often, until fully absorbed, approximately three minutes. Mix in 3½ cups warm broth, bring to simmer, and cook, stirring intermittently, until almost fully absorbed, about fifteen minutes.
4. Carry on cooking rice, stirring often and adding warm broth, 1 cup at a time, every few minutes as liquid is absorbed, until rice is creamy and cooked through but still somewhat firm in center, about fifteen minutes.
5. Mix in shrimp and scallops and cook, stirring often, until opaque throughout, approximately three minutes. Remove pot from

heat, cover, and allow to sit for about five minutes. Adjust consistency with remaining warm broth as required (you may have broth left over). Mix in remaining 3 tablespoons oil, parsley, and lemon juice and sprinkle with salt and pepper to taste. Serve.

Classic Stovetop White Rice

Yield: 4 to 6 Servings

✄ This recipe can be made quickly ✄

Ⓥ This is a Vegetarian Recipe Ⓥ

Ingredients:

- 1 tablespoon extra-virgin olive oil
- 2 cups long-grain white rice, rinsed
- 3 cups water
- Basmati, jasmine, or Texmati rice can be substituted for the long-grain rice.
- Salt and pepper

Directions:

1. Heat oil in a big saucepan on moderate heat until it starts to shimmer. Put in rice and cook, stirring frequently, until grain edges begin to turn translucent, approximately two minutes.
2. Put in water and 1 teaspoon salt and bring to simmer. Cover, decrease the heat to low, and simmer gently until rice becomes soft and water is absorbed, approximately twenty minutes. Remove from the heat, lay clean dish towel underneath lid and let rice sit for about ten minutes. Gently fluff rice with fork. Sprinkle with salt and pepper to taste. Serve.

Classic Tabbouleh

Yield: **4 to 6 Servings**

Ⓥ *This is a Vegetarian Recipe* Ⓥ

Ingredients:

- ⅛ teaspoon cayenne pepper
- ¼ cup lemon juice (2 lemons)
- ½ cup medium-grind bulgur, rinsed
- ½ cup minced fresh mint
- 1½ cups minced fresh parsley
- 2 scallions, sliced thin
- 3 tomatoes, cored and cut into ½-inch pieces
- 6 tablespoons extra-virgin olive oil
- Salt and pepper

Directions:

1. Toss tomatoes with ¼ teaspoon salt using a fine-mesh strainer set over bowl and let drain, tossing occasionally, for 30 minutes; reserve 2 tablespoons drained tomato juice. Toss bulgur with 2 tablespoons lemon juice and reserved tomato juice in a container and allow to sit until grains start to become tender, 30 to 40 minutes.
2. Beat remaining 2 tablespoons lemon juice, oil, cayenne, and ¼ teaspoon salt together in a big container. Put in tomatoes, bulgur, parsley, mint, and scallions and toss gently to combine. Cover and allow to sit at room temperature until flavors have blended and bulgur is tender, about 1 hour. Before serving, toss salad to recombine and sprinkle with salt and pepper to taste.

Farro Cucumber-Mint Salad

Yield: **4 to 6 Servings**

Ⓥ *This is a Vegetarian Recipe* Ⓥ

Ingredients:

- 1 cup baby arugula
- 1 English cucumber, halved along the length, seeded, and cut into ¼-inch pieces
- 1½ cups whole farro
- 2 tablespoons lemon juice
- 2 tablespoons minced shallot
- 2 tablespoons plain Greek yogurt
- 3 tablespoons chopped fresh mint
- 3 tablespoons extra-virgin olive oil
- 6 ounces cherry tomatoes, halved
- Salt and pepper

Directions:

1. Bring 4 quarts water to boil in a Dutch oven. Put in farro and 1 tablespoon salt, return to boil, and cook until grains are soft with slight chew, 15 to 30 minutes. Drain farro, spread in rimmed baking sheet, and allow to cool completely, about fifteen minutes.
2. Beat oil, lemon juice, shallot, yogurt, ¼ teaspoon salt, and ¼ teaspoon pepper together in a big container. Put in farro, cucumber, tomatoes, arugula, and mint and toss gently to combine. Sprinkle with salt and pepper to taste. Serve.

Farro Salad Mix

Yield: 4 to 6 Servings

Ⓥ *This is a Vegetarian Recipe* Ⓥ

Ingredients:

- 1 teaspoon Dijon mustard
- 1½ cups whole farro

- 2 ounces feta cheese, crumbled (½ cup)
- 2 tablespoons lemon juice
- 2 tablespoons minced shallot
- 3 tablespoons chopped fresh dill
- 3 tablespoons extra-virgin olive oil
- 6 ounces asparagus, trimmed and cut into 1-inch lengths
- 6 ounces cherry tomatoes, halved
- 6 ounces sugar snap peas, strings removed, cut into 1-inch lengths
- Salt and pepper

Directions:

1. Bring 4 quarts water to boil in a Dutch oven. Put in asparagus, snap peas, and 1 tablespoon salt and cook until crisp-tender, approximately three minutes. Use a slotted spoon to move vegetables to large plate and allow to cool completely, about fifteen minutes.
2. Put in farro to water, return to boil, and cook until grains are soft with slight chew, 15 to 30 minutes. Drain farro, spread in rimmed baking sheet, and allow to cool completely, about fifteen minutes.
3. Beat oil, lemon juice, shallot, mustard, ¼ teaspoon salt, and ¼ teaspoon pepper together in a big container. Put in vegetables, farro, tomatoes, dill, and ¼ cup feta and toss gently to combine. Sprinkle with salt and pepper to taste. Move to serving platter and drizzle with remaining ¼ cup feta. Serve.

Farrotto Mix

Yield: 6 Servings

Ingredients:

- ½ onion, chopped fine
- 1 cup frozen peas, thawed
- 1 garlic clove, minced

- 1 tablespoon minced fresh chives
- 1 teaspoon grated lemon zest plus 1 teaspoon juice
- 1½ cups whole farro
- 1½ ounces Parmesan cheese, grated (¾ cup)
- 2 tablespoons extra-virgin olive oil
- 2 teaspoons minced fresh tarragon
- 3 cups chicken broth
- 3 cups water
- 4 ounces asparagus, trimmed and cut on bias into 1-inch lengths
- 4 ounces pancetta, cut into ¼-inch pieces
- Salt and pepper

Directions:

1. Pulse farro using a blender until about half of grains are broken into smaller pieces, about 6 pulses.
2. Bring broth and water to boil in moderate-sized saucepan on high heat. Put in asparagus and cook until crisp-tender, 2 to 3 minutes. Use a slotted spoon to move asparagus to a container and set aside. Decrease heat to low, cover broth mixture, and keep warm.
3. Cook pancetta in a Dutch oven on moderate heat until lightly browned and fat has rendered, approximately five minutes. Put in 1 tablespoon oil and onion and cook till they become tender, approximately five minutes. Mix in garlic and cook until aromatic, approximately half a minute. Put in farro and cook, stirring often, until grains are lightly toasted, approximately three minutes.
4. Stir 5 cups warm broth mixture into farro mixture, decrease the heat to low, cover, and cook until almost all liquid has been absorbed and farro is just al dente, about 25 minutes, stirring twice during cooking.
5. Put in peas, tarragon, ¾ teaspoon salt, and ½ teaspoon pepper and cook, stirring continuously, until farro becomes creamy, approximately five minutes. Remove from the heat, mix in Parmesan, chives, lemon zest and juice, remaining 1 tablespoon

oil, and reserved asparagus. Adjust consistency with remaining warm broth mixture as required (you may have broth left over). Sprinkle with salt and pepper to taste. Serve.

Fennel-Parmesan Farro

Yield: 4 to 6 Servings

Ⓥ This is a Vegetarian Recipe Ⓥ

Ingredients:

- ¼ cup minced fresh parsley
- 1 onion, chopped fine
- 1 ounce Parmesan cheese, grated (½ cup)
- 1 small fennel bulb, stalks discarded, bulb halved, cored, and chopped fine
- 1 teaspoon minced fresh thyme or ¼ teaspoon dried
- 1½ cups whole farro
- 2 teaspoons sherry vinegar
- 3 garlic cloves, minced
- 3 tablespoons extra-virgin olive oil
- Salt and pepper

Directions:

1. Bring 4 quarts water to boil in a Dutch oven. Put in farro and 1 tablespoon salt, return to boil, and cook until grains are soft with slight chew, 15 to 30 minutes. Drain farro, return to now-empty pot, and cover to keep warm.
2. Heat 2 tablespoons oil in 12-inch frying pan on moderate heat until it starts to shimmer. Put in onion, fennel, and ¼ teaspoon salt and cook, stirring intermittently, till they become tender, eight to ten minutes. Put in garlic and thyme and cook until aromatic, approximately half a minute.
3. Put in residual 1 tablespoon oil and farro and cook, stirring often, until heated through, approximately two minutes.

Remove from the heat, mix in Parmesan, parsley, and vinegar. Sprinkle with salt and pepper to taste. Serve.

Feta-Grape-Bulgur Salad with Grapes and Feta

Yield: 4 to 6 Servings

Ⓥ This is a Vegetarian Recipe Ⓥ

Ingredients:

- ¼ cup chopped fresh mint
- ¼ cup extra-virgin olive oil
- ¼ teaspoon ground cumin
- ½ cup slivered almonds, toasted
- 1 cup water
- 1½ cups medium-grind bulgur, rinsed
- 2 ounces feta cheese, crumbled (½ cup)
- 2 scallions, sliced thin
- 5 tablespoons lemon juice (2 lemons)
- 6 ounces seedless red grapes, quartered (1 cup)
- Pinch cayenne pepper
- Salt and pepper

Directions:

1. Mix bulgur, water, ¼ cup lemon juice, and ¼ teaspoon salt in a container. Cover and allow to sit at room temperature until grains are softened and liquid is fully absorbed, about 1½ hours.
2. Beat remaining 1 tablespoon lemon juice, oil, cumin, cayenne, and ¼ teaspoon salt together in a big container. Put in bulgur, grapes, ⅓ cup almonds, ⅓ cup feta, scallions, and mint and gently toss to combine. Sprinkle with salt and pepper to taste. Sprinkle with remaining almonds and remaining feta before you serve.

Greek Style Meaty Bulgur

Yield: 4 to 6 Servings

Ingredients:

- ½ cup jarred roasted red peppers, rinsed, patted dry, and chopped
- 1 bay leaf
- 1 cup medium-grind bulgur, rinsed
- 1 onion, chopped fine
- 1 tablespoon chopped fresh dill
- 1 teaspoon extra-virgin olive oil
- 1⅓ cups vegetable broth
- 2 teaspoons minced fresh marjoram or ½ teaspoon dried
- 3 garlic cloves, minced
- 8 ounces ground lamb
- Lemon wedges
- Salt and pepper

Directions:

1. Heat oil in a big saucepan on moderate to high heat until just smoking. Put in lamb, ½ teaspoon salt, and ¼ teaspoon pepper and cook, breaking up meat with wooden spoon, until browned, 3 to 5 minutes. Mix in onion and red peppers and cook until onion is softened, 5 to 7 minutes. Mix in garlic and marjoram and cook until aromatic, approximately half a minute.
2. Mix in bulgur, broth, and bay leaf and bring to simmer. Decrease heat to low, cover, and simmer gently until bulgur is tender, 16 to 18 minutes.
3. Remove from the heat, lay clean dish towel underneath lid and let bulgur sit for about ten minutes. Put in dill and fluff gently with fork to combine. Sprinkle with salt and pepper to taste. Serve with lemon wedges.

Hearty Barley Mix

Yield: 4 Servings

Ⓥ *This is a Vegetarian Recipe* Ⓥ

Ingredients:

- ⅛ teaspoon ground cardamom
- ½ cup plain yogurt
- ½ teaspoon ground cumin
- ⅔ cup raw sunflower seeds
- ¾ teaspoon ground coriander
- 1 cup pearl barley
- 1½ tablespoons minced fresh mint
- 1½ teaspoons grated lemon zest plus 1½ tablespoons juice
- 3 tablespoons extra-virgin olive oil
- 5 carrots, peeled
- 8 ounces snow peas, strings removed, halved along the length
- Salt and pepper

Directions:

1. Beat yogurt, ½ teaspoon lemon zest and 1½ teaspoons juice, 1½ teaspoons mint, ¼ teaspoon salt, and ⅛ teaspoon pepper together in a small-sized container; cover put inside your fridge until ready to serve.
2. Bring 4 quarts water to boil in a Dutch oven. Put in barley and 1 tablespoon salt, return to boil, and cook until tender, 20 to 40 minutes. Drain barley, return to now-empty pot, and cover to keep warm.
3. In the meantime, halve carrots crosswise, then halve or quarter along the length to create uniformly sized pieces. Heat 1 tablespoon oil in 12-inch frying pan on moderate to high heat until just smoking. Put in carrots and ½ teaspoon coriander and cook, stirring intermittently, until mildly charred and just tender, 5 to 7 minutes. Put in snow peas and cook, stirring

intermittently, until spotty brown, 3 to 5 minutes; move to plate.
4. Heat 1½ teaspoons oil in now-empty frying pan on moderate heat until it starts to shimmer. Put in sunflower seeds, cumin, cardamom, remaining ¼ teaspoon coriander, and ¼ teaspoon salt. Cook, stirring continuously, until seeds are toasted, approximately two minutes; move to small-sized container.
5. Beat remaining 1 teaspoon lemon zest and 1 tablespoon juice, remaining 1 tablespoon mint, and remaining 1½ tablespoons oil together in a big container. Put in barley and carrot–snow pea mixture and gently toss to combine. Sprinkle with salt and pepper to taste. Serve, topping individual portions with spiced sunflower seeds and drizzling with yogurt sauce.

Hearty Barley Risotto

Yield: 4 to 6 Servings

Ⓥ This is a Vegetarian Recipe Ⓥ

Ingredients:

- 1 carrot, peeled and chopped fine
- 1 cup dry white wine
- 1 onion, chopped fine
- 1 teaspoon minced fresh thyme or ¼ teaspoon dried
- 1½ cups pearl barley
- 2 ounces Parmesan cheese, grated (1 cup)
- 2 tablespoons extra-virgin olive oil
- 4 cups chicken or vegetable broth
- 4 cups water
- Salt and pepper

Directions:

1. Bring broth and water to simmer in moderate-sized saucepan. Decrease heat to low and cover to keep warm.

2. Heat 1 tablespoon oil in a Dutch oven on moderate heat until it starts to shimmer. Put in onion and carrot and cook till they become tender, 5 to 7 minutes. Put in barley and cook, stirring frequently, until lightly toasted and aromatic, about 4 minutes.
3. Put in wine and cook, stirring often, until fully absorbed, approximately two minutes. Mix in 3 cups warm broth and thyme, bring to simmer, and cook, stirring intermittently, until liquid is absorbed and bottom of pot is dry, 22 to 25 minutes. Mix in 2 cups warm broth, bring to simmer, and cook, stirring intermittently, until liquid is absorbed and bottom of pot is dry, fifteen to twenty minutes.
4. Carry on cooking risotto, stirring frequently and adding warm broth as required to stop pot bottom from becoming dry, until barley is cooked through but still somewhat firm in center, fifteen to twenty minutes. Remove from the heat, adjust consistency with remaining warm broth as required (you may have broth left over). Mix in Parmesan and residual 1 tablespoon oil and sprinkle with salt and pepper to taste. Serve.

Hearty Freekeh Pilaf

Yield: 4 to 6 Servings

Ⓥ This is a Vegetarian Recipe Ⓥ

Ingredients:

- ¼ cup chopped fresh mint
- ¼ cup extra-virgin olive oil, plus extra for serving
- ¼ cup shelled pistachios, toasted and coarsely chopped
- ¼ teaspoon ground coriander
- ¼ teaspoon ground cumin
- 1 head cauliflower (2 pounds), cored and cut into ½-inch florets
- 1 shallot, minced
- 1½ cups whole freekeh
- 1½ tablespoons lemon juice

- 1½ teaspoons grated fresh ginger
- 3 ounces pitted dates, chopped (½ cup)
- Salt and pepper

Directions:

1. Bring 4 quarts water to boil in a Dutch oven. Put in freekeh and 1 tablespoon salt, return to boil, and cook until grains are tender, 30 to 45 minutes. Drain freekeh, return to now-empty pot, and cover to keep warm.
2. Heat 2 tablespoons oil in 12-inch non-stick frying pan on moderate to high heat until it starts to shimmer. Put in cauliflower, ½ teaspoon salt, and ¼ teaspoon pepper, cover, and cook until florets are softened and start to brown, approximately five minutes.
3. Remove lid and continue to cook, stirring intermittently, until florets turn spotty brown, about 10 minutes. Put in remaining 2 tablespoons oil, dates, shallot, ginger, coriander, and cumin and cook, stirring often, until dates and shallot are softened and aromatic, approximately three minutes.
4. Decrease heat to low, put in freekeh, and cook, stirring often, until heated through, about 1 minute. Remove from the heat, mix in pistachios, mint, and lemon juice. Sprinkle with salt and pepper to taste and drizzle with extra oil. Serve.

Herby-Lemony Farro

Yield: 4 to 6 Servings

(V) This is a Vegetarian Recipe (V)

Ingredients:

- ¼ cup chopped fresh mint
- ¼ cup chopped fresh parsley
- 1 garlic clove, minced
- 1 onion, chopped fine

- 1 tablespoon lemon juice
- 1½ cups whole farro
- 3 tablespoons extra-virgin olive oil
- Salt and pepper

Directions:

1. Bring 4 quarts water to boil in a Dutch oven. Put in farro and 1 tablespoon salt, return to boil, and cook until grains are soft with slight chew, 15 to 30 minutes. Drain farro, return to now-empty pot, and cover to keep warm.
2. Heat 2 tablespoons oil in 12-inch frying pan on moderate heat until it starts to shimmer. Put in onion and ¼ teaspoon salt and cook till they become tender, approximately five minutes. Mix in garlic and cook until aromatic, approximately half a minute.
3. Put in residual 1 tablespoon oil and farro and cook, stirring often, until heated through, approximately two minutes. Remove from the heat, mix in parsley, mint, and lemon juice. Sprinkle with salt and pepper to taste. Serve.

Italian Paniscia

Yield: 8 Servings

Ingredients:

BEANS AND BROTH

- 1 carrot, peeled and chopped fine
- 1 celery rib, chopped fine
- 1 cup shredded red cabbage
- 1 leek, white and light green parts only, halved along the length, chopped fine, and washed thoroughly
- 1 small sprig fresh rosemary
- 1 tablespoon extra-virgin olive oil
- 1 zucchini, cut into ½-inch pieces
- 2 ounces pancetta, chopped fine

- 8 ounces (1¼ cups) dried cranberry beans, picked over and rinsed
- Salt and pepper

RISOTTO

- 1 cup dry red wine
- 1 small onion, chopped fine
- 1 tablespoon tomato paste
- 1½ cups carnaroli rice
- 2 (½-inch-thick) slices salami (6 ounces), cut into ½-inch pieces
- 2 tablespoons extra-virgin olive oil
- 2 teaspoons red wine vinegar
- Salt and pepper

Directions:

1. **FOR THE BEANS AND BROTH:** Dissolve 1½ tablespoons salt in 2 quarts cold water in large container. Put in beans and soak at room temperature for minimum 8 hours or for maximum 24 hours. Drain and wash thoroughly.
2. Heat oil in a big saucepan on moderate to high heat until it starts to shimmer. Put in pancetta and cook, stirring intermittently, until starting to brown, 3 to 5 minutes. Mix in leek, carrot, celery, zucchini, and cabbage and cook till they become tender and lightly browned, 5 to 7 minutes. Mix in drained beans, rosemary, and 8 cups water and bring to boil. Decrease heat to moderate to low, cover, and simmer, stirring intermittently, until beans are soft and liquid begins to thicken, forty to sixty minutes. Strain bean-vegetable mixture through fine-mesh strainer into big container. Discard rosemary and move bean-vegetable mixture to different container; set aside. Return broth to now-empty saucepan, cover, and keep warm on low heat.
3. **FOR THE RISOTTO**: Heat 1 tablespoon oil in a Dutch oven on moderate heat until it starts to shimmer. Put in onion, salami, and ½ teaspoon salt and cook until onion is softened, approximately five minutes. Put in rice and cook, stirring often,

until grain edges begin to turn translucent, approximately three minutes.
4. Mix in tomato paste and cook until aromatic, about 1 minute. Put in wine and cook, stirring often, until fully absorbed, approximately two minutes. Mix in 2 cups warm broth, bring to simmer, and cook, stirring intermittently, until almost fully absorbed, approximately five minutes.
5. Carry on cooking rice, stirring often and adding warm broth, 1 cup at a time, every few minutes as liquid is absorbed, until rice is creamy and cooked through but still somewhat firm in center, 14 to 16 minutes.
6. Remove from the heat, mix in bean-vegetable mixture, cover, and allow to sit for about five minutes. Adjust consistency with remaining warm broth as required (you may have broth left over). Mix in residual 1 tablespoon oil and vinegar and sprinkle with salt and pepper to taste. Serve.

Italian Parmesan Farrotto

Yield: 6 Servings

Ⓥ This is a Vegetarian Recipe Ⓥ

Ingredients:

- ½ onion, chopped fine
- 1 garlic clove, minced
- 1½ cups whole farro
- 2 ounces Parmesan cheese, grated (1 cup)
- 2 tablespoons minced fresh parsley
- 2 teaspoons lemon juice
- 2 teaspoons minced fresh thyme
- 3 cups chicken or vegetable broth
- 3 cups water
- 3 tablespoons extra-virgin olive oil
- Salt and pepper

Directions:

1. Pulse farro using a blender until about half of grains are broken into smaller pieces, about 6 pulses.
2. Bring broth and water to boil in moderate-sized saucepan on high heat. Decrease heat to low, cover, and keep warm.
3. Heat 2 tablespoons oil in a Dutch oven over moderate to low heat. Put in onion and cook till they become tender, approximately five minutes. Mix in garlic and cook until aromatic, approximately half a minute. Put in farro and cook, stirring often, until grains are lightly toasted, approximately three minutes.
4. Stir 5 cups warm broth mixture into farro mixture, decrease the heat to low, cover, and cook until almost all liquid has been absorbed and farro is just al dente, about 25 minutes, stirring twice during cooking.
5. Put in thyme, 1 teaspoon salt, and ¾ teaspoon pepper and cook, stirring continuously, until farro becomes creamy, approximately five minutes. Remove from the heat, mix in Parmesan, parsley, lemon juice, and remaining 1 tablespoon oil. Adjust consistency with remaining warm broth mixture as required (you may have broth left over). Sprinkle with salt and pepper to taste. Serve.

Lebanese Herbed Basmati Rice

Yield: 4 to 6 Servings

Ⓥ This is a Vegetarian Recipe Ⓥ

Ingredients:

- 1 garlic clove, minced
- 1 onion, chopped fine
- 1½ cups basmati rice
- 2 ounces vermicelli pasta, broken into 1-inch lengths
- 2½ cups chicken or vegetable broth

- 3 tablespoons extra-virgin olive oil
- 3 tablespoons minced fresh parsley
- Salt and pepper

Directions:

1. Put rice in a moderate-sized container and cover with hot tap water by 2 inches; allow to stand for about fifteen minutes.
2. Use your hands to lightly rinse the grains to eliminate the surplus starch. Cautiously drain water, leaving rice in a container. Pour cold tap water into the rice and drain water. Repeat the process of pouring in and draining cold water 4 to 5 times, until water runs nearly transparent. Drain rice using a fine-mesh strainer.
3. Heat oil in a big saucepan on moderate heat until it starts to shimmer. Put in pasta and cook, stirring intermittently, until browned, approximately three minutes. Put in onion and garlic and cook, stirring intermittently, until onion becomes tender but not browned, about 4 minutes. Put in rice and cook, stirring intermittently, until edges of rice begin to turn translucent, approximately three minutes. Put in broth and 1¼ teaspoons salt and bring to boil. Decrease heat to low, cover, and simmer gently until rice and pasta are soft and broth is absorbed, about 10 minutes. Remove from the heat, lay clean dish towel underneath lid and let pilaf sit for about ten minutes. Put in parsley to pilaf and fluff gently with fork to combine. Sprinkle with salt and pepper to taste. Serve.

Mushroom-Bulgur Pilaf

Yield: 4 Servings

Ⓥ *This is a Vegetarian Recipe* Ⓥ

Ingredients:

- ¼ cup minced fresh parsley

- ¼ ounce dried porcini mushrooms, rinsed and minced
- ¾ cup chicken or vegetable broth
- ¾ cup water
- 1 cup medium-grind bulgur, rinsed
- 1 onion, chopped fine
- 2 garlic cloves, minced
- 2 tablespoons extra-virgin olive oil
- 8 ounces cremini mushrooms, trimmed, halved if small or quartered if large
- Salt and pepper

Directions:

1. Heat oil in a big saucepan on moderate heat until it starts to shimmer. Put in onion, porcini mushrooms, and ½ teaspoon salt and cook until onion is softened, approximately five minutes. Mix in cremini mushrooms, increase heat to medium-high, cover, and cook until cremini release their liquid and begin to brown, about 4 minutes. Mix in garlic and cook until aromatic, approximately half a minute.
2. Mix in bulgur, broth, and water and bring to simmer. Decrease heat to low, cover, and simmer gently until bulgur is tender, 16 to 18 minutes.
3. Remove from the heat, lay clean dish towel underneath lid and let pilaf sit for about ten minutes. Put in parsley to pilaf and fluff gently with fork to combine. Sprinkle with salt and pepper to taste. Serve.

Mushroom-Thyme Farro

Yield: 4 to 6 Servings

Ⓥ This is a Vegetarian Recipe Ⓥ

Ingredients:

- 1 shallot, minced

- 1½ cups whole farro
- 1½ teaspoons minced fresh thyme or ½ teaspoon dried
- 1½ teaspoons sherry vinegar, plus extra for serving
- 12 ounces cremini mushrooms, trimmed and chopped coarse
- 3 tablespoons dry sherry
- 3 tablespoons extra-virgin olive oil
- 3 tablespoons minced fresh parsley
- Salt and pepper

Directions:

1. Bring 4 quarts water to boil in a Dutch oven. Put in farro and 1 tablespoon salt, return to boil, and cook until grains are soft with slight chew, 15 to 30 minutes. Drain farro, return to now-empty pot, and cover to keep warm.
2. Heat 2 tablespoons oil in 12-inch frying pan on moderate heat until it starts to shimmer. Put in mushrooms, shallot, thyme, and ¼ teaspoon salt and cook, stirring intermittently, until moisture has evaporated and vegetables start to brown, eight to ten minutes. Mix in sherry and cook, scraping up any browned bits, until frying pan is almost dry.
3. Put in residual 1 tablespoon oil and farro and cook, stirring often, until heated through, approximately two minutes. Remove from the heat, mix in parsley and vinegar. Sprinkle with salt, pepper, and extra vinegar to taste and serve.

North African Spiced Baked Rice

Yield: 6 to 8 Servings

Ⓥ This is a Vegetarian Recipe Ⓥ

Ingredients:

- ¼ cup extra-virgin olive oil
- ¾ cup large pitted brine-cured green olives, halved

- 1 fennel bulb, stalks discarded, bulb halved, cored, and chopped fine
- 1 small onion, chopped fine
- 1½ cups long-grain white rice, rinsed
- 1½ pounds sweet potatoes, peeled and cut into 1-inch pieces
- 2 tablespoons minced fresh cilantro
- 2 teaspoons ras el hanout
- 2¾ cups chicken or vegetable broth
- 4 garlic cloves, minced
- Lime wedges
- Salt and pepper

Directions:

1. Place the oven rack in the centre of the oven and pre-heat your oven to 400 degrees. Toss potatoes with 2 tablespoons oil and ½ teaspoon salt. Lay out the potatoes in one layer in rimmed baking sheet and roast until soft and browned, about half an hour, stirring potatoes halfway through roasting. Take the potatoes out of the oven and decrease oven temperature to 350 degrees.
2. Heat remaining 2 tablespoons oil in a Dutch oven on moderate heat until it starts to shimmer. Put in fennel and onion and cook till they become tender, 5 to 7 minutes. Mix in rice, garlic, and ras el hanout and cook, stirring often, until grain edges begin to turn translucent, approximately three minutes.
3. Mix in broth and olives and bring to boil. Cover, move pot to oven, and bake until rice becomes soft and liquid is absorbed, 12 to fifteen minutes.
4. Remove pot from oven and allow to sit for about ten minutes. Put in potatoes to rice and fluff gently with fork to combine. Sprinkle with salt and pepper to taste. Sprinkle with cilantro and serve with lime wedges.

Nutty Freekeh Salad

Yield: 4 to 6 Servings

Ⓥ *This is a Vegetarian Recipe* Ⓥ

Ingredients:

- ⅓ cup golden raisins
- ⅓ cup walnuts, toasted and chopped
- ½ cup Tahini-Lemon Dressing
- ½ teaspoon ground fenugreek
- 1 cup coarsely chopped cilantro
- 1 tablespoon extra-virgin olive oil
- 1½ cups whole freekeh
- 1½ pounds butternut squash, peeled, seeded, and cut into ½-inch pieces (4 cups)
- Salt and pepper

Directions:

1. Place oven rack on the lowest position and pre-heat your oven to 450 degrees. Toss squash with oil and fenugreek and sprinkle with salt and pepper. Arrange squash in one layer in rimmed baking sheet and roast until thoroughly browned and tender, 30 to 35 minutes, stirring halfway through roasting; allow to cool to room temperature.
2. In the meantime, bring 4 quarts water to boil in a Dutch oven. Put in freekeh and 1 tablespoon salt, return to boil, and cook until grains are tender, 30 to 45 minutes. Drain freekeh, move to big container, and allow to cool completely, about fifteen minutes.
3. Mix raisins and ¼ cup hot tap water in a small-sized container and allow to sit till they become tender, approximately five minutes; drain raisins. Put in squash, raisins, dressing, cilantro, and walnuts to a container with freekeh and gently toss to combine. Sprinkle with salt and pepper to taste. Serve.

Nutty Wheat Berry Salad

Yield: 4 to 6 Servings

(V) This is a Vegetarian Recipe (V)

Ingredients:

- ¼ cup pine nuts, toasted
- ½ cup fresh parsley leaves
- 1 small shallot, minced
- 1 teaspoon Dijon mustard
- 1 teaspoon honey
- 1½ cups wheat berries
- 2 ounces goat cheese, crumbled (½ cup)
- 2 tablespoons balsamic vinegar
- 3 tablespoons extra-virgin olive oil
- 8 ounces figs, cut into ½-inch pieces
- Salt and pepper

Directions:

1. Bring 4 quarts water to boil in a Dutch oven. Put in wheat berries and 1½ teaspoons salt, return to boil, and cook until soft but still chewy, 60 to 70 minutes. Drain wheat berries, spread onto rimmed baking sheet, and allow to cool completely, about fifteen minutes.
2. Beat vinegar, shallot, mustard, honey, ¼ teaspoon salt, and ¼ teaspoon pepper together in a big container. Whisking continuously, slowly drizzle in oil. Put in wheat berries, figs, parsley, and pine nuts and toss gently to combine. Sprinkle with salt and pepper to taste. Move to serving platter and drizzle with goat cheese. Serve.

Rich Italian Parmesan Polenta

Yield: 4 to 6 Servings

Ⓥ This is a Vegetarian Recipe Ⓥ

Ingredients:

- 1½ cups coarse-ground cornmeal
- 2 ounces Parmesan cheese, grated (1 cup), plus extra for serving
- 2 tablespoons extra-virgin olive oil
- 7½ cups water
- Pinch baking soda
- Salt and pepper

Directions:

1. Bring water to boil in a big saucepan on moderate to high heat. Mix in 1½ teaspoons salt and baking soda. Slowly pour cornmeal into water gradually while stirring back and forth with wooden spoon or rubber spatula. Bring mixture to boil, stirring continuously, about 1 minute. Decrease heat to lowest setting and cover.
2. After 5 minutes, beat polenta to smooth out any lumps that may have formed, approximately fifteen seconds. (Make sure to scrape down sides and bottom of saucepan.) Cover and continue to cook, without stirring, until polenta grains are soft but slightly al dente, about 25 minutes longer. (Polenta should be loose and barely hold its shape; it will continue to thicken as it cools.)
3. Remove from the heat, mix in Parmesan and oil and season with pepper to taste. Cover and allow to sit for about five minutes. Serve, passing extra Parmesan separately.

Sautéed Cherry Tomato and Fresh Mozzarella Polenta Topping

Yield: enough for 4 to 6 servings

Ⓥ This is a Vegetarian Recipe Ⓥ

Ingredients:

- 1½ pounds cherry tomatoes, halved
- 2 garlic cloves, sliced thin
- 2 tablespoons shredded fresh basil
- 3 ounces fresh mozzarella cheese, shredded (¾ cup)
- 3 tablespoons extra-virgin olive oil
- Pinch red pepper flakes
- Pinch sugar
- Salt and pepper

Directions:

1. Cook oil, garlic, pepper flakes, and sugar in 12-inch non-stick frying pan on moderate to high heat until aromatic and sizzling, about 1 minute. Mix in tomatoes and cook until just starting to soften, about 1 minute.
2. Sprinkle with salt and pepper to taste. Spoon mixture over individual portions of polenta and top with mozzarella and basil. Serve.

Broccoli Rabe, Sun-Dried Tomato, and Pine Nut Topping

Yield: enough for 4 to 6 servings

Ⓥ This is a Vegetarian Recipe Ⓥ

Ingredients:

- ¼ cup chicken or vegetable broth
- ¼ cup grated Parmesan cheese
- ½ cup oil-packed sun-dried tomatoes, chopped coarse

- ½ teaspoon red pepper flakes
- 1 pound broccoli rabe, trimmed and cut into 1½-inch pieces
- 2 tablespoons pine nuts, toasted
- 3 tablespoons extra-virgin olive oil
- 6 garlic cloves, minced
- Broccolini can be substituted for the broccoli rabe.
- Salt and pepper

Directions:

1. Cook sun-dried tomatoes, oil, garlic, pepper flakes, and ½ teaspoon salt in 12-inch non-stick frying pan on moderate to high heat, stirring often, until garlic is aromatic and slightly toasted, approximately two minutes. Put in broccoli rabe and broth, cover, and cook until broccoli rabe turns bright green, approximately two minutes. Uncover and cook, stirring often, until most of broth has evaporated and broccoli rabe is just tender, approximately three minutes.
2. Sprinkle with salt and pepper to taste. Spoon mixture over individual portions of polenta and top with pine nuts and Parmesan. Serve.

Rich Spanish Vegetable Paella

Yield: 6 Servings

(V) This is a Vegetarian Recipe (V)

Ingredients:

- ⅓ cup dry white wine
- ½ cup frozen peas, thawed
- ½ cup pitted kalamata olives, chopped
- ½ teaspoon saffron threads, crumbled
- ½ teaspoon smoked paprika
- 1 (14.5-ounce) can diced tomatoes, drained, minced, and drained again

- 1 fennel bulb, stalks discarded, bulb halved, cored, and sliced thin
- 1 onion, chopped fine
- 2 cups Bomba rice
- 2 red bell peppers, stemmed, seeded, and chopped coarse
- 2 tablespoons lemon juice
- 3 cups jarred whole baby artichokes packed in water, quartered, rinsed, and patted dry
- 3 cups vegetable broth
- 3 tablespoons chopped fresh parsley
- 6 tablespoons extra-virgin olive oil
- 9 garlic cloves, peeled (3 whole, 6 minced)
- Salt and pepper

Directions:

1. Place oven rack to lower-middle position, place rimmed baking sheet on rack, and pre-heat your oven to 450 degrees. Toss artichokes and peppers with olives, whole garlic cloves, 2 tablespoons oil, ½ teaspoon salt, and ¼ teaspoon pepper in a container. Lay out vegetables in hot sheet and roast until artichokes become browned around edges and peppers become browned, 20 minutes to half an hour; allow to cool slightly.
2. Mince roasted garlic. In big container, beat 2 tablespoons oil, 2 tablespoons parsley, lemon juice, and minced roasted garlic together. Put in roasted vegetables and toss to combine. Sprinkle with salt and pepper to taste.
3. Reduce oven temperature to 350 degrees. Heat remaining 2 tablespoons oil in a Dutch oven on moderate heat until it starts to shimmer. Put in onion and fennel and cook till they become tender, eight to ten minutes.
4. Mix in remaining minced garlic and paprika and cook until aromatic, approximately half a minute. Mix in tomatoes and cook until mixture begins to darken and thicken slightly, approximately three minutes. Mix in rice and cook until grains are well coated with tomato mixture, approximately two

minutes. Mix in broth, wine, saffron, and 1 teaspoon salt. Increase heat to medium-high and bring to boil, stirring intermittently. Cover, move pot to oven, and bake until liquid is absorbed and rice is tender, 25 to 35 minutes.
5. For optional socarrat, move pot to stovetop and remove lid. Cook on moderate to high heat for approximately five minutes, rotating pot as required, until bottom layer of rice is thoroughly browned and crisp.
6. Sprinkle roasted vegetables and peas over rice, cover, and let paella sit for about five minutes. Sprinkle with remaining 1 tablespoon parsley and serve.

Spanish Broth Rice

Yield: 4 to 6 Servings

Ingredients:

- ¼ cup minced fresh parsley
- 1 (8-ounce) bottle clam juice
- 1 green bell pepper, stemmed, seeded, and chopped fine
- 1 leek, white and light green parts only, halved along the length, chopped fine, and washed thoroughly
- 1 tablespoon white wine vinegar
- 1½ cups Bomba rice
- 2 cups dry white wine
- 2 pounds littleneck clams, scrubbed
- 5 cups water
- 5 tablespoons extra-virgin olive oil
- 6 garlic cloves, minced
- Lemon wedges
- Salt and pepper

Directions:

1. Mix 3 tablespoons oil, parsley, half of garlic, and vinegar in a container; set aside. Bring wine to boil in a big saucepan on high

heat. Put in clams, cover, and cook, stirring intermittently, until clams open, 5 to 7 minutes.
2. Use a slotted spoon to move clams to big container and cover to keep warm; discard any clams that refuse to open. Stir water and clam juice into wine and bring to simmer. Decrease heat to low, cover, and keep warm.
3. Heat remaining 2 tablespoons oil in a Dutch oven on moderate heat until it starts to shimmer. Put in leek, bell pepper, and ½ teaspoon salt and cook till they become tender, eight to ten minutes. Put in rice and remaining garlic and cook, stirring often, until grain edges begin to turn translucent, approximately three minutes.
4. Put in 2 cups warm broth and cook, stirring often, until almost fully absorbed, approximately five minutes. Carry on cooking rice, stirring often and adding warm broth, 1 cup at a time, every few minutes as liquid is absorbed, until rice is creamy and cooked through but still somewhat firm in center, 12 to 14 minutes.
5. Remove from the heat, mix in 1 cup warm broth and adjust consistency with extra broth as required (rice mixture should have thin but creamy consistency; you may have broth left over). Mix in parsley mixture and sprinkle with salt and pepper to taste. Nestle clams into rice along with any accumulated juices, cover, and allow to sit until heated through, 5 to 7 minutes. Serve with lemon wedges.

Spanish Paella

Yield: 6 Servings

Ingredients:

- ⅓ cup dry white wine
- ½ cup frozen peas, thawed
- ½ teaspoon saffron threads, crumbled

- 1 (14.5-ounce) can diced tomatoes, drained, minced, and drained again
- 1 bay leaf
- 1 onion, chopped fine
- 1 pound boneless, skinless chicken thighs, trimmed and halved crosswise
- 1 pound extra-large shrimp (21 to 25 per pound), peeled and deveined
- 1 red bell pepper, stemmed, seeded, and cut into ½-inch-wide strips
- 12 mussels, scrubbed and debearded
- 2 cups Bomba rice
- 2 tablespoons extra-virgin olive oil, plus extra as required
- 2 teaspoons chopped fresh parsley
- 3 cups chicken broth
- 8 garlic cloves, minced
- 8 ounces Spanish-style chorizo sausage, sliced on bias ½ inch thick
- Lemon wedges
- Salt and pepper

Directions:

1. Place oven rack to lower-middle position and pre-heat your oven to 350 degrees. Toss shrimp with 1 tablespoon oil, 1 teaspoon garlic, ¼ teaspoon salt, and ¼ teaspoon pepper in a container until evenly coated. Cover and put in the fridge until needed. Pat chicken dry using paper towels and sprinkle with salt and pepper.
2. Heat 2 teaspoons oil in a Dutch oven on moderate to high heat until it starts to shimmer. Put in bell pepper and cook, stirring intermittently, until skin begins to blister and turn spotty black, about 4 minutes; move to a container.
3. Heat remaining 1 teaspoon oil in now-empty pot until it starts to shimmer. Put in chicken in one layer and cook, without moving, until browned, approximately three minutes. Turn pieces and cook until browned on second side, approximately

three minutes; move to different container. Decrease heat to medium and put in chorizo to now-empty pot. Cook, stirring often, until deeply browned and fat begins to render, approximately five minutes; move to a container with chicken.
4. Put in extra oil to fat left in pot to equal 2 tablespoons and heat on moderate heat until it starts to shimmer. Put in onion and cook till they become tender, approximately three minutes. Mix in remaining garlic and cook until aromatic, about 1 minute. Mix in tomatoes and cook until mixture begins to darken and thicken slightly, approximately three minutes. Mix in rice and cook until grains are well coated with tomato mixture, approximately two minutes.
5. Mix in broth, wine, saffron, bay leaf, and ½ teaspoon salt. Return chicken and chorizo to pot, increase heat to medium-high, and bring to boil, stirring intermittently. Cover, move pot to oven, and bake until almost all liquid is absorbed, fifteen to twenty minutes.
6. Remove pot from oven. Scatter shrimp and mussels evenly over rice and push hinge side of mussels into rice so they stand up. Cover, return pot to oven, and bake until shrimp are opaque throughout and mussels have opened, 10 to fifteen minutes.
7. For optional socarrat, move pot to stovetop and remove lid. Cook on moderate to high heat for approximately five minutes, rotating pot as required, until bottom layer of rice is thoroughly browned and crisp.
8. Discard any mussels that refuse to open and bay leaf, if it can be easily removed. Arrange bell pepper strips in pinwheel pattern over rice and drizzle peas over top. Cover and let paella sit for about five minutes. Sprinkle with parsley and serve with lemon wedges.

Spanish Style Brown Rice

Yield: 6 Servings

Ⓥ This is a Vegetarian Recipe Ⓥ

Ingredients:

- ¼ cup minced fresh cilantro
- 1 cup long-grain brown rice, rinsed
- 1 onion, chopped fine
- 1 tablespoon lime juice
- 12 ounces grape tomatoes, quartered
- 2 (15-ounce) cans chickpeas, rinsed
- 2 red bell peppers, stemmed, seeded, and chopped fine
- 3¼ cups chicken or vegetable broth
- 4 garlic cloves, minced
- 4 teaspoons extra-virgin olive oil
- 5 scallions, sliced thin
- Pinch cayenne pepper
- Pinch saffron threads, crumbled
- Salt and pepper

Directions:

1. Mix tomatoes, scallions, cilantro, 2 teaspoons oil, and lime juice in a container. Sprinkle with salt and pepper to taste; set aside for serving.
2. Heat remaining 2 teaspoons oil in a big saucepan on moderate to high heat until it starts to shimmer. Put in bell peppers and onion and cook till they become tender and lightly browned, eight to ten minutes. Mix in rice, garlic, saffron, and cayenne and cook until aromatic, approximately half a minute.
3. Mix in broth and bring to simmer. Decrease heat to moderate to low, cover, and simmer, stirring intermittently, for 25 minutes.
4. Mix in chickpeas, cover, and simmer until rice becomes soft and broth is almost completely absorbed, about half an hour. Sprinkle with salt and pepper to taste. Serve, topping individual portions with tomato mixture.

Spiced Basmati Rice Mix

Yield: 8 to 10 Servings

(V) This is a Vegetarian Recipe (V)

Ingredients:

- ¼ cup extra-virgin olive oil
- ½ cup pomegranate seeds
- ½ teaspoon ground cinnamon
- ½ teaspoon ground cumin
- ½ teaspoon ground turmeric
- 1 head cauliflower (2 pounds), cored and cut into ¾-inch florets
- 1 onion, chopped coarse
- 1½ cups basmati rice, rinsed
- 2 tablespoons chopped fresh cilantro
- 2 tablespoons chopped fresh mint
- 2¼ cups water
- 4 garlic cloves, minced
- Salt and pepper

Directions:

1. Place oven rack on the lowest position and pre-heat your oven to 475 degrees. Toss cauliflower with 2 tablespoons oil, ½ teaspoon salt, ½ teaspoon pepper, and ¼ teaspoon cumin. Arrange cauliflower in one layer in rimmed baking sheet and roast until just tender, 10 to fifteen minutes; set aside.
2. Heat remaining 2 tablespoons oil in a big saucepan on moderate heat until it starts to shimmer. Put in onion and ¼ teaspoon salt and cook till they become tender and lightly browned, 5 to 7 minutes. Put in rice, garlic, cinnamon, turmeric, and remaining ¼ teaspoon cumin and cook, stirring often, until grain edges begin to turn translucent, approximately three minutes.

3. Mix in water and bring to simmer. Decrease heat to low, cover, and simmer gently until rice becomes soft and water is absorbed, 16 to 18 minutes.
4. Remove from the heat, lay clean dish towel underneath lid and let pilaf sit for about ten minutes. Put in roasted cauliflower to pilaf and fluff gently with fork to combine. Sprinkle with salt and pepper to taste. Move to serving platter and drizzle with pomegranate seeds, cilantro, and mint. Serve.

Tangy Rice Salad

Yield: 4 to 6 Servings

Ⓥ This is a Vegetarian Recipe Ⓥ

Ingredients:

- ⅓ cup large pitted brine-cured green olives, chopped
- ⅓ cup slivered almonds, toasted
- 1 small garlic clove, minced
- 1½ cups basmati rice
- 2 oranges, plus ¼ teaspoon grated orange zest plus 1 tablespoon juice
- 2 tablespoons extra-virgin olive oil
- 2 tablespoons minced fresh oregano
- 2 teaspoons sherry vinegar
- Salt and pepper

Directions:

1. Bring 4 quarts water to boil in a Dutch oven. In the meantime, toast rice in 12-inch frying pan on moderate heat until faintly aromatic and some grains turn opaque, five to ten minutes. Put in rice and 1½ teaspoons salt to boiling water and cook, stirring

intermittently, until rice becomes soft but not soft, about fifteen minutes. Drain rice, spread onto rimmed baking sheet, and allow to cool completely, about fifteen minutes.
2. Cut away peel and pith from oranges. Holding fruit over bowl, use paring knife to slice between membranes to release segments. Beat oil, vinegar, garlic, orange zest and juice, 1 teaspoon salt, and ½ teaspoon pepper together in a big container. Put in rice, orange segments, olives, almonds, and oregano, gently toss to combine, and allow to sit for 20 minutes. Serve.

Tangy Wheat Berry Salad

Yield: 4 to 6 Servings

Ⓥ This is a Vegetarian Recipe Ⓥ

Ingredients:

- ⅛ teaspoon grated orange zest
- 1 garlic clove, minced
- 1 orange
- 1 small shallot, minced
- 1 tablespoon minced fresh tarragon
- 1½ cups wheat berries
- 1½ tablespoons Dijon mustard
- 1½ teaspoons honey
- 2 tablespoons extra-virgin olive oil
- 3 carrots, peeled and shredded
- 3 tablespoons red wine vinegar
- Salt and pepper

Directions:

1. Bring 4 quarts water to boil in a Dutch oven. Put in wheat berries and 1½ teaspoons salt, return to boil, and cook until soft but still chewy, 60 to 70 minutes. Drain wheat berries, spread in

rimmed baking sheet, and allow to cool completely, about fifteen minutes.
2. Cut away peel and pith from orange. Quarter orange, then slice crosswise into ¼-inch-thick pieces. Beat vinegar, mustard, shallot, garlic, orange zest, honey, and ¼ teaspoon salt together in a big container until combined. Whisking continuously, slowly drizzle in oil. Put in wheat berries, carrots, tarragon, and orange pieces and gently toss to coat. Sprinkle with salt and pepper to taste. Serve.

Ultimate Barley Mix

Yield: **4 Servings**

Ⓥ This is a Vegetarian Recipe Ⓥ

Ingredients:

- ½ cup black lentils, picked over and rinsed
- ½ cup Tahini-Yogurt Sauce
- ½ ounce dried porcini mushrooms, rinsed
- ¾ teaspoon ground coriander
- 1 cup pearl barley
- 1 onion, chopped fine
- 2 large portobello mushroom caps, cut into 1-inch pieces
- 2 tablespoons chopped fresh dill
- 2 tablespoons extra-virgin olive oil
- 3 (2-inch) strips lemon zest, sliced thin along the length
- Salt and pepper

Directions:

1. Microwave 1½ cups water and porcini mushrooms in covered bowl until steaming, about 1 minute. Allow to sit till they become tender, approximately five minutes. Drain mushrooms using a fine-mesh strainer lined with coffee filter, reserving soaking liquid, and chop mushrooms.

2. Bring 4 quarts water to boil in a Dutch oven. Put in barley, lentils, and 1 tablespoon salt, return to boil, and cook until tender, 20 to 40 minutes. Drain barley and lentils, return to now-empty pot, and cover to keep warm.
3. In the meantime, heat oil in 12-inch non-stick frying pan on moderate heat until it starts to shimmer. Put in onion and cook till they become tender, approximately five minutes. Mix in portobello mushrooms, cover, and cook until portobellos have released their liquid and begin to brown, about 4 minutes.
4. Uncover, mix in lemon zest, coriander, ½ teaspoon salt, and ¼ teaspoon pepper, and cook until aromatic, approximately half a minute. Mix in porcini and porcini soaking liquid, bring to boil, and cook, stirring intermittently, until liquid becomes thick slightly and reduced to ½ cup, approximately five minutes. Stir mushroom mixture and dill into barley-lentil mixture and sprinkle with salt and pepper to taste. Serve, drizzling individual portions with Tahini-Yogurt Sauce.

Vibrant Egyptian Barley Salad

Yield: 6 to 8 Servings

Ⓥ This is a Vegetarian Recipe Ⓥ

Ingredients:

- ¼ cup shelled pistachios, toasted and chopped coarse
- ¼ teaspoon ground cumin
- ⅓ cup golden raisins
- ½ cup coarsely chopped cilantro
- ½ cup pomegranate seeds
- ½ teaspoon ground cinnamon
- 1½ cups pearl barley
- 2 tablespoons pomegranate molasses
- 3 ounces feta cheese, cut into ½-inch cubes (¾ cup)
- 3 tablespoons extra-virgin olive oil, plus extra for serving

- 6 scallions, green parts only, sliced thin
- Salt and pepper

Directions:

1. Bring 4 quarts water to boil in a Dutch oven. Put in barley and 1 tablespoon salt, return to boil, and cook until tender, 20 to 40 minutes. Drain barley, spread onto rimmed baking sheet, and allow to cool completely, about fifteen minutes.
2. Beat oil, molasses, cinnamon, cumin, and ½ teaspoon salt together in a big container. Put in barley, raisins, cilantro, and pistachios and gently toss to combine. Sprinkle with salt and pepper to taste. Lay out barley salad uniformly serving platter and arrange feta, scallions, and pomegranate seeds in separate diagonal rows on top. Sprinkle with extra oil and serve.

Vibrant Spanish Grilled Paella

Yield: 8 Servings

Ingredients:

- ½ cup jarred roasted red peppers, rinsed, patted dry, and chopped fine
- ⅔ cup dry sherry
- 1 (8-ounce) bottle clam juice
- 1 cup frozen peas, thawed
- 1 onion, chopped fine
- 1 pound littleneck clams, scrubbed
- 1½ pounds boneless, skinless chicken thighs, trimmed and halved crosswise
- 1¾ teaspoons hot smoked paprika
- 12 ounces jumbo shrimp (16 to 20 per pound), peeled and deveined
- 3 cups Bomba rice
- 3 tablespoons tomato paste
- 4½ cups chicken broth

- 5 tablespoons extra-virgin olive oil
- 6 garlic cloves, minced
- 8 ounces Spanish-style chorizo sausage, cut into ½-inch pieces
- Lemon wedges
- Pinch saffron threads, crumbled (optional)
- Salt and pepper

Directions:

1. Pat chicken dry using paper towels and season both sides with 1 teaspoon salt and 1 teaspoon pepper. Toss shrimp with 1½ teaspoons oil, ½ teaspoon garlic, ¼ teaspoon paprika, and ¼ teaspoon salt in a container until evenly coated. Set aside.
2. Heat 1½ teaspoons oil in moderate-sized saucepan on moderate heat until it starts to shimmer. Put in remaining garlic and cook, stirring continuously, until garlic sticks to bottom of saucepan and begins to brown, about 1 minute. Put in tomato paste and remaining 1½ teaspoons paprika and continue to cook, stirring continuously, until dark brown bits form on bottom of saucepan, about 1 minute. Mix in 4 cups broth, sherry, clam juice, and saffron, if using. Increase heat to high and bring to boil. Remove saucepan from heat and set aside.
3. FOR A CHARCOAL GRILL: Open bottom vent fully. Light large chimney starter mounded with charcoal briquettes (7 quarts). When top coals are partially covered with ash, pour uniformly over grill. Using tongs, arrange 20 unlit briquettes evenly over coals. Set cooking grate in place, cover, and open lid vent fully. Heat grill until hot, approximately five minutes.
4. FOR A GAS GRILL: Turn all burners to high, cover, and heat grill until hot, about fifteen minutes. Leave all burners on high.
5. Clean and oil cooking grate. Place chicken on grill and cook until both sides are lightly browned, 5 to 7 minutes; move chicken to plate and clean cooking grate.
6. Place roasting pan on grill (turning burners to medium-high if using gas) and put in remaining ¼ cup oil. When oil begins to shimmer, put in onion, red peppers, and ½ teaspoon salt. Cook, stirring often, until onion begins to brown, four to eight

minutes. Mix in rice (turning burners to medium if using gas) until grains are well coated with oil.
7. Place the chicken around the perimeter of the pan. Pour chicken broth mixture and any accumulated chicken juices over rice. Level the rice into a uniform layer, making sure nothing sticks to sides of pan and no rice rests atop chicken. When liquid starts to mildly simmer, place shrimp in center of pan in one layer. Arrange clams in center of pan, evenly dispersing with shrimp and pushing hinge side of clams into rice slightly so they stand up. Distribute chorizo uniformly on the surface of rice. Cook, moving and rotating pan to maintain mild simmer across entire surface of pan, until rice is almost cooked through, about 12 to 18 minutes. Regulate the gas heat to maintain the simmer if you're using gas.
8. Sprinkle peas evenly over paella, cover grill, and cook until liquid is fully absorbed and rice on bottom of pan sizzles, five to ten minutes. Carry on cooking, uncovered, checking often, until an evenly golden-brown crust is achieved on the bottom of pan, about eight to fifteen minutes longer. (Rotate and slide pan around grill as necessary to ensure even crust formation.) Remove from grill, cover with aluminium foil, and allow to sit for about ten minutes. Serve with lemon wedges.

Wheat Berry Mix

Yield: 4 to 6 Servings

Ⓥ This is a Vegetarian Recipe Ⓥ

Ingredients:

- 1 garlic clove, minced
- 1 red bell pepper, stemmed, seeded, and cut into ½-inch pieces
- 1 red onion, chopped
- 1 tablespoon grated lemon zest

- 1 tablespoon minced fresh oregano or 1½ teaspoons dried
- 1 zucchini, cut into ½-inch pieces
- 1½ cups wheat berries
- 2 tablespoons extra-virgin olive oil
- 3 tablespoons red wine vinegar
- Salt and pepper

Directions:

1. Bring 4 quarts water to boil in a Dutch oven. Put in wheat berries and 1½ teaspoons salt, return to boil, and cook until soft but still chewy, 60 to 70 minutes.
2. In the meantime, beat 1 tablespoon oil, vinegar, garlic, lemon zest, and oregano together in a big container. Drain wheat berries, put in to a container with dressing, and toss gently to coat.
3. Heat 2 teaspoons oil in 12-inch non-stick frying pan on moderate to high heat until just smoking. Put in zucchini and ¼ teaspoon salt and cook, stirring intermittently, until deep golden brown and starting to char in spots, six to eight minutes; move to a container with wheat berries.
4. Return now-empty frying pan to medium-high heat and put in remaining 1 teaspoon oil, onion, bell pepper, and ¼ teaspoon salt. Cook, stirring intermittently, until onion is charred at edges and pepper skin is charred and blistered, eight to ten minutes. Put in wheat berry–zucchini mixture and cook, stirring often, until heated through, approximately two minutes. Sprinkle with salt and pepper to taste. Serve.

Pasta and Couscous

When you think Pasta, Italy is the first thing that comes to mind. However, pasta is highly popular is other Mediterranean countries too. Various versions of pasta are a staple all across the Mediterranean, and we will take a look at a few of the best recipes in this section.

Pasta Sauces

The sauce is the life of the pasta!

Classic Marinara Sauce

Ⓥ This is a Vegetarian Recipe Ⓥ

This sauce works well with any type of pasta. If you prefer a chunkier sauce, give it just three or four pulses in the food processor in step 4.

Ingredients:

- ⅓ cup dry red wine
- 1 onion, chopped fine
- 2 (28-ounce) cans whole peeled tomatoes
- 2 garlic cloves, minced
- 2 teaspoons minced fresh oregano or ½ teaspoon dried
- 3 tablespoons chopped fresh basil
- 3 tablespoons extra-virgin olive oil
- Salt and pepper
- Sugar

Directions:

1. Drain tomatoes using a fine-mesh strainer set over big container. Using hands, open tomatoes and remove and discard seeds and fibrous cores; let tomatoes drain, approximately five

minutes. Reserve ¾ cup tomatoes separately. Reserve 2½ cups drained tomato juice; discard extra juice.

2. Heat 2 tablespoons oil in 12-inch frying pan on moderate heat until it starts to shimmer. Put in onion and cook till they become tender and lightly browned, 5 to 7 minutes. Mix in garlic and oregano and cook until aromatic, approximately half a minute. Mix in remaining drained tomatoes and increase heat to medium-high. Cook, stirring frequently, until liquid has evaporated and tomatoes begin to brown and stick to pan, 10 to 12 minutes.
3. Mix in wine and cook until thick and syrupy, about 1 minute. Mix in reserved tomato juice, scraping up any browned bits. Bring to simmer and cook, stirring intermittently, until sauce is thickened, eight to ten minutes.
4. Move sauce to your food processor, put in reserved ¾ cup tomatoes, and pulse until slightly chunky, approximately 8 pulses. Return sauce to now-empty skillet, mix in basil and remaining 1 tablespoon oil, and season with salt, pepper, and sugar to taste. While you toss sauce with cooked pasta, gradually pour in some pasta cooking water as required to regulate consistency.

Fresh & Raw Tomato Sauce

This recipe can be made quickly

Ⓥ This is a Vegetarian Recipe Ⓥ

Make sure the tomatoes are in season, and ripe.

Ingredients:

- ¼ cup extra-virgin olive oil
- 1 garlic clove, minced
- 1 shallot, minced
- 2 pounds very ripe tomatoes, cored and cut into ½-inch pieces
- 2 teaspoons lemon juice, plus extra as required

- 3 tablespoons chopped fresh basil
- Salt and pepper
- Sugar

Directions:

1. Stir oil, lemon juice, shallot, garlic, 1 teaspoon salt, ¼ teaspoon pepper, and pinch sugar together in a big container. Mix in tomatoes and allow to marinate until very soft and flavorful, approximately half an hour.
2. Before you serve, mix in basil and season with salt, pepper, sugar, and extra lemon juice to taste. While you toss sauce with cooked pasta, gradually pour in some pasta cooking water as required to regulate consistency.

Quick Tomato Sauce

This recipe can be made quickly

(V) This is a Vegetarian Recipe (V)

This sauce works well with any type of pasta.

Ingredients:

- ¼ teaspoon sugar
- 1 (14.5-ounce) can diced tomatoes
- 1 (28-ounce) can crushed tomatoes
- 3 garlic cloves, minced
- 3 tablespoons chopped fresh basil
- 3 tablespoons extra-virgin olive oil
- Salt and pepper

Directions:

1. Cook oil and garlic in moderate-sized saucepan on moderate heat, stirring frequently, until aromatic but not browned, approximately two minutes. Mix in tomatoes and their juice.

Bring to simmer and cook until slightly thickened, fifteen to twenty minutes. Remove from the heat, mix in basil and sugar.
2. Sprinkle with salt and pepper to taste. While you toss sauce with cooked pasta, gradually pour in some pasta cooking water as required to regulate consistency.

Pesto Sauces

Pesto is a versatile Italian condiment that goes great with pasta, and can also be used for garnishing your favourite recipes!

Classic Basil Pesto

Yield: ¾ cup

This recipe can be made quickly

(V) This is a Vegetarian Recipe (V)

Ingredients:

- ¼ cup grated Parmesan cheese
- ¼ cup pine nuts, toasted
- 2 cups fresh basil leaves, lightly bruised
- 2 tablespoons fresh parsley leaves (optional)
- 3 garlic cloves, toasted and minced
- 7 tablespoons extra-virgin olive oil

Directions:

1. Process all ingredients except oil and cheese using a food processor until smooth, scraping down bowl as required. While your food processor runs slowly put in oil until incorporated.
2. Move pesto to a container, mix in cheese, and sprinkle with salt and pepper to taste. When tossing pesto with cooked pasta, put

in some of pasta cooking water as required (up to ½ cup) to loosen consistency of pesto.
3. Pesto will keep safely in a fridge for maximum 3 days or frozen for maximum 3 months. To stop browning, press plastic wrap flush to surface, or top with thin layer of olive oil.

Green Olive and Orange Pesto

Yield: 1½ cups

This recipe can be made quickly

Ⓥ This is a Vegetarian Recipe Ⓥ

Ingredients:

- ½ cup extra-virgin olive oil
- ½ cup pitted green olives
- ½ cup slivered almonds, toasted
- ½ teaspoon grated orange zest plus 2 tablespoons juice
- 1½ cups fresh parsley leaves
- 1½ ounces Parmesan cheese, grated (¾ cup)
- 2 garlic cloves, toasted and minced

Directions:

1. Process all ingredients except oil and cheese using a food processor until smooth, scraping down bowl as required. While your food processor runs slowly put in oil until incorporated.
2. Move pesto to a container, mix in cheese, and sprinkle with salt and pepper to taste. When tossing pesto with cooked pasta, put in some of pasta cooking water as required (up to ½ cup) to loosen consistency of pesto.
3. Pesto will keep safely in a fridge for maximum 3 days or frozen for maximum 3 months. To stop browning, press plastic wrap flush to surface, or top with thin layer of olive oil.

Roasted Red Pepper Pesto

Yield: 1½ cups

This recipe can be made quickly

Ⓥ This is a Vegetarian Recipe Ⓥ

Ingredients:

- ¼ cup fresh parsley leaves
- ¼ cup grated Parmesan cheese
- ½ cup extra-virgin olive oil
- 1 shallot, chopped
- 1 tablespoon fresh thyme leaves
- 2 roasted red bell peppers, peeled and chopped (1 cup)
- 3 garlic cloves, toasted and minced

Directions:

1. Process all ingredients except oil and cheese using a food processor until smooth, scraping down bowl as required. While your food processor runs slowly put in oil until incorporated.
2. Move pesto to a container, mix in cheese, and sprinkle with salt and pepper to taste. When tossing pesto with cooked pasta, put in some of pasta cooking water as required (up to ½ cup) to loosen consistency of pesto.
3. Pesto will keep safely in a fridge for maximum 3 days or frozen for maximum 3 months. To stop browning, press plastic wrap flush to surface, or top with thin layer of olive oil.

Tomato and Almond Pesto

Yield: 1½ cups

This recipe can be made quickly

Ⓥ *This is a Vegetarian Recipe* Ⓥ

Ingredients:

- ¼ cup slivered almonds, toasted
- ⅓ cup extra-virgin olive oil
- ½ cup fresh basil leaves
- 1 garlic clove, toasted and minced
- 1 ounce Parmesan cheese, grated (½ cup)
- 1 small pepperoncini, stemmed, seeded, and minced
- 12 ounces cherry or grape tomatoes
- Pinch red pepper flakes (optional)

Directions:

1. Process all ingredients except oil and cheese using a food processor until smooth, scraping down bowl as required. While your food processor runs slowly put in oil until incorporated.
2. Move pesto to a container, mix in cheese, and sprinkle with salt and pepper to taste. When tossing pesto with cooked pasta, put in some of pasta cooking water as required (up to ½ cup) to loosen consistency of pesto.
3. Pesto will keep safely in a fridge for maximum 3 days or frozen for maximum 3 months. To stop browning, press plastic wrap flush to surface, or top with thin layer of olive oil.

Pasta

And now to the Pasta recipes! You don't have to stick to the sauce suggestion given in the recipe. Feel free to experiment with one of the sauces you've already seen above! This section covers all the popular versions of pasta in the Mediterranean.

Briny Italian Spaghetti

Yield: 6 Servings

This recipe can be made quickly

Ingredients:

- ½ cup dry white wine
- ½ teaspoon red pepper flakes
- 1 pound mussels, scrubbed and debearded
- 1 pound spaghetti or linguine
- 1 tablespoon extra-virgin olive oil
- 1 teaspoon grated lemon zest plus 2 tablespoons juice
- 2 garlic cloves, minced
- 2 tablespoons minced fresh parsley
- Salt and pepper

Directions:

1. Bring mussels and wine to boil in 12-inch straight-sided sauté pan, cover, and cook, shaking pan occasionally, until mussels open, approximately five minutes. As mussels open, remove them using a slotted spoon and move to a container. Discard any mussels that refuse to open. (If desired, remove mussels from shells.) Drain steaming liquid through fine-mesh strainer lined with coffee filter into a container, avoiding any gritty sediment that has settled on bottom of pan. Wipe frying pan clean using paper towels.
2. Cook oil, garlic, and pepper flakes in now-empty pan on moderate heat, stirring often, until garlic turns golden but not brown, approximately three minutes. Mix in reserved mussel steaming liquid and lemon zest and juice, bring to simmer, and cook until flavours blend, about 4 minutes. Mix in mussels, cover, and cook until heated through, approximately two minutes.
3. In the meantime, bring 4 quarts water to boil in large pot. Put in pasta and 1 tablespoon salt and cook, stirring frequently, until al dente. Reserve ½ cup cooking water, then drain pasta and return it to pot. Put in sauce and parsley and toss to combine. Sprinkle with salt and pepper to taste and regulate consistency with reserved cooking water as required. Serve.

Cheesy Penne with Roasted Cherry Tomatoes

Yield: 6 Servings

Ⓥ This is a Vegetarian Recipe Ⓥ

Ingredients:

- ¼ cup extra-virgin olive oil
- ¼ teaspoon red pepper flakes
- 1 pound penne
- 1 shallot, sliced thin
- 1 tablespoon sherry or red wine vinegar
- 1½ teaspoons sugar, or to taste
- 2 pounds cherry tomatoes, halved
- 3 large garlic cloves, sliced thin
- 4 ounces (4 cups) baby arugula
- 4 ounces goat cheese, crumbled (1 cup)
- Salt and pepper

Directions:

1. Place the oven rack in the centre of the oven and pre-heat your oven to 350 degrees. Toss shallot with 1 teaspoon oil in a container. In a different container, gently toss tomatoes with remaining oil, garlic, vinegar, sugar, ½ teaspoon salt, ¼ teaspoon pepper, and pepper flakes. Lay out tomato mixture in a uniform layer in rimmed baking sheet, scatter shallot over tomatoes, and roast until edges of shallot begin to brown and tomato skins are slightly shrivelled, 35 to 40 minutes. (Do not stir tomatoes during roasting.) Allow it to cool for 5 to 10 minutes.
2. In the meantime, bring 4 quarts water to boil in large pot. Put in pasta and 1 tablespoon salt and cook, stirring frequently, until al dente. Reserve ½ cup cooking water, then drain pasta and

return it to pot. Put in arugula to pasta and toss until wilted. Using rubber spatula, scrape tomato mixture onto pasta and toss to combine. Sprinkle with salt and pepper to taste and regulate consistency with reserved cooking water as required. Serve, passing goat cheese separately.

Classic Clammed Italian Spaghetti

Yield: 6 Servings

Ingredients:

- ⅛ teaspoon red pepper flakes
- ⅓ cup chopped fresh mint or parsley
- ½ cup dry white wine
- 1 pound spaghetti or linguine
- 1 shallot, sliced thin
- 12 cloves garlic, peeled (8 smashed, 4 minced)
- 2 tablespoons tomato paste
- 2 teaspoons minced fresh thyme or ½ teaspoon dried
- 3 pounds ripe tomatoes, cored and halved
- 3 tablespoons extra-virgin olive oil, plus extra for serving
- 4 pounds littleneck clams, scrubbed
- Salt and pepper

Directions:

1. Place the oven rack in the centre of the oven and pre-heat your oven to 475 degrees. Mix tomato paste, 1 tablespoon oil, thyme, ¼ teaspoon salt, and ¼ teaspoon pepper in a big container. Put in tomatoes and smashed garlic and gently toss to coat. Place 4-inch square of aluminium foil in center of wire rack set in rimmed baking sheet lined with aluminium foil. Place smashed garlic cloves on foil and arrange tomatoes, cut side down, around garlic. Roast until tomatoes are soft and skins are well charred, 45 to 55 minutes.

2. Heat remaining 2 tablespoons oil in a Dutch oven on moderate heat until it starts to shimmer. Put in shallot, pepper flakes, and minced garlic and cook until aromatic, about 1 minute. Mix in wine and cook until almost completely evaporated, about 1 minute. Mix in roasted tomatoes and garlic and bring to boil. Put in clams, cover, and cook, shaking pot occasionally, until clams open, about four to eight minutes. As clams open, remove them using a slotted spoon and move to a container. Discard any clams that refuse to open. (If desired, remove clams from shells.)
3. In the meantime, bring 4 quarts water to boil in large pot. Put in pasta and 1 tablespoon salt and cook, stirring frequently, until al dente. Reserve ½ cup cooking water, then drain pasta and put in to pot with sauce. Put in mint and toss to combine. Sprinkle with salt and pepper to taste and regulate consistency with reserved cooking water as required. Move pasta to serving bowl, top with clams, and drizzle with extra oil. Serve.

Classic Italian Linguine ai Frutti di Mare

Yield: 6 Servings

Ingredients:

- ⅛ teaspoon red pepper flakes
- ⅛ teaspoon saffron threads, crumbled
- ⅓ cup minced fresh parsley
- 1 (28-ounce) can whole peeled tomatoes, drained
- 1 (8-ounce) bottle clam juice
- 1 anchovy fillet, rinsed and minced
- 1 cup dry white wine
- 1 cup Lemon-Chili Bread Crumbs
- 1 pound linguine
- 2 shallots, sliced thin
- 2 tablespoons tomato paste
- 3 tablespoons extra-virgin olive oil, plus extra for serving

- 6 garlic cloves, sliced thin
- 8 ounces large sea scallops, tendons removed
- 8 ounces large shrimp (26 to 30 per pound), peeled and deveined, shells reserved
- 8 ounces mussels, scrubbed and debearded
- 8 ounces squid, bodies sliced crosswise into ¼-inch-thick rings, tentacles halved

Directions:

1. Heat 1 tablespoon oil in a Dutch oven on moderate heat until it starts to shimmer. Put in shrimp shells and cook, stirring often, until starting to turn spotty brown and pot starts to brown, 2 to 4 minutes. Put in wine and simmer, stirring intermittently, for about five minutes. Strain mixture through fine-mesh strainer into a container, pressing on solids to extract as much liquid as possible; discard solids.
2. Pulse tomatoes using a food processor until finely ground, approximately ten pulses. Heat remaining 2 tablespoons oil in now-empty pot on moderate heat until it starts to shimmer. Put in shallots and cook till they become tender and lightly browned, 2 to 3 minutes. Mix in garlic, tomato paste, anchovy, pepper flakes, and saffron and cook until aromatic, about 1 minute. Mix in wine mixture, scraping up any browned bits, and cook until nearly evaporated, approximately half a minute. Mix in tomatoes and clam juice, bring to simmer, and cook, stirring intermittently, until thickened and flavours blend, approximately twenty minutes.
3. Put in mussels, bring to boil, cover, and cook, shaking pot occasionally, until mussels open, 3 to 6 minutes. As mussels open, remove them using a slotted spoon and move to a container. Discard any mussels that refuse to open.
4. Reduce sauce to simmer, gently mix in scallops, and cook for 2 minutes. Gently mix in shrimp and cook until just opaque throughout, approximately two minutes. Remove from the heat, mix in squid, cover, and allow to sit until just opaque and tender, 1 to 2 minutes.

5. In the meantime, bring 4 quarts water to boil in large pot. Put in pasta and 1 tablespoon salt and cook, stirring frequently, until al dente. Reserve ½ cup cooking water, then drain pasta and put in to pot with sauce. Put in mussels and parsley and toss to combine. Sprinkle with salt and pepper to taste and regulate consistency with reserved cooking water as required. Serve, sprinkling individual portions with bread crumbs and drizzling with extra oil.

Classic Italian Spaghetti al Limone

Yield: 6 Servings

This recipe can be made quickly

This is a Vegetarian Recipe

Ingredients:

- ½ cup extra-virgin olive oil
- 1 pound spaghetti
- 1 small garlic clove, minced to paste
- 2 ounces Parmesan cheese, grated (1 cup)
- 2 teaspoons grated lemon zest plus ⅓ cup lemon juice (2 lemons)
- 6 tablespoons shredded fresh basil
- Salt and pepper

Directions:

1. Beat oil, lemon zest and juice, garlic, ½ teaspoon salt, and ¼ teaspoon pepper together in a small-sized container, then mix in Parmesan until thick and creamy.
2. In the meantime, bring 4 quarts water to boil in large pot. Put in pasta and 1 tablespoon salt and cook, stirring frequently, until al dente. Reserve ½ cup cooking water, then drain pasta and return it to pot. Put in oil mixture and basil and toss to combine.

Sprinkle with salt and pepper to taste and regulate consistency with reserved cooking water as required. Serve.

Colourful & Nutty Farfalle

Yield: 6 Servings

Ⓥ This is a Vegetarian Recipe Ⓥ

Ingredients:

- ¼ cup pine nuts, toasted
- ½ cup chopped fresh basil
- ½ teaspoon red pepper flakes
- 1 pound farfalle
- 12 ounces grape tomatoes, halved
- 2 pounds zucchini and/or summer squash, halved along the length and sliced ½ inch thick
- 2 tablespoons balsamic vinegar
- 3 garlic cloves, minced
- 5 tablespoons extra-virgin olive oil
- Grated Parmesan cheese
- Kosher salt and pepper

Directions:

1. Toss squash with 1 tablespoon salt and allow to drain using a colander for 30 minutes. Pat squash dry using paper towels and carefully wipe away any residual salt.
2. Heat 1 tablespoon oil in 12-inch non-stick frying pan on high heat until just smoking. Put in half of squash and cook, stirring intermittently, until golden brown and mildly charred, 5 to 7 minutes, reducing heat if frying pan begins to scorch; move to large plate. Repeat with 1 tablespoon oil and remaining squash; move to plate.
3. Heat 1 tablespoon oil in now-empty frying pan on moderate heat until it starts to shimmer. Put in garlic and pepper flakes

and cook until aromatic, approximately half a minute. Mix in squash and cook until heated through, approximately half a minute.

4. In the meantime, bring 4 quarts water to boil in large pot. Put in pasta and 1 tablespoon salt and cook, stirring frequently, until al dente. Reserve ½ cup cooking water, then drain pasta and return it to pot. Put in squash mixture, tomatoes, basil, pine nuts, vinegar, and remaining 2 tablespoons oil and toss to combine. Sprinkle with salt and pepper to taste and regulate consistency with reserved cooking water as required. Serve with Parmesan.

Flavourful Italian Spaghetti Mix

Yield: 6 Servings

Ingredients:

- ¼–½ teaspoon red pepper flakes
- 1 (15-ounce) can cannellini beans, rinsed
- 1 cup Parmesan Bread Crumbs
- 1 onion, chopped fine
- 1 pound whole-wheat spaghetti
- 1 tablespoon extra-virgin olive oil
- 1½ cups chicken broth
- 1½ pounds kale or collard greens, stemmed and cut into 1-inch pieces
- 3 garlic cloves, minced
- 3 ounces pancetta, cut into ½-inch pieces
- 4 ounces fontina cheese, shredded (1 cup)
- Salt and pepper

Directions:

1. Heat oil in 12-inch straight-sided sauté pan on moderate heat until it starts to shimmer. Put in pancetta and cook, stirring

intermittently, until crisp, 5 to 7 minutes. Use a slotted spoon to move pancetta to paper towel–lined plate.
2. Put in onion to fat left in pan and cook on moderate heat till they become tender and lightly browned, 5 to 7 minutes. Mix in garlic and pepper flakes and cook until aromatic, approximately half a minute. Put in half of greens and cook, tossing occasionally, until starting to wilt, approximately two minutes. Put in remaining greens, broth, and ¾ teaspoon salt and bring to simmer. Decrease heat to medium, cover (pan will be very full), and cook, tossing occasionally, until greens are tender, about fifteen minutes (mixture will be somewhat soupy). Remove from the heat, mix in beans and pancetta.
3. In the meantime, bring 4 quarts water to boil in large pot. Put in pasta and 1 tablespoon salt and cook, stirring frequently, until just shy of al dente. Reserve ½ cup cooking water, then drain pasta and return it to pot. Put in greens mixture and cook on moderate heat, tossing to combine, until pasta absorbs most of liquid, approximately two minutes.
4. Remove from the heat, mix in fontina. Sprinkle with salt and pepper to taste and regulate consistency with reserved cooking water as required. Serve, sprinkling individual portions with bread crumbs.

Flavourful Italian Tagliatelle

Yield: 6 Servings

Ingredients:

- ⅛ teaspoon red pepper flakes
- ¼ cup extra-virgin olive oil, plus extra for serving
- ¼ cup minced fresh parsley
- ½ cup dry white wine
- 1 ounce Parmesan cheese, grated (½ cup), plus extra for serving
- 1 pound tagliatelle
- 1 recipe Parmesan Bread Crumbs

- 1 tablespoon minced fresh oregano or 1 teaspoon dried
- 1½ teaspoons grated lemon zest
- 2 anchovy fillets, rinsed, patted dry, and minced
- 4 cups jarred whole baby artichoke hearts packed in water
- 4 garlic cloves, minced
- Salt and pepper

Directions:

1. Cut leaves from artichoke hearts. Cut hearts in half and dry using paper towels. Place leaves in a container and cover with water. Let leaves sit for about fifteen minutes. Drain well.
2. Heat 1 tablespoon oil in 12-inch non-stick frying pan on moderate to high heat until it starts to shimmer. Put in artichoke hearts and ⅛ teaspoon salt and cook, stirring often, until spotty brown, seven to nine minutes. Mix in garlic, anchovies, oregano, and pepper flakes and cook, stirring continuously, until aromatic, approximately half a minute. Mix in wine and bring to simmer. Remove from the heat, mix in artichoke leaves.
3. In the meantime, bring 4 quarts water to boil in large pot. Put in pasta and 1 tablespoon salt and cook, stirring frequently, until al dente. Reserve 1½ cups cooking water, then drain pasta and return it to pot. Put in 1 cup reserved cooking water, artichoke mixture, Parmesan, parsley, lemon zest, and remaining 3 tablespoons oil and toss to combine. Sprinkle with salt and pepper to taste and regulate consistency with remaining ½ cup reserved cooking water as required. Serve, sprinkling individual portions with bread crumbs and extra Parmesan (recipe belo) and drizzling with extra oil.

Parmesan Bread Crumbs
Yield: 1 cup

This recipe can be made quickly

(V) This is a Vegetarian Recipe (V)

Ingredients:

- ¼ cup grated Parmesan cheese
- 2 slices hearty white sandwich bread
- 2 tablespoons extra-virgin olive oil
- Salt and pepper

Directions:

1. Pulse bread using a food processor until finely ground, 10 to 15 pulses. Heat oil in 12-inch non-stick frying pan on moderate heat until it starts to shimmer.
2. Put in bread crumbs and cook, stirring continuously, until crumbs begin to brown, 3 to 5 minutes. Put in Parmesan and continue to cook, stirring continuously, until crumbs start to look golden brown, 1 to 2 minutes. Move crumbs to a container and sprinkle with salt and pepper to taste. Serve.

Flavourful Toasted Orzo Mix

Yield: 6 to 8 Servings

Ⓥ This is a Vegetarian Recipe Ⓥ

Ingredients:

- ½ cup pitted kalamata olives, chopped
- ¾ cup dry white wine
- ¾ teaspoon fennel seeds
- 1 fennel bulb, stalks discarded, bulb halved, cored, and chopped fine
- 1 onion, chopped fine
- 1 teaspoon grated orange zest
- 1½ cups water
- 1½ ounces Parmesan cheese, grated (¾ cup)
- 2 cups chicken or vegetable broth
- 2 garlic cloves, minced

- 2 tablespoons extra-virgin olive oil
- 2⅔ cups orzo
- Pinch ground nutmeg
- Pinch red pepper flakes
- Salt and pepper

Directions:

1. Heat oil in 12-inch non-stick frying pan on moderate heat until it starts to shimmer. Put in fennel, onion, and ¾ teaspoon salt and cook till they become tender and lightly browned, 5 to 7 minutes. Mix in garlic, orange zest, fennel seeds, and pepper flakes and cook until aromatic, approximately half a minute. Put in orzo and cook, stirring often, until orzo is coated with oil and lightly browned, approximately five minutes.
2. Mix in broth, water, and wine and bring to boil. Cook, stirring intermittently, until all liquid has been absorbed and orzo is tender, 10 to fifteen minutes. Mix in olives, Parmesan, and nutmeg and sprinkle with salt and pepper to taste. Serve.

Greek Crunchy Orzo Salad

Yield: 4 to 6 Servings

(V) This is a Vegetarian Recipe (V)

Ingredients:

- ¼ cup extra-virgin olive oil, plus extra for serving
- ¼ cup pine nuts, toasted
- ½ cup chopped fresh basil
- ½ cup oil-packed sun-dried tomatoes, minced
- ½ cup pitted kalamata olives, halved
- 1 ounce Parmesan cheese, grated (½ cup)
- 1¼ cups orzo
- 2 garlic cloves, minced
- 2 ounces (2 cups) baby arugula, chopped

- 3 tablespoons balsamic vinegar
- Salt and pepper

Directions:

1. Bring 2 quarts water to boil in large pot. Put in orzo and 1½ teaspoons salt and cook, stirring frequently, until al dente. Drain orzo and move to rimmed baking sheet. Toss with 1 tablespoon oil and allow to cool completely, about fifteen minutes.
2. Beat remaining 3 tablespoons oil, vinegar, garlic, ½ teaspoon salt, and ½ teaspoon pepper together in a big container. Put in arugula, Parmesan, tomatoes, olives, basil, pine nuts, and orzo and gently toss to combine. Sprinkle with salt and pepper to taste. Let salad sit until flavours blend, approximately half an hour. Serve, drizzled with extra oil. (Salad will keep safely in a fridge for maximum 2 days.)

Greek Manestra

Yield: 6 Servings

Ⓥ This is a Vegetarian Recipe Ⓥ

Ingredients:

- 1 onion, chopped fine
- 1 ounce Parmesan cheese, grated (½ cup)
- 1 pound eggplant, cut into ½-inch pieces
- 1¼ cups chicken or vegetable broth
- 1¼ cups water
- 2 anchovy fillets, rinsed, patted dry, and minced
- 2 cups orzo
- 2 tablespoons capers, rinsed and minced
- 2 teaspoons tomato paste
- 3 garlic cloves, minced
- 3 ounces feta cheese, crumbled (¾ cup)

- 3 tablespoons extra-virgin olive oil, plus extra for serving
- 4 teaspoons minced fresh oregano or 1 teaspoon dried
- 4 tomatoes, cored and sliced ¼ inch thick
- Salt and pepper

Directions:

1. Place oven rack to upper-middle position and pre-heat your oven to 400 degrees. Line large plate using double layer of coffee filters and spray using vegetable oil spray. Toss eggplant with ½ teaspoon salt and spread uniformly coffee filters. Microwave eggplant, uncovered, until dry to touch and slightly shriveled, 7 to 10 minutes, tossing halfway through microwaving.
2. Toast orzo in 12-inch non-stick frying pan on moderate to high heat until lightly browned, 3 to 5 minutes; move to a container. Heat 1 tablespoon oil in now-empty frying pan on moderate to high heat until it starts to shimmer. Put in eggplant and cook, stirring intermittently, until well browned, 5 to 7 minutes; move to different container.
3. Heat remaining 2 tablespoons oil in again-empty frying pan on moderate heat until it starts to shimmer. Put in onion and cook till they become tender and lightly browned, 5 to 7 minutes. Mix in garlic, 1 tablespoon oregano, tomato paste, and anchovies and cook until aromatic, approximately half a minute. Remove from the heat, mix in orzo, eggplant, broth, water, Parmesan, capers, and ¼ teaspoon pepper. Move to greased 13 by 9-inch baking dish and spread into even layer.
4. Shingle tomatoes beautifully over top, then drizzle with ¼ teaspoon salt. Bake until all liquid has been absorbed and orzo is tender, 30 to 35 minutes. Allow it to cool for about five minutes. Sprinkle feta and remaining 1 teaspoon oregano over tomatoes and drizzle with extra oil. Serve.

Greek Spicy Orzo

Yield: 4 to 6 Servings

Ingredients:

- ⅛ teaspoon red pepper flakes
- ¼ cup chopped fresh mint
- ¼ cup plain whole-milk Greek yogurt
- ¼ teaspoon ground cinnamon
- ½ cup dry white wine
- 1 onion, chopped fine
- 1 red bell pepper, stemmed, seeded, and chopped fine
- 1 tablespoon extra-virgin olive oil
- 1 tablespoon tomato paste
- 1 teaspoon paprika
- 1½ cups orzo
- 1½ teaspoons grated lemon zest
- 2 garlic cloves, minced
- 2½ cups chicken broth
- 4 ounces loukaniko sausage, chopped fine
- Salt and pepper

Directions:

1. Toast orzo in 12-inch frying pan on moderate to high heat until lightly browned, 3 to 5 minutes; move to a container. Heat oil in now-empty frying pan on moderate heat until it starts to shimmer. Put in sausage and cook until browned and fat is rendered, four to eight minutes.
2. Mix in onion and bell pepper and cook till they become tender, 5 to 7 minutes. Mix in tomato paste, garlic, paprika, cinnamon, and pepper flakes and cook until aromatic, about 1 minute. Mix in wine, scraping up any browned bits. Mix in broth and orzo and bring to simmer. Decrease heat to low, cover, and simmer gently until most of liquid is absorbed, about 10 minutes, stirring once halfway through simmering.

3. Uncover and continue to cook, stirring intermittently, until orzo is al dente and creamy, about 4 minutes. Remove from the heat, mix in yogurt and lemon zest. Sprinkle with salt and pepper to taste and regulate consistency with hot water as required. Sprinkle with mint and serve.

Green Penne and Fresh Tomato Sauce

Yield: 6 Servings

✤ This recipe can be made quickly ✤

Ⓥ This is a Vegetarian Recipe Ⓥ

Ingredients:

- 1 pound penne
- 2 garlic cloves, minced
- 2 tablespoons chopped fresh mint or oregano
- 2 tablespoons lemon juice
- 3 pounds ripe tomatoes, cored, peeled, seeded, and cut into ½-inch pieces
- 3 tablespoons extra-virgin olive oil
- 4 ounces feta cheese, crumbled (1 cup)
- 5 ounces (5 cups) baby spinach
- Salt and pepper
- Sugar
- The success of this recipe depends on ripe, in-season tomatoes.

Directions:

1. Cook 2 tablespoons oil and garlic in 12-inch frying pan on moderate heat, stirring frequently, until garlic turns golden but not brown, approximately three minutes. Mix in tomatoes and cook until tomato pieces begin to lose their shape, approximately eight minutes. Mix in spinach, 1 handful at a

time, and cook until spinach is wilted and tomatoes have made chunky sauce, approximately two minutes.
2. In the meantime, bring 4 quarts water to boil in large pot. Put in pasta and 1 tablespoon salt and cook, stirring frequently, until al dente. Reserve ½ cup cooking water, then drain pasta and return it to pot.
3. Stir mint, lemon juice, ¼ teaspoon salt, and ⅛ teaspoon pepper into sauce and season with sugar to taste. Put in sauce and residual 1 tablespoon oil to pasta and toss to combine. Sprinkle with salt and pepper to taste and regulate consistency with reserved cooking water as required. Serve, passing feta separately.

Lemony Shrimp Orzo

Yield: 4 Servings

Ingredients:

- ½ cup pitted kalamata olives, chopped coarse
- 1 onion, chopped fine
- 1 tablespoon grated lemon zest plus 1 tablespoon juice
- 1½ pounds extra-large shrimp (21 to 25 per pound), peeled and deveined
- 2 cups chicken broth
- 2 cups orzo
- 2 cups water
- 2 garlic cloves, minced
- 2 ounces feta cheese, crumbled (½ cup)
- 2 tablespoons chopped fresh parsley
- 2 tablespoons extra-virgin olive oil, plus extra for serving
- Salt and pepper

Directions:

1. Mix lemon zest, ½ teaspoon salt, and ½ teaspoon pepper in medium bowl. Put in shrimp, toss to coat, put inside your fridge until ready to use.
2. Heat 1 tablespoon oil in 12-inch non-stick frying pan on moderate to high heat until just smoking. Put in onion and cook till they become tender, approximately five minutes. Mix in garlic and cook until aromatic, approximately half a minute. Put in orzo and cook, stirring often, until orzo is coated with oil and lightly browned, approximately five minutes. Mix in broth and water and bring to boil. Cook, stirring intermittently, until orzo is al dente, about 6 minutes. Mix in olives, ¼ cup feta, and lemon juice. Sprinkle with salt and pepper to taste.
3. Decrease heat to moderate to low, nestle shrimp into orzo, cover, and cook until shrimp are opaque throughout, approximately five minutes. Sprinkle with parsley and remaining ¼ cup feta and drizzle with extra oil. Serve.

Nutty Penne with Roasted Cherry Tomatoes

Yield: **6 Servings**

(V) This is a Vegetarian Recipe (V)

Ingredients:

- ¼ cup capers, rinsed
- ¼ cup extra-virgin olive oil
- ¼ cup pine nuts, toasted
- ½ cup pitted kalamata olives, chopped
- ½ teaspoon red pepper flakes
- 1 pound penne
- 1½ teaspoons sugar, or to taste
- 2 pounds cherry tomatoes, halved
- 3 large garlic cloves, sliced thin

- 3 tablespoons chopped fresh oregano
- Grated Pecorino Romano cheese
- Salt and pepper

Directions:

1. Place the oven rack in the centre of the oven and pre-heat your oven to 350 degrees. Gently toss tomatoes with oil, capers, garlic, sugar, ½ teaspoon salt, pepper flakes, and ¼ teaspoon pepper in a container. Lay out tomato mixture in a uniform layer in rimmed baking sheet and roast until tomato skins are slightly shriveled, 35 to 40 minutes. (Do not stir tomatoes during roasting.) Allow it to cool for 5 to 10 minutes.
2. In the meantime, bring 4 quarts water to boil in large pot. Put in pasta and 1 tablespoon salt and cook, stirring frequently, until al dente. Reserve ½ cup cooking water, then drain pasta and return it to pot. Using rubber spatula, scrape tomato mixture onto pasta. Put in olives, pine nuts, and oregano and toss to combine. Sprinkle with salt and pepper to taste and regulate consistency with reserved cooking water as required. Serve with Pecorino Romano.

Penne with Cherry Tomato Sauce

Yield: 6 Servings

Ⓥ This is a Vegetarian Recipe Ⓥ

Ingredients:

- ¼ cup coarsely chopped fresh basil
- ¼ cup extra-virgin olive oil
- ¼ teaspoon red pepper flakes
- 1 pound penne
- 1 shallot, sliced thin
- 1 tablespoon balsamic vinegar
- 1½ teaspoons sugar, or to taste

- 2 pounds cherry tomatoes, halved
- 3 large garlic cloves, sliced thin
- Grated Parmesan cheese
- Salt and pepper

Directions:

1. Place the oven rack in the centre of the oven and pre-heat your oven to 350 degrees. Toss shallot with 1 teaspoon oil in a container. In a different container, gently toss tomatoes with remaining oil, garlic, vinegar, sugar, ½ teaspoon salt, ¼ teaspoon pepper, and pepper flakes. Lay out tomato mixture in a uniform layer in rimmed baking sheet, scatter shallot over tomatoes, and roast until edges of shallot begin to brown and tomato skins are slightly shriveled, 35 to 40 minutes. (Do not stir tomatoes during roasting.) Allow it to cool for 5 to 10 minutes.
2. In the meantime, bring 4 quarts water to boil in large pot. Put in pasta and 1 tablespoon salt and cook, stirring frequently, until al dente. Reserve ½ cup cooking water, then drain pasta and return it to pot. Using rubber spatula, scrape tomato mixture onto pasta. Put in basil and toss to combine. Sprinkle with salt and pepper to taste and regulate consistency with reserved cooking water as required. Serve with Parmesan.

Puglia-Style Orecchiette

Yield: 6 Servings

✔ This recipe can be made quickly ✔

Ⓥ This is a Vegetarian Recipe Ⓥ

Ingredients:

- ¼ cup extra-virgin olive oil
- ¼ teaspoon red pepper flakes

- ½ teaspoon fennel seeds, crushed
- 1 (15-ounce) can cannellini beans, rinsed
- 1 pound broccoli rabe, trimmed and cut into 1½-inch pieces
- 1 pound orecchiette
- 1 shallot, minced
- 1 teaspoon minced fresh oregano or ¼ teaspoon dried
- 2 ounces Parmesan or Asiago cheese, grated (1 cup)
- 6 garlic cloves, minced
- Salt and pepper

Directions:

1. Heat oil in 12-inch non-stick frying pan on moderate heat until it starts to shimmer. Put in shallot and cook till they become tender, approximately two minutes. Mix in garlic, oregano, fennel seeds, and pepper flakes and cook until aromatic, approximately half a minute. Mix in beans and cook until heated through, approximately two minutes; set aside.
2. In the meantime, bring 4 quarts water to boil in large pot. Put in broccoli rabe and 1 tablespoon salt and cook, stirring frequently, until crisp-tender, approximately two minutes. Use a slotted spoon to move broccoli rabe to frying pan with bean mixture.
3. Return water to boil, put in pasta, and cook, stirring frequently, until al dente. Reserve 1 cup cooking water, then drain pasta and return it to pot. Put in bean–broccoli rabe mixture, Parmesan, and ⅓ cup reserved cooking water and toss to combine. Sprinkle with salt and pepper to taste and regulate consistency with remaining ⅔ cup reserved cooking water as required. Serve.

Rustic Italian Whole-Wheat Spaghetti

Yield: 6 Servings

Ingredients:

- ¼ cup chopped fresh parsley
- ¼ cup dry white wine
- ¼ cup extra-virgin olive oil
- ¾ cup lentilles du Puy, picked over and rinsed
- 1 head escarole (1 pound), trimmed and sliced ½ inch thick
- 1 onion, chopped fine
- 1 pound whole-wheat spaghetti
- 1½ cups water
- 2 carrots, peeled, halved along the length, and sliced ¼ inch thick
- 2 cups chicken broth
- 2 garlic cloves, minced
- 4 ounces pancetta, cut into ¼-inch pieces
- Grated Parmesan cheese
- Salt and pepper

Directions:

1. Heat 2 tablespoons oil in a big saucepan on moderate heat until it starts to shimmer. Put in pancetta and cook, stirring intermittently, until starting to brown, 3 to 5 minutes. Put in onion and carrots and cook till they become tender, 5 to 7 minutes. Mix in garlic and cook until aromatic, approximately half a minute. Mix in lentils, broth, and water and bring to simmer. Decrease heat to moderate to low, cover, and simmer until lentils are fully cooked and tender, 30 to 40 minutes.
2. Mix in wine and simmer, uncovered, for 2 minutes. Mix in escarole, 1 handful at a time, and cook until completely wilted, approximately five minutes.
3. In the meantime, bring 4 quarts water to boil in large pot. Put in pasta and 1 tablespoon salt and cook, stirring frequently, until al dente. Reserve ¾ cup cooking water, then drain pasta and return it to pot. Put in ½ cup reserved cooking water, lentil mixture, parsley, and remaining 2 tablespoons oil and toss to combine. Sprinkle with salt and pepper to taste and regulate

consistency with remaining ¼ cup reserved cooking water as required. Serve with Parmesan.

Spanish Toasted Shrimpy Pasta

Yield: 4 Servings

Ingredients:

- ¼ cup dry white wine
- ½ teaspoon anchovy paste
- 1 (14.5-ounce) can diced tomatoes, drained and chopped fine
- 1 bay leaf
- 1 cup chicken broth
- 1 onion, chopped fine
- 1 tablespoon chopped fresh parsley
- 1 teaspoon paprika
- 1 teaspoon smoked paprika
- 1½ pounds extra-large shrimp (21 to 25 per pound), peeled and deveined, shells reserved
- 2¾ cups water
- 3 garlic cloves, minced
- 3 tablespoons plus 2 teaspoons extra-virgin olive oil
- 8 ounces vermicelli pasta or thin spaghetti, broken into 1- to 2-inch lengths
- Lemon wedges
- Salt and pepper

Directions:

1. Mix 1 tablespoon oil, 1 teaspoon garlic, ¼ teaspoon salt, and ⅛ teaspoon pepper in medium bowl. Put in shrimp, toss to coat, put inside your fridge until ready to use.
2. Place reserved shrimp shells, water, broth, and bay leaf in medium bowl. Cover and microwave until liquid is hot and shells have turned pink, about 6 minutes. Set aside until ready to use.

3. Toss pasta with 2 teaspoons oil in broiler-safe 12-inch frying pan until evenly coated. Toast pasta on moderate to high heat, stirring often, until browned and nutty in aroma (pasta should be color of peanut butter), 6 to 10 minutes. Move pasta to a container. Wipe out frying pan using paper towels.
4. Heat remaining 2 tablespoons oil in now-empty frying pan on moderate to high heat until it starts to shimmer. Put in onion and ¼ teaspoon salt and cook till they become tender and starting to brown around edges, four to eight minutes. Put in tomatoes and cook, stirring intermittently, until mixture is thick, dry, and slightly darkened in color, four to eight minutes. Decrease heat to medium, put in remaining garlic, paprika, smoked paprika, and anchovy paste, and cook until aromatic, about 1½ minutes. Mix in pasta until combined. Place oven rack 5 to 6 inches from broiler element and heat broiler.
5. Pour shrimp broth through fine-mesh strainer into skillet; discard shells. Put in wine, ¼ teaspoon salt, and ½ teaspoon pepper and stir well. Increase heat to medium-high and bring to simmer. Cook, stirring intermittently, until liquid is slightly thickened and pasta is just tender, eight to ten minutes. Scatter shrimp over pasta and stir to partially submerge. Move frying pan to oven and broil until shrimp are opaque and surface of pasta is dry with crisped, browned spots, 5 to 7 minutes. Remove from oven and let sit, uncovered, for about five minutes. Sprinkle with parsley and serve instantly with lemon wedges.

Spicy Beefy Rigatoni

Yield: 6 Servings

Ingredients:

- ½ cup dry red wine
- ½ teaspoon ground cinnamon

- 1 (28-ounce) can whole peeled tomatoes, drained with juice reserved, chopped fine
- 1 onion, chopped fine
- 1 pound rigatoni
- 1 tablespoon extra-virgin olive oil
- 1 teaspoon minced fresh thyme or ¼ teaspoon dried
- 1½ pounds bone-in English-style short ribs, trimmed
- 2 tablespoons minced fresh parsley
- 3 garlic cloves, minced
- Grated Parmesan cheese
- Pinch ground cloves
- Salt and pepper

Directions:

1. Pat ribs dry using paper towels and sprinkle with salt and pepper. Heat oil in 12-inch frying pan on moderate to high heat until just smoking. Brown ribs on all sides, eight to ten minutes; move to plate.
2. Pour off all but 1 teaspoon fat from skillet, put in onion, and cook on moderate heat till they become tender, approximately five minutes. Mix in garlic, thyme, cinnamon, and cloves and cook until aromatic, approximately half a minute. Mix in wine, scraping up any browned bits, and simmer until nearly evaporated, approximately two minutes.
3. Mix in tomatoes and reserved juice. Nestle ribs into sauce along with any accumulated juices and bring to simmer. Decrease heat to low, cover, and simmer gently, turning ribs occasionally, until meat is very soft and falling off bones, about 2 hours.
4. Move ribs to slicing board, allow to cool slightly, then shred meat into bite-size pieces using 2 forks; discard excess fat and bones. Using wide, shallow spoon, skim excess fat from surface of sauce. Stir shredded meat and any accumulated juices into sauce and bring to simmer on moderate heat. Sprinkle with salt and pepper to taste.
5. In the meantime, bring 4 quarts water to boil in large pot. Put in pasta and 1 tablespoon salt and cook, stirring frequently, until

al dente. Reserve ½ cup cooking water, then drain pasta and return it to pot. Put in sauce and parsley and toss to combine. Sprinkle with salt and pepper to taste and regulate consistency with reserved cooking water as required. Serve with Parmesan.

Tangy Penne with Fresh Tomato Sauce

Yield: 6 Servings

This recipe can be made quickly

Ⓥ *This is a Vegetarian Recipe* Ⓥ

Ingredients:

- ⅛ teaspoon red pepper flakes
- ¼ cup extra-virgin olive oil
- ½ teaspoon fennel seeds, crushed
- 1 fennel bulb, stalks discarded, bulb halved, cored, and cut into ¼-inch pieces
- 1 pound penne
- 2 (3-inch) strips orange zest plus 3 tablespoons juice
- 2 garlic cloves, minced
- 3 pounds ripe tomatoes, cored, peeled, seeded, and cut into ½-inch pieces
- 3 tablespoons chopped fresh basil
- Pinch saffron threads, crumbled (optional)
- Salt and pepper
- Sugar

Directions:

1. Heat 2 tablespoons oil in 12-inch frying pan on moderate heat until it starts to shimmer. Put in fennel and cook till they become tender and lightly browned, 5 to 7 minutes. Mix in garlic, orange zest, fennel seeds, pepper flakes, and saffron, if using, and cook until aromatic, approximately half a minute.

Mix in tomatoes and cook until tomato pieces lose their shape and make chunky sauce, about 10 minutes. Discard orange zest.
2. In the meantime, bring 4 quarts water to boil in large pot. Put in pasta and 1 tablespoon salt and cook, stirring frequently, until al dente. Reserve ½ cup cooking water, then drain pasta and return it to pot.
3. Stir orange juice, basil, ¼ teaspoon salt, and ⅛ teaspoon pepper into sauce and season with sugar to taste. Put in sauce and remaining 2 tablespoons oil to pasta and toss to combine. Sprinkle with salt and pepper to taste and regulate consistency with reserved cooking water as required. Serve.

Whole-Wheat Spaghetti Mix

Yield: 6 Servings

(V) This is a Vegetarian Recipe (V)

Ingredients:

- ¼–½ teaspoon red pepper flakes
- ¾ cup pitted kalamata olives, chopped coarse
- ¾ cup vegetable broth
- 1 (14.5-ounce) can diced tomatoes, drained
- 1 (15-ounce) can cannellini beans, rinsed
- 1 onion, chopped fine
- 1 pound whole-wheat spaghetti
- 1¼ pounds curly-leaf spinach, stemmed and cut into 1-inch pieces
- 2 ounces Parmesan cheese, grated (1 cup), plus extra for serving
- 3 tablespoons extra-virgin olive oil, plus extra for serving
- 8 garlic cloves, peeled (5 sliced thin along the length, 3 minced)
- Salt and pepper

Directions:

1. Cook oil and sliced garlic in 12-inch straight-sided sauté pan on moderate heat, stirring frequently, until garlic turns golden but not brown, approximately three minutes. Use a slotted spoon to move garlic to plate coated using paper towels and season lightly with salt; set aside.
2. Put in onion to oil left in pan and cook on moderate heat till they become tender and lightly browned, 5 to 7 minutes. Mix in minced garlic and pepper flakes and cook until aromatic, approximately half a minute. Put in half of spinach and cook, tossing occasionally, until starting to wilt, approximately two minutes. Put in remaining spinach, broth, tomatoes, and ¾ teaspoon salt and bring to simmer. Decrease heat to medium, cover (pan will be very full), and cook, tossing occasionally, until spinach is completely wilted, about 10 minutes (mixture will be somewhat soupy). Remove from the heat, mix in beans and olives.
3. In the meantime, bring 4 quarts water to boil in large pot. Put in pasta and 1 tablespoon salt and cook, stirring frequently, until just shy of al dente. Reserve ½ cup cooking water, then drain pasta and return it to pot. Put in greens mixture and cook on moderate heat, tossing to combine, until pasta absorbs most of liquid, approximately two minutes.
4. Remove from the heat, mix in Parmesan. Sprinkle with salt and pepper to taste and regulate consistency with reserved cooking water as required. Serve, sprinkling individual portions with garlic chips and extra Parmesan and drizzling with extra oil.

Zucchini-Tomatoes Farfalle

Yield: 6 Servings

Ⓥ This is a Vegetarian Recipe Ⓥ

Ingredients:

- ¼ cup chopped fresh mint
- ½ cup pitted kalamata olives, quartered

- 1 pound farfalle
- 1 red onion, chopped fine
- 1 teaspoon grated lemon zest plus 1 tablespoon juice
- 12 ounces grape tomatoes, halved
- 2 pounds zucchini and/or summer squash, halved along the length and sliced ½ inch thick
- 2 teaspoons red wine vinegar
- 3 garlic cloves, minced
- 4 ounces feta cheese, crumbled (1 cup)
- 5 tablespoons extra-virgin olive oil
- Kosher salt and pepper

Directions:

1. Toss squash with 1 tablespoon salt and allow to drain using a colander for 30 minutes. Pat squash dry using paper towels and carefully wipe away any residual salt.
2. Heat 1 tablespoon oil in 12-inch non-stick frying pan on high heat until just smoking. Put in half of squash and cook, stirring intermittently, until golden brown and mildly charred, 5 to 7 minutes, reducing heat if frying pan begins to scorch; move to large plate. Repeat with 1 tablespoon oil and remaining squash; move to plate.
3. Heat 1 tablespoon oil in now-empty frying pan on moderate heat until it starts to shimmer. Put in onion and cook till they become tender and lightly browned, 5 to 7 minutes. Mix in garlic, lemon zest, and ½ teaspoon pepper and cook until aromatic, approximately half a minute. Mix in squash and cook until heated through, approximately half a minute.
4. In the meantime, bring 4 quarts water to boil in large pot. Put in pasta and 1 tablespoon salt and cook, stirring frequently, until al dente. Reserve ½ cup cooking water, then drain pasta and return it to pot. Put in squash mixture, tomatoes, olives, mint, vinegar, lemon juice, and remaining 2 tablespoons oil and toss to combine. Sprinkle with salt and pepper to taste and regulate consistency with reserved cooking water as required. Serve, passing feta seperately.

Couscous

Couscous is a staple food throughout the North African cuisines of Morocco, Algeria, Tunisia, Mauritania, and Libya.

Basic Couscous

Yield: 6 Servings

This recipe can be made quickly

Ⓥ This is a Vegetarian Recipe Ⓥ

Ingredients:

- 1 cup chicken or vegetable broth
- 1 cup water
- 2 cups couscous
- 2 tablespoons extra-virgin olive oil
- Salt and pepper

Directions:

1. Heat oil in moderate-sized saucepan on moderate to high heat until it starts to shimmer. Put in couscous and cook, stirring often, until grains are just starting to brown, 3 to 5 minutes.
2. Mix in water, broth, and 1 teaspoon salt. Cover, remove saucepan from heat, and allow to sit until couscous is tender, approximately seven minutes. Gently fluff couscous with fork and season with pepper to taste. Serve.

Basic Couscous with Carrots, Raisins, and Pine Nuts

This recipe can be made quickly

Ⓥ This is a Vegetarian Recipe Ⓥ

Increase oil to 3 tablespoons. Before adding couscous to saucepan, put in 2 peeled and grated carrots and ½ teaspoon ground cinnamon and cook till they become tender, approximately two minutes. Put in ½ cup raisins to saucepan with couscous and increase water to 1¼ cups. Before you serve, mix in ⅓ cup toasted pine nuts, 3 tablespoons minced fresh cilantro, ½ teaspoon grated orange zest, and 1 tablespoon orange juice.

Basic Couscous with Dates and Pistachios

This recipe can be made quickly

Ⓥ This is a Vegetarian Recipe Ⓥ

Increase oil to 3 tablespoons. Put in ½ cup chopped pitted dates, 1 tablespoon grated fresh ginger, and ½ teaspoon ground cardamom to saucepan with couscous. Increase water to 1¼ cups. Before you serve, mix in ¾ cup coarsely chopped toasted pistachios, 3 tablespoons minced fresh cilantro, and 2 teaspoons lemon juice.

Basic Pearl Couscous

Yield: 6 Servings

This recipe can be made quickly

Ⓥ *This is a Vegetarian Recipe* Ⓥ

Ingredients:

- ½ teaspoon salt
- 1 tablespoon extra-virgin olive oil
- 2 cups pearl couscous
- 2½ cups water

Directions:

1. Heat couscous and oil in moderate-sized saucepan on moderate heat, stirring often, until about half of grains start to look golden brown, approximately five minutes.
2. Mix in water and salt, increase heat to high, and bring to boil. Decrease heat to moderate to low, cover, and simmer, stirring intermittently, until water is absorbed and couscous is tender, 9 to 12 minutes. Remove from the heat, let couscous sit, covered, for about three minutes. Serve.

Basic Pearl Couscous Wholesome Mix

Yield: 6 Servings

Ⓥ *This is a Vegetarian Recipe* Ⓥ

Ingredients:

- ¼ teaspoon ground cardamom
- 1 (15-ounce) can great Northern beans, rinsed
- 1 onion, chopped
- 1 pound eggplant, cut into ½-inch pieces
- 1 tablespoon tomato paste
- 1 teaspoon ground fenugreek
- 1 teaspoon ground sumac
- 1½ cups pearl couscous

- 2 cups chicken or vegetable broth
- 3 garlic cloves, minced
- 3 ounces (3 cups) baby spinach
- 5 tablespoons extra-virgin olive oil, plus extra for serving
- Salt and pepper

Directions:

1. Mix sumac, fenugreek, ½ teaspoon salt, ½ teaspoon pepper, and cardamom in a small-sized container. Line large plate using double layer of coffee filters and spray using vegetable oil spray. Toss eggplant with ½ teaspoon spice mixture and spread uniformly coffee filters. Microwave eggplant, uncovered, until dry to touch and slightly shriveled, 7 to 10 minutes, tossing halfway through microwaving.
2. Heat couscous and 2 tablespoons oil in 12-inch non-stick frying pan on moderate heat, stirring often, until about half of grains start to look golden brown, approximately five minutes. Move to a container and wipe frying pan clean using paper towels.
3. Toss eggplant with 1 teaspoon spice mixture. Heat 1 tablespoon oil in now-empty frying pan on moderate to high heat until it starts to shimmer. Put in eggplant and cook, stirring intermittently, until well browned, 5 to 7 minutes. Move to different container.
4. Heat remaining 2 tablespoons oil in again-empty frying pan on moderate heat until it starts to shimmer. Put in onion and cook till they become tender and lightly browned, 5 to 7 minutes. Mix in garlic, tomato paste, and remaining spice mixture and cook until aromatic, about 1 minute.
5. Mix in broth, beans, and couscous and bring to simmer. Decrease heat to moderate to low, cover, and simmer, stirring intermittently, until broth is absorbed and couscous is tender, 9 to 12 minutes. Remove from the heat, mix in spinach and eggplant, cover, and allow to sit for about three minutes. Sprinkle with salt and pepper to taste and drizzle with extra oil. Serve.

Basic Pearl Couscous with Peas, Feta, and Pickled Shallots

Yield: 6 Servings

Ⓥ *This is a Vegetarian Recipe* Ⓥ

Ingredients:

- ⅛ teaspoon red pepper flakes
- ¼ cup extra-virgin olive oil
- ⅓ cup red wine vinegar
- ½ cup frozen peas, thawed
- ½ cup shelled pistachios, toasted and chopped
- 1 cup fresh mint leaves, torn
- 1 teaspoon Dijon mustard
- 2 cups pearl couscous
- 2 shallots, sliced thin
- 2 tablespoons sugar
- 2½ cups water
- 3 ounces feta cheese, crumbled (¾ cup)
- 3 tablespoons lemon juice
- 4 ounces (4 cups) baby arugula, coarsely chopped
- Salt and pepper

Directions:

1. Heat 1 tablespoon oil and couscous in moderate-sized saucepan on moderate heat, stirring often, until about half of grains start to look golden brown, approximately five minutes. Mix in water and ½ teaspoon salt, increase heat to high, and bring to boil. Decrease heat to moderate to low, cover, and simmer, stirring intermittently, until water is absorbed and couscous is tender, 9 to 12 minutes. Remove from the heat, let couscous sit, covered, for about three minutes. Move couscous to rimmed baking sheet and allow to cool completely, about fifteen minutes.

2. In the meantime, bring vinegar, sugar, and pinch salt to simmer in small saucepan on moderate to high heat, stirring intermittently, until sugar dissolves. Put in shallots and stir to combine. Remove from heat, cover, and allow to cool completely, approximately half an hour. Drain and discard liquid.
3. Beat remaining 3 tablespoons oil, lemon juice, mustard, pepper flakes, and ⅛ teaspoon salt together in a big container. Put in couscous, arugula, mint, peas, 6 tablespoons pistachios, ½ cup feta, and shallots and gently toss to combine. Sprinkle with salt and pepper to taste and move to serving bowl. Allow to sit for about five minutes. Sprinkle with remaining ¼ cup feta and remaining 2 tablespoons pistachios and serve.

Basic Pearl Couscous with Radishes and Watercress

Yield: 6 Servings

Ⓥ This is a Vegetarian Recipe Ⓥ

Ingredients:

- ¼ cup extra-virgin olive oil
- ¼ teaspoon sugar
- ½ cup walnuts, toasted and chopped coarse
- 1 teaspoon Dijon mustard
- 1 teaspoon smoked paprika
- 1½ cups coarsely chopped parsley
- 2 cups pearl couscous
- 2 ounces (2 cups) watercress, torn into bite-size pieces
- 2½ cups water
- 3 tablespoons sherry vinegar
- 4 ounces goat cheese, crumbled (1 cup)
- 6 radishes, trimmed and cut into matchsticks

- 6 scallions, sliced thin
- Salt and pepper

Directions:

1. Heat 1 tablespoon oil and couscous in moderate-sized saucepan on moderate heat, stirring often, until about half of grains start to look golden brown, approximately five minutes. Mix in water and ½ teaspoon salt, increase heat to high, and bring to boil. Decrease heat to moderate to low, cover, and simmer, stirring intermittently, until water is absorbed and couscous is tender, 9 to 12 minutes. Remove from the heat, let couscous sit, covered, for about three minutes. Move couscous to rimmed baking sheet and allow to cool completely, about fifteen minutes.
2. Beat vinegar, mustard, paprika, sugar, ⅛ teaspoon salt, and remaining 3 tablespoons oil together in a big container. Put in couscous, watercress, scallions, radishes, parsley, and 6 tablespoons walnuts and gently toss to combine. Sprinkle with salt and pepper to taste and move to serving bowl. Allow to sit for about five minutes. Sprinkle with goat cheese and remaining 2 tablespoons walnuts and serve.

Basic Pearl Couscous with Tomatoes, Olives, and Ricotta Salata

Yield: 6 Servings

(V) This is a Vegetarian Recipe (V)

Ingredients:

- ¼ cup extra-virgin olive oil
- ¼ cup minced fresh chives
- ½ cup pine nuts, toasted
- ⅔ cup pitted kalamata olives, sliced
- 1 teaspoon Dijon mustard

- 1½ cups coarsely chopped fresh basil
- 12 ounces grape tomatoes, quartered
- 2 cups pearl couscous
- 2 ounces (2 cups) baby spinach, sliced ¼ inch thick
- 2½ cups water
- 3 ounces ricotta salata cheese, crumbled (¾ cup)
- 3 tablespoons red wine vinegar
- Salt and pepper

Directions:

1. Heat 1 tablespoon oil and couscous in moderate-sized saucepan on moderate heat, stirring often, until about half of grains start to look golden brown, approximately five minutes. Mix in water and ½ teaspoon salt, increase heat to high, and bring to boil. Decrease heat to moderate to low, cover, and simmer, stirring intermittently, until water is absorbed and couscous is tender, 9 to 12 minutes. Remove from the heat, let couscous sit, covered, for about three minutes. Move couscous to rimmed baking sheet and allow to cool completely, about fifteen minutes.
2. Beat vinegar, mustard, ⅛ teaspoon salt, and remaining 3 tablespoons oil together in a big container. Put in couscous, tomatoes, spinach, basil, ½ cup ricotta salata, olives, 6 tablespoons pine nuts, and chives and gently toss to combine. Sprinkle with salt and pepper to taste and move to serving bowl. Allow to sit for about five minutes. Sprinkle with remaining ¼ cup ricotta salata and remaining 2 tablespoons pine nuts and serve.

Lemony Sujuk Couscous

Yield: 6 Servings

✄ This recipe can be made quickly ✄

Feel free to substitute Sujuk with any other dry-cured meat if you cannot find it.

Ingredients:

- ¼ cup chopped fresh cilantro
- ¼ preserved lemon, pulp and white pith removed, rind rinsed and minced (1 tablespoon)
- ¼ teaspoon ground cardamom
- ½ cup golden raisins
- 1 onion, chopped fine
- 1½ cups couscous
- 1¾ cups vegetable broth
- 2 carrots, peeled and chopped fine
- 3 garlic cloves, minced
- 3 tablespoons extra-virgin olive oil
- 4 ounces sujuk (Turkish dry-cured beef sausage) sausage, chopped fine
- Salt and pepper

Directions:

1. Heat 2 tablespoons oil in 12-inch frying pan on moderate to high heat until it starts to shimmer. Put in couscous and cook, stirring often, until grains are just starting to brown, 3 to 5 minutes. Move to a container and wipe frying pan clean using paper towels.
2. Heat residual 1 tablespoon oil in now-empty frying pan on moderate heat until it starts to shimmer. Put in sujuk, onion, carrots, ¼ teaspoon salt, and ¼ teaspoon pepper and cook until vegetables are softened and lightly browned, six to eight minutes. Mix in preserved lemon, garlic, and cardamom and cook until aromatic, approximately half a minute. Mix in broth and bring to simmer.
3. Mix in raisins and couscous. Cover, remove frying pan from heat, and allow to sit until couscous is tender, approximately seven minutes. Put in cilantro to couscous and gently fluff with fork to combine. Sprinkle with salt and pepper to taste. Serve.

Moroccan Chickpea Couscous

Yield: 6 Servings

⁄ This recipe can be made quickly ⁄

Ⓥ This is a Vegetarian Recipe Ⓥ

Ingredients:

- ¼ cup extra-virgin olive oil, plus extra for serving
- ¼ teaspoon ground anise seed
- ½ cup chopped fresh parsley, cilantro, and/or mint
- 1 (15-ounce) can chickpeas, rinsed
- 1 onion, chopped fine
- 1 teaspoon ground coriander
- 1 teaspoon ground ginger
- 1½ cups couscous
- 1½ cups frozen peas
- 1¾ cups chicken or vegetable broth
- 2 carrots, peeled and chopped fine
- 3 garlic cloves, minced
- Lemon wedges
- Salt and pepper

Directions:

1. Heat 2 tablespoons oil in 12-inch frying pan on moderate to high heat until it starts to shimmer. Put in couscous and cook, stirring often, until grains are just starting to brown, 3 to 5 minutes. Move to a container and wipe frying pan clean using paper towels.
2. Heat remaining 2 tablespoons oil in now-empty frying pan on moderate heat until it starts to shimmer. Put in carrots, onion, and 1 teaspoon salt and cook till they become tender and lightly browned, 5 to 7 minutes. Mix in garlic, coriander, ginger, and anise and cook until aromatic, approximately half a minute. Mix in broth and chickpeas and bring to simmer.

3. Mix in peas and couscous. Cover, remove frying pan from heat, and allow to sit until couscous is tender, approximately seven minutes. Put in parsley to couscous and gently fluff with fork to combine. Sprinkle with salt and pepper to taste and drizzle with extra oil. Serve with lemon wedges.

Spicy Vegge Couscous

Yield: 6 Servings

(V) This is a Vegetarian Recipe (V)

Ingredients:

- 1 head cauliflower (2 pounds), cored and cut into 1-inch florets
- 1 red bell pepper, stemmed, seeded, and cut into ½-inch pieces
- 1 tablespoon minced fresh marjoram
- 1 teaspoon grated lemon zest, plus lemon wedges for serving
- 1 zucchini, cut into ½-inch pieces
- 1½ cups couscous
- 1¾ cups chicken or vegetable broth
- 2 teaspoons ras el hanout
- 4 garlic cloves, minced
- 6 tablespoons extra-virgin olive oil, plus extra for serving
- Salt and pepper

Directions:

1. Toss cauliflower with 2 tablespoons oil, ¾ teaspoon salt, and ½ teaspoon pepper in 12-inch non-stick skillet. Cover and cook on moderate to high heat until florets start to brown and edges just start to become translucent (do not lift lid), approximately five minutes.
2. Remove lid and continue to cook, stirring every 2 minutes, until florets turn golden brown in several spots, about 10 minutes. Move to a container and wipe frying pan clean using paper towels.

3. Heat 2 tablespoons oil in now-empty frying pan on moderate to high heat until it starts to shimmer. Put in couscous and cook, stirring often, until grains are just starting to brown, 3 to 5 minutes. Move to different container and wipe frying pan clean using paper towels.
4. Heat remaining 2 tablespoons oil in again-empty frying pan on moderate to high heat until just smoking. Put in zucchini, bell pepper, and ½ teaspoon salt and cook until tender, six to eight minutes. Mix in garlic, ras el hanout, and lemon zest and cook until aromatic, approximately half a minute. Mix in broth and bring to simmer.
5. Mix in couscous. Cover, remove frying pan from heat, and allow to sit until couscous is tender, approximately seven minutes. Put in cauliflower and marjoram to couscous and gently fluff with fork to combine. Sprinkle with salt and pepper to taste and drizzle with extra oil. Serve with lemon wedges.

Tangy Lamb-Chickpea Couscous

Yield: 6 Servings

Ingredients:

- ⅛ teaspoon cayenne pepper
- ¼ teaspoon ground cinnamon
- ⅓ cup minced fresh parsley
- ½ cup dry white wine
- ½ cup raisins
- ½ cup sliced almonds, toasted
- 1 (15-ounce) can chickpeas, rinsed
- 1 onion, chopped fine
- 1 pound lamb shoulder chops (blade or round bone), 1 to 1½ inches thick, trimmed and halved
- 1 teaspoon grated fresh ginger
- 1 teaspoon ground coriander
- 10 (2-inch) strips orange zest (1 orange)

- 1½ cups couscous
- 2½ cups chicken broth
- 3 tablespoons extra-virgin olive oil, plus extra for serving
- Salt and pepper

Directions:

1. Place oven rack to lower-middle position and pre-heat your oven to 325 degrees. Heat 2 tablespoons oil in a Dutch oven on moderate to high heat until it starts to shimmer. Put in couscous and cook, stirring often, until grains are just starting to brown, 3 to 5 minutes. Move to a container and wipe pot clean using paper towels.
2. Pat lamb dry using paper towels and sprinkle with salt and pepper. Heat residual 1 tablespoon oil in now-empty pot on moderate to high heat until just smoking. Brown lamb, about 4 minutes each side; move to plate.
3. Put in onion to fat left in pot and cook on moderate heat till they become tender, approximately five minutes. Mix in orange zest, ginger, coriander, cinnamon, cayenne, and ⅛ teaspoon pepper and cook until aromatic, approximately half a minute. Mix in wine, scraping up any browned bits. Mix in broth and chickpeas and bring to boil.
4. Nestle lamb into pot along with any accumulated juices. Cover, place pot in oven, and cook until fork slips easily in and out of lamb, about 1 hour.
5. Move lamb to slicing board, allow to cool slightly, then shred into bite-size pieces using 2 forks, discarding excess fat and bones. Strain cooking liquid through fine mesh strainer set over bowl. Return solids and 1½ cups cooking liquid to now-empty pot and bring to simmer on moderate heat; discard remaining liquid.
6. Mix in couscous and raisins. Cover, remove pot from heat, and allow to sit until couscous is tender, approximately seven minutes. Put in shredded lamb, almonds, and parsley to couscous and gently fluff with fork to combine. Sprinkle with salt and pepper to taste and drizzle with extra oil. Serve.

Beans

Chickpea Mix 1

Yield: 4 to 6 Servings

This recipe can be made quickly

(V) *This is a Vegetarian Recipe* (V)

Ingredients:

- ⅛ teaspoon red pepper flakes
- ¼ cup extra-virgin olive oil
- 1 cup chicken or vegetable broth
- 1 onion, chopped fine
- 2 (15-ounce) cans chickpeas, rinsed
- 2 tablespoons minced fresh parsley
- 2 teaspoons lemon juice
- 4 garlic cloves, sliced thin
- Salt and pepper

Directions:

1. Cook 3 tablespoons oil, garlic, and pepper flakes in 12-inch frying pan on moderate heat, stirring often, until garlic turns golden but not brown, approximately three minutes. Mix in onion and ¼ teaspoon salt and cook till they become tender and lightly browned, 5 to 7 minutes. Mix in chickpeas and broth and bring to simmer. Decrease heat to moderate to low, cover, and cook until chickpeas are heated through and flavours blend, approximately seven minutes.
2. Uncover, increase heat to high, and carry on cooking until nearly all liquid has evaporated, approximately three minutes. Remove from the heat, mix in parsley and lemon juice. Sprinkle with salt and pepper to taste and drizzle with remaining 1 tablespoon oil. Serve.

Chickpea Mix 2

This recipe can be made quickly

Ⓥ *This is a Vegetarian Recipe* Ⓥ

Refer to Chickpea Mix 1. Put in 1 chopped red bell pepper to frying pan with onion. Substitute 2 tablespoons chopped fresh basil for parsley and mix in 2 thinly sliced scallions before you serve.

Chickpea Mix 3

This recipe can be made quickly

Ⓥ *This is a Vegetarian Recipe* Ⓥ

Refer to Chickpea Mix 1. Omit red pepper flakes. Put in ½ teaspoon smoked paprika to frying pan before chickpeas and cook until aromatic, approximately half a minute. Substitute 2 tablespoons minced fresh cilantro for parsley and 2 teaspoons sherry vinegar for lemon juice.

Chickpea Mix 4

This recipe can be made quickly

Ⓥ *This is a Vegetarian Recipe* Ⓥ

Refer to Chickpea Mix 1. Omit red pepper flakes. Put in ⅛ teaspoon crumbled saffron threads to frying pan before chickpeas and cook until aromatic, approximately half a minute. Put in ⅓ cup raisins to frying pan with chickpeas. Substitute 2 tablespoons minced fresh mint for parsley and mix in ¼ cup plain yogurt before you serve.

Chickpea Salad 1

Yield: 6 Servings

This recipe can be made quickly

Ⓥ *This is a Vegetarian Recipe* Ⓥ

Ingredients:

- ¼ cup extra-virgin olive oil
- ½ cup pitted kalamata olives, chopped coarse
- 1 cup baby arugula, chopped coarse
- 2 (15-ounce) cans chickpeas, rinsed
- 2 tablespoons lemon juice
- 3 carrots, peeled and shredded
- Pinch cayenne pepper
- Salt and pepper

Directions:

1. Microwave chickpeas in a moderate-sized container until hot, approximately two minutes. Mix in oil, lemon juice, ¾ teaspoon salt, ½ teaspoon pepper, and cayenne and allow to sit for 30 minutes.
2. Put in carrots, arugula, and olives and toss to combine. Sprinkle with salt and pepper to taste. Serve.

Chickpea Salad 2

This recipe can be made quickly

Ⓥ *This is a Vegetarian Recipe* Ⓥ

Refer to Chickpea Salad 1 and substitute 1 fennel bulb, stalks discarded, bulb halved, cored, and cut into ¼-inch pieces, for carrots and olives.

Chickpea Salad 3

This recipe can be made quickly

Ⓥ This is a Vegetarian Recipe Ⓥ

Refer to Chickpea Salad 1 and substitute ½ cup chopped jarred roasted red peppers, ½ cup crumbled feta cheese, and ¼ cup chopped fresh parsley for carrots, arugula, and olives.

Classis Levantine Mujaddara

Yield: 4 to 6 Servings

Ⓥ This is a Vegetarian Recipe Ⓥ

Ingredients:

YOGURT SAUCE

- ½ teaspoon minced garlic
- ½ teaspoon salt
- 1 cup plain whole-milk yogurt
- 2 tablespoons lemon juice

RICE AND LENTILS

- ⅛ teaspoon cayenne pepper
- ½ teaspoon ground allspice
- ½ teaspoon ground cinnamon
- 1 recipe Crispy Onions, plus 3 tablespoons reserved oil (see below)
- 1 teaspoon ground coriander
- 1 teaspoon ground cumin
- 1 teaspoon sugar
- 1¼ cups basmati rice
- 3 garlic cloves, minced
- 3 tablespoons minced fresh cilantro

- 8¾ ounces (1¼ cups) green or brown lentils, picked over and rinsed
- Salt and pepper

Directions:

1. **FOR THE YOGURT SAUCE:** Beat all ingredients together in a container put inside your fridge until ready to serve.
2. **FOR THE RICE AND LENTILS:** Bring lentils, 4 cups water, and 1 teaspoon salt to boil in moderate-sized saucepan on high heat. Decrease heat to low and cook until lentils are just tender, 15 to 17 minutes. Drain and set aside.
3. In the meantime, place rice in medium bowl, cover with hot tap water by 2 inches, and allow to sit for about fifteen minutes. Use your hands to lightly rinse the grains to eliminate the surplus starch. Cautiously drain water, leaving rice in a container. Repeat the process of pouring in and draining cold water 4 to 5 times, until water runs nearly transparent. Drain rice using a fine-mesh strainer.
4. Cook reserved onion oil, garlic, coriander, cumin, cinnamon, allspice, ¼ teaspoon pepper, and cayenne in a Dutch oven on moderate heat until aromatic, approximately two minutes. Put in rice and cook, stirring intermittently, until grain edges begin to turn translucent, approximately three minutes. Mix in 2¼ cups water, sugar, and 1 teaspoon salt and bring to boil. Mix in lentils, decrease the heat to low, cover, and simmer gently until all liquid is absorbed, about 12 minutes.
5. Remove from the heat, cover, laying clean dish towel underneath lid, and allow to sit for about ten minutes. Fluff rice and lentils with fork and mix in cilantro and half of onions. Move to serving platter and top with remaining onions. Serve with yogurt sauce.

CRISPY ONIONS

Yield: 1½ cups

Ⓥ This is a Vegetarian Recipe Ⓥ

Ingredients:

- 1½ cups vegetable oil
- 2 pounds onions, halved and sliced crosswise into ¼-inch-thick pieces
- 2 teaspoons salt

Directions:

1. Toss onions and salt together in a big container. Microwave for about five minutes. Wash comprehensively, move to paper towel–lined baking sheet, and dry well.
2. Heat onions and oil in a Dutch oven on high heat, stirring often, until onions start to look golden brown, about half an hour. Drain onions using a colander set in a big container. Move onions to paper towel–lined baking sheet to drain. Serve.

Eastern Mediterranean Falafel

Yield: Approximately 24

Ⓥ This is a Vegetarian Recipe Ⓥ

Ingredients:

- ⅛ teaspoon ground cinnamon
- ½ teaspoon ground cumin
- 1 cup fresh cilantro leaves
- 1 cup fresh parsley leaves
- 10 scallions, chopped coarse
- 12 ounces (2 cups) dried chickpeas, picked over and rinsed
- 2 cups vegetable oil
- 6 garlic cloves, minced
- Salt and pepper

Directions:

1. Dissolve 3 tablespoons salt in 4 quarts cold water in large container. Put in chickpeas and soak at room temperature for minimum 8 hours or for maximum 24 hours. Drain and wash thoroughly.
2. Process chickpeas, scallions, parsley, cilantro, garlic, 1 teaspoon salt, 1 teaspoon pepper, cumin, and cinnamon using a food processor until smooth, approximately one minute, scraping down sides of the container as required. Pinch off and shape chickpea mixture into 2-tablespoon-size disks, about 1½ inches wide and 1 inch thick, and place on parchment paper–lined baking sheet. (Falafel will keep safely in a fridge for maximum 2 hours.)
3. Place the oven rack in the centre of the oven and pre-heat your oven to 200 degrees. Set wire rack in rimmed baking sheet. Heat oil in 12-inch frying pan on moderate to high heat to 375 degrees. Fry half of falafel until deep golden brown, 2 to 3 minutes each side. Adjust burner, if needed, to maintain oil temperature of 375 degrees. Use a slotted spoon to move falafel to readied sheet and keep warm in oven. Return oil to 375 degrees and repeat with remaining falafel. Serve.

Pink Pickled Turnips

Yield: 4 cups

Ⓥ *This is a Vegetarian Recipe* Ⓥ

These go great with falafel!

Ingredients:

- ¾ teaspoon black peppercorns
- ¾ teaspoon whole allspice berries
- 1 pound turnips, peeled and cut into 2 by ½-inch sticks
- 1 small beet, trimmed, peeled, and cut into 1-inch pieces
- 1¼ cups water
- 1¼ cups white wine vinegar
- 1½ tablespoons canning and pickling salt

- 2½ tablespoons sugar
- 3 garlic cloves, smashed and peeled

Directions:

1. Bring vinegar, water, sugar, salt, garlic, allspice, and peppercorns to boil in moderate-sized saucepan. Cover, remove from heat, and allow to steep for about ten minutes. Strain brine through fine-mesh strainer, then return to saucepan.
2. Place two 1-pint jars in a container and place under hot running water until heated through, 1 to 2 minutes; shake dry. Pack turnips vertically into hot jars with beet pieces evenly distributed throughout.
3. Return brine to brief boil. Using funnel and ladle, pour hot brine over vegetables to cover. Let jars cool to room temperature, cover with lids, put inside your fridge for minimum 2 days before you serve. (Pickled turnips will keep safely in a fridge for maximum 1 month; turnips will soften over time.)

Egyptian Black-Eyed Pea Salad Mix

Yield: 4 to 6 Servings

✎ This recipe can be made quickly ✎

Ⓥ This is a Vegetarian Recipe Ⓥ

Ingredients:

- ½ cup minced fresh parsley
- ½ cup pomegranate seeds
- ½ cup walnuts, toasted and chopped
- 2 (15-ounce) cans black-eyed peas, rinsed
- 2 tablespoons lemon juice
- 2 tablespoons pomegranate molasses
- 3 tablespoons dukkah
- 3 tablespoons extra-virgin olive oil

- 4 scallions, sliced thin
- Salt and pepper

Directions:

1. Beat oil, 2 tablespoons dukkah, lemon juice, pomegranate molasses, ¼ teaspoon salt, and ⅛ teaspoon pepper together in a big container until smooth.
2. Put in peas, walnuts, pomegranate seeds, parsley, and scallions and toss to combine. Sprinkle with salt and pepper to taste. Sprinkle with remaining 1 tablespoon dukkah and serve.

Egyption Koshari

Yield: 4 to 6 Servings

Ⓥ This is a Vegetarian Recipe Ⓥ

Ingredients:

- ¼ teaspoon cayenne pepper
- ¼ teaspoon ground nutmeg
- ¾ teaspoon ground cinnamon
- 1 (15-ounce) can chickpeas, rinsed
- 1 (28-ounce) can tomato sauce
- 1 cup basmati rice
- 1 cup elbow macaroni
- 1 cup green or brown lentils, picked over and rinsed
- 1 recipe Crispy Onions, plus ¼ cup reserved oil
- 1 tablespoon red wine vinegar
- 1½ teaspoons ground coriander
- 1½ teaspoons ground cumin
- 3 tablespoons minced fresh parsley
- 4 garlic cloves, minced
- Salt and pepper

Directions:

1. Bring 2 quarts water to boil in a Dutch oven. Put in pasta and 1½ teaspoons salt and cook, stirring frequently, until al dente. Drain pasta, rinse with water, then drain again. Move to a container and set aside.
2. In the meantime, bring lentils, 4 cups water, and 1 teaspoon salt to boil in moderate-sized saucepan on high heat. Decrease heat to low and cook until lentils are just tender, 15 to 17 minutes. Drain and set aside.
3. Cook 1 tablespoon reserved onion oil, 1 teaspoon garlic, ½ teaspoon salt, ½ teaspoon coriander, ½ teaspoon cumin, ¼ teaspoon cinnamon, ⅛ teaspoon nutmeg, and ⅛ teaspoon cayenne in now-empty saucepan on moderate heat until aromatic, approximately one minute. Mix in tomato sauce and chickpeas, bring to simmer, and cook until slightly thickened, about 10 minutes. Cover and keep warm.
4. While sauce cooks, place rice in medium bowl, cover with hot tap water by 2 inches, and allow to sit for about fifteen minutes. Use your hands to lightly rinse the grains to eliminate the surplus starch. Cautiously drain water, leaving rice in a container. Repeat the process of pouring in and draining cold water 4 to 5 times, until water runs nearly transparent. Drain rice using a fine-mesh strainer.
5. Cook remaining 3 tablespoons reserved onion oil, remaining garlic, remaining 1 teaspoon coriander, remaining 1 teaspoon cumin, remaining ½ teaspoon cinnamon, remaining ⅛ teaspoon nutmeg, and remaining ⅛ teaspoon cayenne in now-empty pot on moderate heat until aromatic, approximately two minutes. Put in rice and cook, stirring intermittently, until grain edges begin to turn translucent, approximately three minutes. Mix in 2 cups water and ½ teaspoon salt and bring to boil. Mix in lentils, decrease the heat to low, cover, and simmer gently until all liquid is absorbed, about 12 minutes.
6. Remove from the heat, drizzle pasta over rice mixture. Cover, laying clean dish towel underneath lid, and allow to sit for about ten minutes.
7. Return sauce to simmer on moderate heat. Mix in vinegar and sprinkle with salt and pepper to taste. Fluff rice and lentils with

fork and mix in parsley and half of onions. Move to serving platter and top with half of sauce and remaining onions. Serve, passing remaining sauce separately.

Flavourful Winter Squash Lentil Salad

Yield: 6 Servings

Ⓥ This is a Vegetarian Recipe Ⓥ

Ingredients:

- ⅛ teaspoon ground cinnamon
- ¼ cup thinly sliceped red onion
- ¼ teaspoon ground cumin
- ¼ teaspoon ground ginger
- ½ cup fresh parsley leaves
- ½ teaspoon ground coriander
- 1 cup black lentils, picked over and rinsed
- 1 garlic clove, minced
- 1 pound butternut squash, peeled, seeded, and cut into ½-inch pieces (3 cups)
- 1 tablespoon raw pepitas, toasted
- 1 teaspoon Dijon mustard
- 2 tablespoons balsamic vinegar
- 5 tablespoons extra-virgin olive oil
- Salt and pepper

Directions:

1. Dissolve 1 teaspoon salt in 4 cups warm water (about 110 degrees) in a container. Put in lentils and soak at room temperature for about one hour. Drain well.
2. In the meantime, adjust oven racks to middle and lowest positions and pre-heat your oven to 450 degrees. Toss squash with 1 tablespoon oil, 1½ teaspoons vinegar, ¼ teaspoon salt, and ¼ teaspoon pepper. Arrange squash in one layer in rimmed

baking sheet and roast on lower rack until thoroughly browned and tender, 20 minutes to half an hour, stirring halfway through roasting. Allow it to cool slightly. Reduce oven temperature to 325 degrees.
3. Cook 1 tablespoon oil, garlic, coriander, cumin, ginger, and cinnamon in medium oven-safe saucepan on moderate heat until aromatic, approximately one minute. Mix in 4 cups water and lentils. Cover, move saucepan to upper rack in oven, and cook until lentils are soft but remain undamaged, forty minutes to one hour.
4. Drain lentils well. Beat remaining 3 tablespoons oil, remaining 1½ tablespoons vinegar, and mustard together in a big container. Put in squash, lentils, parsley, and onion and toss to combine. Sprinkle with salt and pepper to taste. Move to serving platter and drizzle with pepitas. Serve warm or at room temperature.

French Lentils with Carrots and Parsley

Yield: 4 to 6 Servings

(V) This is a Vegetarian Recipe (V)

Ingredients:

- 1 celery rib, chopped fine
- 1 cup lentilles du Puy, picked over and rinsed
- 1 onion, chopped fine
- 1 teaspoon minced fresh thyme or ¼ teaspoon dried
- 2 carrots, peeled and chopped fine
- 2 garlic cloves, minced
- 2 tablespoons extra-virgin olive oil
- 2 tablespoons minced fresh parsley
- 2 teaspoons lemon juice
- 2½ cups water
- Salt and pepper

Directions:

1. Mix carrots, onion, celery, 1 tablespoon oil, and ½ teaspoon salt in a big saucepan. Cover and cook over moderate to low heat, stirring intermittently, until vegetables are softened, eight to ten minutes. Mix in garlic and thyme and cook until aromatic, approximately half a minute.
2. Mix in water and lentils and bring to simmer. Decrease heat to low, cover, and simmer gently, stirring intermittently, until lentils are mostly tender, forty to fifty minutes.
3. Uncover and continue to cook, stirring intermittently, until lentils are completely tender, approximately eight minutes. Mix in remaining 1 tablespoon oil, parsley, and lemon juice. Sprinkle with salt and pepper to taste and serve.

French Lentils with Swiss Chard

Ⓥ This is a Vegetarian Recipe Ⓥ

Follow the recipe just above this one, except you will need to omit carrots, celery, and parsley. Separate stems and leaves from 12 ounces Swiss chard; thinly slice stems and chop leaves into ½-inch pieces. Put in chard stems to pot with onion and stir chard leaves into pot after uncovering in step 3.

Greek Chickpea Cakes

Yield: 6 Servings

This recipe can be made quickly

Ⓥ This is a Vegetarian Recipe Ⓥ

Ingredients:

- ⅛ teaspoon cayenne pepper

- ⅛ teaspoon salt
- ½ cup plain Greek yogurt
- 1 cup panko bread crumbs
- 1 recipe Cucumber-Yogurt Sauce
- 1 shallot, minced
- 1 teaspoon ground coriander
- 2 (15-ounce) cans chickpeas, rinsed
- 2 large eggs
- 2 scallions, sliced thin
- 3 tablespoons minced fresh cilantro
- 6 tablespoons extra-virgin olive oil

Directions:

1. Pulse chickpeas using a food processor until coarsely ground, approximately 8 pulses. Beat yogurt, eggs, 2 tablespoons oil, coriander, cayenne, and salt together in medium bowl. Gently mix in chickpeas, panko, scallions, cilantro, and shallot until just combined. Divide mixture into 6 equal portions and gently pack into 1-inch-thick patties.
2. Heat 2 tablespoons oil in 12-inch non-stick frying pan on moderate heat until it starts to shimmer. Cautiously lay 3 patties in frying pan and cook until thoroughly browned and firm, 4 to 5 minutes each side.
3. Move cakes to plate coated using paper towels and tent loosely with aluminium foil. Replicate the process with the rest of the 2 tablespoons oil and remaining 3 patties. Serve with yogurt sauce.

Greek Gigante Bean Mix

Yield: 6 to 8 Servings

Ⓥ *This is a Vegetarian Recipe* Ⓥ

Ingredients:

- ¼ cup minced fresh dill
- 2 (14.5-ounce) cans diced tomatoes, drained
- 2 onions, chopped fine
- 2 slices hearty white sandwich bread, torn into quarters
- 20 ounces curly-leaf spinach, stemmed
- 3 garlic cloves, minced
- 6 ounces feta cheese, crumbled (1½ cups)
- 6 tablespoons extra-virgin olive oil
- 8 ounces (1½ cups) dried gigante beans, picked over and rinsed
- Lemon wedges
- Salt and pepper

Directions:

1. Dissolve 3 tablespoons salt in 4 quarts cold water in large container. Put in beans and soak at room temperature for minimum 8 hours or for maximum 24 hours. Drain and wash thoroughly.
2. Bring beans and 2 quarts water to boil in a Dutch oven. Decrease the heat to a simmer and cook, stirring intermittently, until beans are tender, 1 to 1½ hours. Drain beans and set aside.
3. Wipe Dutch oven clean using paper towels. Heat 2 tablespoons oil in now-empty pot on moderate heat until it starts to shimmer. Put in onions and ½ teaspoon salt and cook till they become tender, approximately five minutes. Mix in garlic and cook until aromatic, approximately half a minute. Mix in half of spinach, cover, and cook until starting to wilt, approximately two minutes. Mix in remaining spinach, cover, and cook until wilted, approximately two minutes. Remove from the heat, gently mix in beans, tomatoes, dill, and 2 tablespoons oil. Sprinkle with salt and pepper to taste.
4. In the meantime, adjust oven rack to middle position and preheat your oven to 400 degrees. Pulse bread and remaining 2 tablespoons oil using a food processor to coarse crumbs, about 5 pulses. Move bean mixture to 13 by 9-inch baking dish and drizzle with feta, then bread crumbs. Bake until bread crumbs

start to look golden brown and edges are bubbling, approximately twenty minutes. Serve with lemon wedges.

Greek Stewed

Yield: 6 Servings

Ⓥ *This is a Vegetarian Recipe* Ⓥ

Ingredients:

- ¼ cup extra-virgin olive oil
- 1 (28-ounce) can whole peeled tomatoes, drained with juice reserved, chopped coarse
- 1 green bell pepper, stemmed, seeded, and chopped fine
- 1 pound eggplant, cut into 1-inch pieces
- 1 tablespoon minced fresh oregano or 1 teaspoon dried
- 2 (15-ounce) cans chickpeas, drained with 1 cup liquid reserved
- 2 bay leaves
- 2 onions, chopped
- 3 garlic cloves, minced
- Salt and pepper

Directions:

1. Place oven rack to lower-middle position and pre-heat your oven to 400 degrees. Heat oil in a Dutch oven on moderate heat until it starts to shimmer. Put in onions, bell pepper, ½ teaspoon salt, and ¼ teaspoon pepper and cook till they become tender, approximately five minutes. Mix in garlic, 1 teaspoon oregano, and bay leaves and cook until aromatic, approximately half a minute.
2. Mix in eggplant, tomatoes and reserved juice, and chickpeas and reserved liquid and bring to boil. Move pot to oven and cook, uncovered, until eggplant is very tender, forty minutes to one hour, stirring twice during cooking.

3. Discard bay leaves. Mix in remaining 2 teaspoons oregano and sprinkle with salt and pepper to taste. Serve.

Italian Sweet and Sour Cranberry Bean Sauce

Yield: 6 to 8 Servings

Ⓥ *This is a Vegetarian Recipe* Ⓥ

Ingredients:

- ½ cup pine nuts, toasted
- ½ cup sugar
- ½ fennel bulb, 2 tablespoons fronds chopped, stalks discarded, bulb cored and chopped
- 1 cup plus 2 tablespoons red wine vinegar
- 1 pound (2½ cups) dried cranberry beans, picked over and rinsed
- 1 teaspoon fennel seeds
- 3 tablespoons extra-virgin olive oil
- 6 ounces seedless red grapes, halved (1 cup)
- Salt and pepper

Directions:

1. Dissolve 3 tablespoons salt in 4 quarts cold water in large container. Put in beans and soak at room temperature for minimum 8 hours or for maximum 24 hours. Drain and wash thoroughly.
2. Bring beans, 4 quarts water, and 1 teaspoon salt to boil in a Dutch oven. Decrease the heat to a simmer and cook, stirring intermittently, until beans are tender, 1 to 1½ hours. Drain beans and set aside.
3. Wipe Dutch oven clean using paper towels. Heat oil in now-empty pot on moderate heat until it starts to shimmer. Put in

fennel, ¼ teaspoon salt, and ¼ teaspoon pepper and cook till they become tender, approximately five minutes. Mix in 1 cup vinegar, sugar, and fennel seeds until sugar is dissolved. Bring to simmer and cook until liquid becomes thick to syrupy glaze and edges of fennel are starting to brown, about 10 minutes.
4. Put in beans to vinegar-fennel mixture and toss to coat. Move to big container and allow to cool to room temperature. Put in grapes, pine nuts, fennel fronds, and remaining 2 tablespoons vinegar and toss to combine. Sprinkle with salt and pepper to taste and serve.

Lentil Salad Mix 1

Yield: 4 to 6 Servings

Ⓥ This is a Vegetarian Recipe Ⓥ

Ingredients:

- ½ cup chopped fresh mint
- ½ cup pitted kalamata olives, chopped coarse
- 1 bay leaf
- 1 cup lentilles du Puy, picked over and rinsed
- 1 large shallot, minced
- 1 ounce feta cheese, crumbled (¼ cup)
- 3 tablespoons white wine vinegar
- 5 garlic cloves, lightly crushed and peeled
- 5 tablespoons extra-virgin olive oil
- Salt and pepper

Directions:

1. Dissolve 1 teaspoon salt in 4 cups warm water (about 110 degrees) in a container. Put in lentils and soak at room temperature for about one hour. Drain well.
2. Place the oven rack in the centre of the oven and pre-heat your oven to 325 degrees. Mix lentils, 4 cups water, garlic, bay leaf,

and ½ teaspoon salt in medium oven-safe saucepan. Cover, move saucepan to oven, and cook until lentils are soft but remain undamaged, forty minutes to one hour.
3. Drain lentils well, discarding garlic and bay leaf. In big container, beat oil and vinegar together. Put in lentils, olives, mint, and shallot and toss to combine. Sprinkle with salt and pepper to taste. Move to serving dish and drizzle with feta. Serve warm or at room temperature.

Lentil Salad Mix 2

Ⓥ This is a Vegetarian Recipe Ⓥ

Refer to Lentil Salad Mix 1. Substitute 3 tablespoons red wine vinegar for white wine vinegar and put in 2 teaspoons Dijon mustard to dressing. Omit olives and substitute ¼ cup chopped fresh parsley for mint. Substitute ¼ cup crumbled goat cheese for feta and drizzle salad with ¼ cup coarsely chopped toasted hazelnuts before you serve.

Lentil Salad Mix 3

Ⓥ This is a Vegetarian Recipe Ⓥ

Refer to Lentil Salad Mix 1. Omit shallot and feta. Toss 2 carrots, peeled and cut into 2-inch-long matchsticks, with 1 teaspoon ground cumin, ½ teaspoon ground cinnamon, and ⅛ teaspoon cayenne pepper in a container; cover and microwave until carrots are soft but still crisp, 2 to 4 minutes. Substitute 3 tablespoons lemon juice for white wine vinegar, carrots for olives, and ¼ cup chopped fresh cilantro for mint.

Lentil Salad Mix 4

Ⓥ This is a Vegetarian Recipe Ⓥ

Refer to Lentil Salad Mix 1. Substitute 3 tablespoons sherry vinegar for white wine vinegar. Place 4 cups baby spinach and 2 tablespoons water in a container. Cover and microwave until spinach is wilted and volume is halved, about 4 minutes. Remove bowl from microwave and keep covered for about sixty seconds. Move spinach to colander and gently press to release liquid. Move spinach to slicing board and chop coarse. Return to colander and press again. Substitute chopped spinach for olives and mint and ¼ cup coarsely grated Parmesan cheese for feta. Sprinkle salad with ¼ cup coarsely chopped toasted walnuts before you serve.

Lentils with Spinach and Garlic Chips

Yield: 6 Servings

(V) This is a Vegetarian Recipe (V)

Ingredients:

- 1 cup green or brown lentils, picked over and rinsed
- 1 onion, chopped fine
- 1 tablespoon red wine vinegar
- 1 teaspoon ground coriander
- 1 teaspoon ground cumin
- 2 tablespoons extra-virgin olive oil
- 2½ cups water
- 4 garlic cloves, sliced thin
- 8 ounces curly-leaf spinach, stemmed and chopped coarse
- Salt and pepper

Directions:

1. Cook oil and garlic in a big saucepan over moderate to low heat, stirring frequently, until garlic turns crisp and golden but not brown, approximately five minutes. Use a slotted spoon to move garlic to plate coated using paper towels and season lightly with salt; set aside.

2. Put in onion and ½ teaspoon salt to oil left in saucepan and cook on moderate heat till they become tender and lightly browned, 5 to 7 minutes. Mix in coriander and cumin and cook until aromatic, approximately half a minute.
3. Mix in water and lentils and bring to simmer. Decrease heat to low, cover, and simmer gently, stirring intermittently, until lentils are mostly soft but still undamaged, 45 to 55 minutes.
4. Mix in spinach, 1 handful at a time. Cook, uncovered, stirring intermittently, until spinach is wilted and lentils are completely tender, approximately eight minutes. Mix in vinegar and sprinkle with salt and pepper to taste. Move to serving dish, drizzle with toasted garlic, and serve.

Moroccan Loubia

Yield: 6 to 8 Servings

Ingredients:

- ¼ teaspoon cayenne pepper
- ½ cup dry white wine
- 1 (12- to 16-ounce) lamb shank
- 1 onion, chopped
- 1 pound (2½ cups) dried great Northern beans, picked over and rinsed
- 1 red bell pepper, stemmed, seeded, and chopped fine
- 1 tablespoon extra-virgin olive oil, plus extra for serving
- 1½ teaspoons ground ginger
- 2 tablespoons minced fresh parsley
- 2 tablespoons tomato paste
- 2 teaspoons ground cumin
- 2 teaspoons paprika
- 3 garlic cloves, minced
- 4 cups chicken broth

- Salt and pepper

Directions:

1. Dissolve 3 tablespoons salt in 4 quarts cold water in large container. Put in beans and soak at room temperature for minimum 8 hours or for maximum 24 hours. Drain and wash thoroughly.
2. Place oven rack to lower-middle position and pre-heat your oven to 350 degrees. Pat lamb dry using paper towels and sprinkle with salt and pepper. Heat oil in a Dutch oven on moderate to high heat until just smoking. Brown lamb on all sides, 10 to fifteen minutes; move to plate. Pour off all but 2 tablespoons fat from pot.
3. Put in onion and bell pepper to fat left in pot and cook on moderate heat till they become tender and lightly browned, 5 to 7 minutes. Mix in tomato paste, garlic, paprika, cumin, ginger, cayenne, and ⅛ teaspoon pepper and cook until aromatic, approximately half a minute. Mix in wine, scraping up any browned bits. Mix in broth, 1 cup water, and beans and bring to boil.
4. Nestle lamb into beans along with any accumulated juices. Cover, move pot to oven, and cook until fork slips easily in and out of lamb and beans are tender, 1½ to 1¾ hours, stirring every 30 minutes.
5. Move lamb to slicing board, allow to cool slightly, then shred into bite-size pieces using 2 forks; discard excess fat and bone. Stir shredded lamb and parsley into beans and sprinkle with salt and pepper to taste. Adjust consistency with extra hot water as required. Serve, drizzling individual portions with extra oil.

North African Veggie Bean Stew

Yield: 6 to 8 Servings

Ⓥ *This is a Vegetarian Recipe* Ⓥ

Ingredients:

- ¼ teaspoon ground cinnamon
- ⅓ cup minced fresh parsley
- ½ cup small pasta, such as ditalini, tubettini, or elbow macaroni
- ½ teaspoon ground coriander
- ½ teaspoon paprika
- 1 (15-ounce) can butter beans, rinsed
- 1 (15-ounce) can chickpeas, rinsed
- 1 onion, chopped fine
- 1 tablespoon extra-virgin olive oil
- 1 teaspoon ground cumin
- 2 carrots, peeled and cut into ½-inch pieces
- 2 tablespoons all-purpose flour
- 2 tablespoons tomato paste
- 4 garlic cloves, minced
- 6 tablespoons harissa
- 7 cups vegetable broth
- 8 ounces Swiss chard, stems chopped fine, leaves cut into ½-inch pieces
- Salt and pepper

Directions:

1. Heat oil in a Dutch oven on moderate heat until it starts to shimmer. Put in onion and chard stems and cook till they become tender, approximately five minutes. Mix in garlic, cumin, paprika, coriander, and cinnamon and cook until aromatic, approximately half a minute. Mix in tomato paste and flour and cook for about sixty seconds.
2. Slowly mix in broth and carrots, scraping up any browned bits and smoothing out any lumps, and bring to boil. Reduce to mild simmer and cook for about ten minutes. Mix in chard leaves, chickpeas, beans, and pasta and simmer until vegetables and pasta are tender, 10 to fifteen minutes. Mix in parsley and ¼ cup harissa. Sprinkle with salt and pepper to taste. Serve, passing remaining harissa separately.

Sicilian White Beans with Escarole

Yield: 4 Servings

This recipe can be made quickly

Ⓥ *This is a Vegetarian Recipe* Ⓥ

Ingredients:

- ⅛ teaspoon red pepper flakes
- 1 (15-ounce) can cannellini beans, rinsed
- 1 cup chicken or vegetable broth
- 1 cup water
- 1 head escarole (1 pound), trimmed and sliced 1 inch thick
- 1 tablespoon extra-virgin olive oil, plus extra for serving
- 2 onions, chopped fine
- 2 teaspoons lemon juice
- 4 garlic cloves, minced
- Salt and pepper

Directions:

1. Heat oil in a Dutch oven on moderate heat until it starts to shimmer. Put in onions and ½ teaspoon salt and cook till they become tender and lightly browned, 5 to 7 minutes. Mix in garlic and pepper flakes and cook until aromatic, approximately half a minute.
2. Mix in escarole, beans, broth, and water and bring to simmer. Cook, stirring intermittently, until escarole is wilted, approximately five minutes. Increase heat to high and cook until liquid is nearly evaporated, 10 to fifteen minutes. Mix in lemon juice and sprinkle with salt and pepper to taste. Sprinkle with extra oil and serve.

Spanish Espinacas

Yield: 4 to 6 Servings

✎This recipe can be made quickly✎

Ingredients:

- 1 recipe Picada
- 1 tablespoon sherry vinegar
- 1 tablespoon smoked paprika
- 1 teaspoon ground cumin
- 2 (15-ounce) cans chickpeas
- 2 teaspoons extra-virgin olive oil
- 3 ounces Spanish-style chorizo sausage, chopped fine
- 5 garlic cloves, sliced thin
- 8 ounces curly-leaf spinach, stemmed
- Pinch saffron threads, crumbled
- Salt and pepper

Directions:

1. Mix 2 tablespoons boiling water and saffron in a small-sized container and allow to steep for about five minutes.
2. Heat 1 teaspoon oil in a Dutch oven on moderate heat until it starts to shimmer. Put in spinach and 2 tablespoons water, cover, and cook, stirring intermittently, until spinach is wilted but still bright green, approximately one minute. Move spinach to colander and gently press to release liquid. Move spinach to slicing board and chop coarse. Return to colander and press again.
3. Heat remaining 1 teaspoon oil in now-empty pot on moderate heat until it starts to shimmer. Put in chorizo and cook until lightly browned, approximately five minutes. Mix in garlic, paprika, cumin, and ¼ teaspoon pepper and cook until aromatic, approximately half a minute. Mix in chickpeas and their liquid, 1 cup water, and saffron mixture and bring to

simmer. Cook, stirring intermittently, until chickpeas are soft and liquid has thickened slightly, 10 to fifteen minutes.
4. Remove from the heat, mix in picada, spinach, and vinegar and allow to sit until heated through, approximately two minutes. Adjust sauce consistency with hot water as required. Sprinkle with salt and pepper to taste and serve.

Spiced Cranberry Beans

Yield: 6 to 8 Servings

Ⓥ This is a Vegetarian Recipe Ⓥ

Ingredients:

- ¼ cup extra-virgin olive oil
- ½ cup dry white wine
- ½ teaspoon ground cinnamon
- 1 onion, chopped fine
- 1 pound (2½ cups) dried cranberry beans, picked over and rinsed
- 1 tablespoon tomato paste
- 2 carrots, peeled and chopped fine
- 2 tablespoons lemon juice, plus extra for seasoning
- 2 tablespoons minced fresh mint
- 4 cups chicken or vegetable broth
- 4 garlic cloves, sliced thin
- Salt and pepper

Directions:

1. Dissolve 3 tablespoons salt in 4 quarts cold water in large container. Put in beans and soak at room temperature for minimum 8 hours or for maximum 24 hours. Drain and wash thoroughly.
2. Place oven rack to lower-middle position and pre-heat your oven to 350 degrees. Heat oil in a Dutch oven on moderate heat

until it starts to shimmer. Put in onion and carrots and cook till they become tender, approximately five minutes. Mix in garlic, tomato paste, cinnamon, and ¼ teaspoon pepper and cook until aromatic, approximately one minute. Mix in wine, scraping up any browned bits. Mix in broth, ½ cup water, and beans and bring to boil. Cover, move pot to oven, and cook until beans are tender, about 1½ hours, stirring every 30 minutes.
3. Mix in lemon juice and mint. Sprinkle with salt, pepper, and extra lemon juice to taste. Adjust consistency with extra hot water as required. Serve.

Squashed Fava Beans Basic Mix

Yield: 4 to 6 Servings

✍ This recipe can be made quickly ✍

Ⓥ This is a Vegetarian Recipe Ⓥ

Ingredients:

- 1 small onion, chopped fine
- 1 tablespoon extra-virgin olive oil, plus extra for serving
- 1 teaspoon ground cumin
- 1 tomato, cored and cut into ½-inch pieces
- 2 (15-ounce) cans fava beans
- 2 hard-cooked large eggs, chopped (optional)
- 2 tablespoons lemon juice, plus lemon wedges for serving
- 2 tablespoons minced fresh parsley
- 3 tablespoons tahini
- 4 garlic cloves, minced
- Salt and pepper

Directions:

1. Cook garlic, oil, and cumin in moderate-sized saucepan on moderate heat until aromatic, approximately two minutes. Mix

in beans and their liquid and tahini. Bring to simmer and cook until liquid thickens slightly, eight to ten minutes.
2. Remove from the heat, mash beans to coarse consistency using potato masher. Mix in lemon juice and 1 teaspoon pepper. Sprinkle with salt and pepper to taste. Move to serving dish, top with tomato, onion, parsley, and eggs, if using, and drizzle with extra oil. Serve with lemon wedges.

Squashed Fava Beans Mix 2

This recipe can be made quickly

(V) This is a Vegetarian Recipe (V)

Refer to the Recipe "Squashed Fava Beans basic mix". Omit onion and egg. Sprinkle ½ cucumber, peeled, halved along the length, seeded, and cut into ½-inch pieces, ¼ cup pitted kalamata olives, halved, and ¼ cup crumbled feta cheese over beans along with tomatoes and parsley.

Squashed Fava Beans Mix 3

This recipe can be made quickly

(V) This is a Vegetarian Recipe (V)

Refer to the Recipe "Squashed Fava Beans basic mix". Omit parsley and egg. Put in 1 thinly sliced jalapeño chile and ¼ teaspoon cayenne pepper to saucepan with garlic. Substitute 3 chopped scallions for onion. Mix ⅓ cup plain yogurt with additional 1 tablespoon lemon juice and drizzle over beans before you serve.

Squashed Fava Beans with Sautéed Escarole and Parmesan

Yield: 4 Servings

Ⓥ *This is a Vegetarian Recipe* Ⓥ

Ingredients:

- ¼ teaspoon red pepper flakes
- 1 head escarole (1 pound), cored and cut into 1-inch pieces
- 1 ounce Parmesan cheese, shaved
- 1 tablespoon grated lemon zest
- 1 Yukon Gold potato, peeled and cut into 1-inch pieces
- 2½ cups chicken or vegetable broth
- 2½ cups water, plus extra as required
- 3 garlic cloves, minced
- 3 tablespoons extra-virgin olive oil, plus extra for serving
- 8 ounces (1½ cups) dried split fava beans
- Salt and pepper

Directions:

1. Bring broth, water, and beans to boil in a big saucepan. Decrease the heat to a simmer and cook until beans are softened and starting to break down, about fifteen minutes. Mix in potato, return to simmer, and cook until potato becomes soft and almost all liquid is absorbed, about half an hour. Process bean-potato mixture through food mill or ricer into medium bowl. Mix in 2 tablespoons oil and sprinkle with salt and pepper to taste. Adjust consistency with extra hot water as required. (Mixture should be consistency of thin mashed potatoes.) Cover to keep warm.
2. In the meantime, heat residual 1 tablespoon oil in 12-inch frying pan on moderate heat until it starts to shimmer. Put in garlic, pepper flakes, and ¼ teaspoon salt and cook until aromatic, approximately half a minute. Mix in escarole, cover, and cook

until wilted, 3 to 5 minutes. Mix in lemon zest and sprinkle with salt and pepper to taste.
3. Lay out fava bean mixture into even layer on serving platter and arrange escarole on top. Sprinkle with Parmesan and drizzle with extra oil. Serve.

Tunisian Chickpea Spice

Yield: 4 to 6 Servings

Ⓥ This is a Vegetarian Recipe Ⓥ

Ingredients:

- ¼ cup chopped fresh parsley
- ¼ cup tomato paste
- ¼ teaspoon cayenne pepper
- ¾ cup water, plus extra as required
- ¾ teaspoon ground cumin
- 1 jalapeño chile, stemmed, seeded, and minced
- 12 ounces turnips, peeled and cut into ½-inch pieces
- 2 (15-ounce) cans chickpeas
- 2 onions, chopped
- 2 red bell peppers, stemmed, seeded, and chopped
- 2 tablespoons extra-virgin olive oil
- 2 tablespoons lemon juice, plus extra for seasoning
- 5 garlic cloves, minced
- Salt and pepper

Directions:

1. Heat oil in a Dutch oven on moderate heat until it starts to shimmer. Put in onions, bell peppers, ½ teaspoon salt, and ¼ teaspoon pepper and cook till they become tender and lightly browned, 5 to 7 minutes. Mix in tomato paste, jalapeño, garlic, cumin, and cayenne and cook until aromatic, approximately half a minute.

2. Mix in chickpeas and their liquid, turnips, and water. Bring to simmer and cook until turnips are soft and sauce has thickened, 25 to 35 minutes.
3. Mix in parsley and lemon juice. Sprinkle with salt, pepper, and extra lemon juice to taste. Adjust consistency with extra hot water as required. Serve.

Turkish Fasulye piyazi Salad

Yield: 4 to 6 Servings

This recipe can be made quickly

Ⓥ *This is a Vegetarian Recipe* Ⓥ

Ingredients:

- ¼ cup extra-virgin olive oil
- ¼ cup tahini
- ¼ red onion, sliced thin
- ½ cup fresh parsley leaves
- 1 tablespoon ground dried Aleppo pepper, plus extra for serving
- 1 tablespoon toasted sesame seeds
- 2 (15-ounce) cans pinto beans, rinsed
- 2 hard-cooked large eggs, quartered
- 3 garlic cloves, lightly crushed and peeled
- 3 tablespoons lemon juice
- 8 ounces cherry tomatoes, halved
- Salt and pepper

Directions:

1. Cook 1 tablespoon oil and garlic in moderate-sized saucepan on moderate heat, stirring frequently, until garlic turns golden but not brown, approximately three minutes. Put in beans, 2 cups water, and 1 teaspoon salt and bring to simmer. Turn off the heat, cover, and allow to sit for 20 minutes.

2. Drain beans and discard garlic. Beat remaining 3 tablespoons oil, tahini, lemon juice, Aleppo, 1 tablespoon water, and ¼ teaspoon salt together in a big container. Put in beans, tomatoes, onion, and parsley and gently toss to combine. Sprinkle with salt and pepper to taste. Move to serving platter and arrange eggs on top. Sprinkle with sesame seeds and extra Aleppo and serve.

EASY-PEEL HARD-COOKED EGGS

Yield: 6 eggs

Ⓥ This is a Vegetarian Recipe Ⓥ

Ingredients:

- 6 large eggs

Directions:

1. Bring 1 inch water to rolling boil in moderate-sized saucepan on high heat. Place eggs in steamer basket. Move basket to saucepan. Cover, decrease the heat to moderate to low, and cook eggs for 13 minutes.
2. When eggs are almost finished cooking, combine 2 cups ice cubes and 2 cups cold water in medium bowl. Using tongs or spoon, move eggs to ice bath; allow to sit for about fifteen minutes. Peel before using.

White Bean Salad Basic

Yield: 6 to 8 Servings

Ⓥ This is a Vegetarian Recipe Ⓥ

Ingredients:

- ¼ cup chopped fresh parsley

- ¼ cup extra-virgin olive oil
- 1 red bell pepper, stemmed, seeded, and cut into ¼-inch pieces
- 1 small shallot, minced
- 2 (15-ounce) cans cannellini beans, rinsed
- 2 teaspoons chopped fresh chives
- 2 teaspoons sherry vinegar
- 3 garlic cloves, peeled and smashed
- Salt and pepper

Directions:

1. Cook 1 tablespoon oil and garlic in moderate-sized saucepan on moderate heat, stirring frequently, until garlic turns golden but not brown, approximately three minutes. Put in beans, 2 cups water, and 1 teaspoon salt and bring to simmer. Turn off the heat, cover, and allow to sit for 20 minutes.
2. In the meantime, combine vinegar and shallot in a big container and allow to sit for 20 minutes. Drain beans and remove garlic. Put in beans, remaining 3 tablespoons oil, bell pepper, parsley, and chives to shallot mixture and gently toss to combine. Sprinkle with salt and pepper to taste. Allow to sit for 20 minutes. Serve.

White Bean Salad Mix 1

Ⓥ This is a Vegetarian Recipe Ⓥ

Refer to the recipe "White Bean Salad Basic". Substitute 1 cup quartered cherry tomatoes for bell pepper and ½ cup chopped fresh basil for parsley and chives. Put in ⅓ cup chopped kalamata olives to salad before tossing to combine.

White Bean Salad Squid-Pepperoncini Mix

Yield: 4 to 6 Servings

Ingredients:

- ⅓ cup pepperoncini, stemmed and sliced into ¼-inch-thick rings, plus 2 tablespoons brine
- ½ cup fresh parsley leaves
- 1 pound squid, bodies sliced crosswise into ½-inch-thick rings, tentacles halved
- 1 red onion, chopped fine
- 1 tablespoon baking soda
- 2 (15-ounce) cans cannellini beans, rinsed
- 2 tablespoons sherry vinegar
- 3 garlic cloves, minced
- 3 scallions, green parts only, sliced thin
- 6 tablespoons extra-virgin olive oil
- Salt and pepper

Directions:

1. Dissolve baking soda and 1 tablespoon salt in 3 cups cold water in medium container. Put in squid, cover, put inside your fridge for about fifteen minutes. Dry squid thoroughly using paper towels and toss with 1 tablespoon oil.
2. Heat 1 tablespoon oil in moderate-sized saucepan on moderate heat until it starts to shimmer. Put in onion and ¼ teaspoon salt and cook, stirring intermittently, till they become tender and lightly browned, 5 to 7 minutes. Mix in garlic and cook until aromatic, approximately half a minute. Mix in beans and ¼ cup water and bring to simmer. Decrease heat to low, cover, and continue to simmer, stirring intermittently, for 2 to 3 minutes; set aside.
3. Heat 1 tablespoon oil in 12-inch non-stick frying pan on high heat until just smoking. Put in half of squid in one layer and

cook, without moving, until well browned, approximately three minutes. Flip squid and continue to cook, without moving, until thoroughly browned on second side, approximately two minutes; move to a container. Wipe frying pan clean using paper towels and repeat with 1 tablespoon oil and remaining squid.
4. Beat remaining 2 tablespoons oil, pepperoncini brine, and vinegar together in a big container. Put in beans and any remaining cooking liquid, squid, parsley, scallions, and pepperoncini and toss to combine. Sprinkle with salt and pepper to taste. Serve.

Wholesome Tuscan Bean Stew

Yield: 8 Servings

Ingredients:

- 1 (14.5-ounce) can diced tomatoes, drained
- 1 large onion, chopped
- 1 pound (2½ cups) dried cannellini beans, picked over and rinsed
- 1 pound kale or collard greens, stemmed and chopped
- 1 sprig fresh rosemary
- 1 tablespoon extra-virgin olive oil, plus extra for serving
- 2 bay leaves
- 2 carrots, peeled and cut into ½-inch pieces
- 2 celery ribs, cut into ½-inch pieces
- 3 cups water
- 4 cups chicken broth
- 6 ounces pancetta, cut into ¼-inch pieces
- 8 garlic cloves, peeled and smashed
- Salt and pepper

Directions:

1. Dissolve 3 tablespoons salt in 4 quarts cold water in large container. Put in beans and soak at room temperature for minimum 8 hours or for maximum 24 hours. Drain and wash thoroughly.
2. Place oven rack to lower-middle position and pre-heat your oven to 250 degrees. Heat oil and pancetta in a Dutch oven on moderate heat. Cook, stirring intermittently, until pancetta is lightly browned and fat has rendered, 6 to 10 minutes. Put in onion, carrots, and celery and cook, stirring intermittently, till they become tender and lightly browned, 10 to 16 minutes. Mix in garlic and cook until aromatic, approximately one minute. Mix in broth, water, bay leaves, and beans and bring to boil. Cover, move pot to oven, and cook until beans are almost soft (very center of beans will still be firm), forty to sixty minutes.
3. Mix in kale and tomatoes, cover, and cook until beans and greens are fully tender, 30 to 40 minutes.
4. Remove pot from oven and submerge rosemary sprig in stew. Cover and allow to sit for about fifteen minutes. Discard bay leaves and rosemary sprig and season stew with salt and pepper to taste. If desired, use back of spoon to press some beans against side of pot to thicken stew. Serve, drizzling individual portions with extra oil.

Vegetable Recipes

The recipes in this section will form the basis of your Mediterranean diet, and will make up the bulk of your main courses every week.

Braised Asparagus Mix

Yield: 4 to 6 Servings

This recipe can be made quickly

(V) This is a Vegetarian Recipe (V)

Ingredients:

- ¼ cup extra-virgin olive oil
- 1 bay leaf
- 1 pound asparagus, trimmed and cut into 2-inch lengths
- 1 shallot, sliced into thin rounds
- 10 radishes, trimmed and quartered along the length
- 1¼ cups water
- 2 cups frozen peas
- 2 garlic cloves, sliced thin
- 2 teaspoons grated lemon zest
- 2 teaspoons grated orange zest
- 3 fresh thyme sprigs
- 4 teaspoons chopped fresh tarragon
- Pinch red pepper flakes
- Salt and pepper

Directions:

1. Cook oil, shallot, garlic, thyme sprigs, and pepper flakes in a Dutch oven on moderate heat until shallot is just softened, approximately two minutes. Mix in radishes, water, lemon zest, orange zest, bay leaf, and 1 teaspoon salt and bring to simmer. Decrease heat to moderate to low, cover, and cook until

radishes can be easily pierced with tip of paring knife, 3 to 5 minutes. Mix in asparagus, cover, and cook until tender, 3 to 5 minutes.
2. Remove from the heat, mix in peas, cover, and allow to sit until heated through, approximately five minutes. Discard thyme sprigs and bay leaf. Mix in tarragon and sprinkle with salt and pepper to taste. Serve.

Braised Cauliflower Mix 1

Yield: 4 to 6 Servings

This recipe can be made quickly

Ⓥ This is a Vegetarian Recipe Ⓥ

Ingredients:

- ⅛ teaspoon red pepper flakes
- ⅓ cup chicken or vegetable broth
- ⅓ cup dry white wine
- 1 head cauliflower (2 pounds), cored and cut into 1½-inch florets
- 2 tablespoons minced fresh parsley
- 3 garlic cloves, minced
- 3 tablespoons plus 1 teaspoon extra-virgin olive oil
- Salt and pepper

Directions:

1. Mix 1 teaspoon oil, garlic, and pepper flakes in a small-sized container. Heat remaining 3 tablespoons oil in 12-inch frying pan on moderate to high heat until it starts to shimmer. Put in cauliflower and ¼ teaspoon salt and cook, stirring intermittently, until florets start to look golden brown, seven to nine minutes.

2. Push cauliflower to sides of skillet. Put in garlic mixture to center and cook, mashing mixture into skillet, until aromatic, approximately half a minute. Stir garlic mixture into cauliflower.
3. Mix in broth and wine and bring to simmer. Decrease heat to moderate to low, cover, and cook until cauliflower is crisp-tender, four to eight minutes. Remove from the heat, mix in parsley and sprinkle with salt and pepper to taste. Serve.

Braised Cauliflower Mix 2

✎ This recipe can be made quickly ✎

Refer to the recipe "Braised Cauliflower Mix 1. Put in 2 anchovy fillets, rinsed and minced, and 1 tablespoon rinsed and minced capers to oil mixture in step 1. Stir 1 tablespoon lemon juice into cauliflower with parsley.

Braised Cauliflower Mix 3

✎ This recipe can be made quickly ✎

Ⓥ This is a Vegetarian Recipe Ⓥ

Refer to the recipe "Braised Cauliflower Mix 1. Omit wine. Substitute 2 teaspoons ground sumac for pepper flakes and increase broth to ½ cup. In step 3, once cauliflower is crisp-tender, uncover and carry on cooking until liquid is almost evaporated, approximately one minute. Substitute 2 tablespoons chopped fresh mint for parsley and stir ¼ cup plain yogurt into cauliflower with mint.

Braised Green Beans Mix 3

Refer to the recipe "Roasted Green Beans Mix 1. For velvety green beans, simmer them with a little baking soda, then put in canned tomatoes partway through cooking.

Broiled Eggplant

Yield: 4 to 6 Servings

This recipe can be made quickly

Ⓥ This is a Vegetarian Recipe Ⓥ

Ingredients:

- 1½ pounds eggplant, sliced into ¼-inch-thick rounds
- 2 tablespoons chopped fresh basil
- 3 tablespoons extra-virgin olive oil
- Kosher salt and pepper

Directions:

1. Lay out eggplant on paper towel–lined baking sheet, drizzle both sides with 1½ teaspoons salt, and allow to sit for 30 minutes.
2. Place oven rack 4 inches from broiler element and heat broiler. Comprehensively pat eggplant dry using paper towels, arrange on aluminium foil–lined rimmed baking sheet in one layer, and brush both sides with oil. Broil eggplant until mahogany brown and mildly charred, about 4 minutes each side. Move eggplant to serving platter, season with pepper to taste, and drizzle with basil. Serve.

Ciambotta

Yield: 6 Servings

Ⓥ This is a Vegetarian Recipe Ⓥ

Ingredients:

PESTO

- ¼ teaspoon red pepper flakes
- ⅓ cup chopped fresh basil
- ⅓ cup fresh oregano leaves
- 2 tablespoons extra-virgin olive oil
- 6 garlic cloves, minced

STEW

- ¼ cup extra-virgin olive oil
- 1 (28-ounce) can whole peeled tomatoes, drained with juice reserved, chopped coarse
- 1 cup shredded fresh basil
- 1 large onion, chopped
- 1 pound russet potatoes, peeled and cut into ½-inch pieces
- 12 ounces eggplant, peeled and cut into ½-inch pieces
- 2 red or yellow bell peppers, stemmed, seeded, and cut into ½-inch pieces
- 2 tablespoons tomato paste
- 2 zucchinis, halved along the length, seeded, and cut into ½-inch pieces
- 2¼ cups water
- Salt

Directions:

1. **FOR THE PESTO:** Process all ingredients using a food processor until finely ground, approximately one minute, scraping down sides of the container as required; set aside.

2. **FOR THE STEW:** Line large plate using double layer of coffee filters and spray using vegetable oil spray. Toss eggplant with 1½ teaspoons salt and spread uniformly coffee filters. Microwave eggplant, uncovered, until dry to touch and slightly shrivelled, 8 to 12 minutes, tossing halfway through microwaving.
3. Heat 2 tablespoons oil in a Dutch oven on high heat until it starts to shimmer. Put in eggplant, onion, and potatoes and cook, stirring often, until eggplant is browned, approximately two minutes.
4. Push vegetables to sides of pot. Put in 1 tablespoon oil and tomato paste to center and cook, stirring frequently, until brown fond develops on bottom of pot, approximately two minutes. Mix in 2 cups water and tomatoes and their juice, scraping up any browned bits, and bring to simmer. Decrease heat to moderate to low, cover, and simmer gently until eggplant is completely broken down and potatoes are tender, 20 minutes to half an hour.
5. In the meantime, heat residual 1 tablespoon oil in 12-inch frying pan on high heat until just smoking. Put in zucchini, bell peppers, and ½ teaspoon salt and cook, stirring intermittently, until vegetables become browned and tender, 10 to 12 minutes. Push vegetables to sides of skillet. Put in pesto to center and cook until aromatic, approximately one minute. Stir pesto into vegetables and move to a container. Remove from the heat, put in remaining ¼ cup water to frying pan and scrape up any browned bits.
6. Remove from the heat, stir vegetable mixture and water from frying pan into pot. Cover and allow to sit until flavours blend, approximately twenty minutes. Mix in basil and sprinkle with salt to taste. Serve.

Classic French Vegetable Gratin

Yield: **6 to 8 Servings**

Ⓥ This is a Vegetarian Recipe Ⓥ

Ingredients:

- ¼ cup chopped fresh basil
- 1 pound yellow summer squash, sliced ¼ inch thick
- 1 pound zucchini, sliced ¼ inch thick
- 1 slice hearty white sandwich bread, torn into quarters
- 1 tablespoon minced fresh thyme
- 1½ pounds ripe tomatoes, cored and sliced ¼ inch thick
- 2 garlic cloves, minced
- 2 onions, halved and sliced thin
- 2 ounces Parmesan cheese, grated (1 cup)
- 2 shallots, minced
- 6 tablespoons extra-virgin olive oil
- Salt and pepper

Directions:

1. Toss zucchini and summer squash with 1 teaspoon salt and allow to drain using a colander set over bowl until vegetables release at least 3 tablespoons liquid, about 45 minutes. Comprehensively pat zucchini and summer squash dry using paper towels.
2. In the meantime, spread tomatoes on paper towel–lined baking sheet, drizzle with ½ teaspoon salt, and allow to sit for 30 minutes. Comprehensively pat tomatoes dry using paper towels.
3. Heat 1 tablespoon oil in 12-inch non-stick frying pan on moderate heat until it starts to shimmer. Put in onions and ½ teaspoon salt and cook, stirring intermittently, till they become tender and dark golden brown, 20 minutes to half an hour; set aside.
4. Place oven rack to upper-middle position and pre-heat your oven to 400 degrees. Coat bottom of 13 by 9-inch baking dish with 1 tablespoon oil. Mix 3 tablespoons oil, garlic, thyme, and ½ teaspoon pepper in a container. Process bread using a food processor until finely ground, about 10 seconds, then combine

with remaining 1 tablespoon oil, Parmesan, and shallots in different container.

5. Toss zucchini and summer squash with half of garlic-oil mixture and lay out on prepared dish. Sprinkle evenly with onions, then arrange tomatoes on top, overlapping them slightly. Spoon remaining garlic-oil mixture uniformly tomatoes. Bake until vegetables are soft and tomatoes are starting to brown on edges, 40 to 45 minutes.
6. Remove dish from oven and increase oven temperature to 450 degrees. Sprinkle bread-crumb mixture evenly over top and continue to bake gratin until bubbling and cheese is lightly browned, 5 to 10 minutes. Allow it to cool for about ten minutes, then drizzle with basil. Serve.

Eastern Cauliflower Cakes

Yield: 4 Servings

Ⓥ This is a Vegetarian Recipe Ⓥ

Ingredients:

- ¼ cup all-purpose flour
- ¼ cup extra-virgin olive oil
- ¼ teaspoon pepper
- ½ teaspoon ground ginger
- 1 head cauliflower (2 pounds), cored and cut into 1-inch florets
- 1 large egg, lightly beaten
- 1 teaspoon grated lemon zest, plus lemon wedges for serving
- 1 teaspoon ground coriander
- 1 teaspoon ground turmeric
- 1 teaspoon salt
- 2 garlic cloves, minced
- 2 scallions, sliced thin
- 4 ounces goat cheese, softened

Directions:

1. Place the oven rack in the centre of the oven and pre-heat your oven to 450 degrees. Toss cauliflower with 1 tablespoon oil, turmeric, coriander, salt, ginger, and pepper. Move to aluminium foil–lined rimmed baking sheet and spread into one layer. Roast until cauliflower is thoroughly browned and tender, about 25 minutes. Allow it to cool slightly, then move to big container.
2. Line clean rimmed baking sheet with parchment paper. Mash cauliflower coarsely with potato masher. Mix in goat cheese, scallions, egg, garlic, and lemon zest until thoroughly mixed. Sprinkle flour over cauliflower mixture and stir to incorporate. Using wet hands, divide mixture into 4 equal portions, pack gently into ¾-inch-thick cakes, and place on readied sheet. Refrigerate cakes until chilled and firm, approximately half an hour.
3. Line large plate using paper towels. Heat remaining 3 tablespoons oil in 12-inch non-stick frying pan on moderate heat until it starts to shimmer. Gently lay cakes in frying pan and cook until deep golden brown and crisp, 5 to 7 minutes each side. Drain cakes briefly on prepared plate. Serve with lemon wedges.

Enhanced Pan-Roasted Asparagus Mix 1

Yield: 6 Servings

✒ This recipe can be made quickly ✒

Ⓥ This is a Vegetarian Recipe Ⓥ

Ingredients:

- ¼ cup grated Parmesan cheese
- ½ cup pitted kalamata olives, chopped coarse
- 12 ounces cherry tomatoes, halved
- 2 garlic cloves, minced
- 2 pounds thick asparagus, trimmed

- 2 tablespoons extra-virgin olive oil
- 2 tablespoons shredded fresh basil
- Salt and pepper

Directions:

1. Cook 1 tablespoon oil and garlic in 12-inch frying pan on moderate heat, stirring frequently, until garlic turns golden but not brown, approximately three minutes. Put in tomatoes and olives and cook until tomatoes begin to break down, approximately three minutes; move to a container.
2. Heat residual 1 tablespoon oil in now-empty frying pan on moderate to high heat until it starts to shimmer. Put in half of asparagus with tips pointed in 1 direction and remaining asparagus with tips pointed in opposite direction. Shake frying pan gently to help distribute spears evenly (they will not quite fit in one layer). Put in 1 teaspoon water, cover, and cook until asparagus is bright green and still crisp, approximately five minutes.
3. Uncover, increase heat to high, and cook, moving spears around with tongs as required, until asparagus is thoroughly browned on 1 side and tip of paring knife inserted at base of largest spear meets little resistance, 5 to 7 minutes. Sprinkle with salt and pepper to taste. Move asparagus to serving platter, top with tomato mixture, and drizzle with basil and Parmesan. Serve.

Enhanced Pan-Roasted Asparagus Mix 2

✔ This recipe can be made quickly ✔

Ⓥ *This is a Vegetarian Recipe* Ⓥ

Refer to Enhanced Pan-Roasted Asparagus Mix 1. Omit tomatoes, olives, and basil. Increase garlic to 3 cloves and slice thin. Before cooking asparagus, cook 2 tablespoons extra-virgin olive oil and sliced garlic in 12-inch frying pan over moderate to low heat, stirring frequently, until garlic turns crisp and golden but not brown, approximately five minutes. Use a slotted spoon to move garlic to plate coated using paper towels and season lightly with salt. Put in asparagus to oil left in frying pan and cook as directed. Sprinkle asparagus with toasted garlic and Parmesan before you serve.

Fava Beans Mix

Yield: 6 Servings

(V) This is a Vegetarian Recipe (V)

Ingredients:

- 1 cup chicken or vegetable broth
- 1 leek, white and light green parts only, halved along the length, sliced thin, and washed thoroughly
- 1 pound asparagus, trimmed and cut on bias into 2-inch lengths
- 1 pound fava beans, shelled (1 cup)
- 1 pound fresh peas, shelled (1¼ cups)
- 1 tablespoon chopped fresh mint
- 1 tablespoon extra-virgin olive oil, plus extra for serving
- 1 teaspoon baking soda
- 2 tablespoons shredded fresh basil
- 2 teaspoons grated lemon zest, plus 1 lemon
- 3 garlic cloves, minced
- 4 baby artichokes (3 ounces each)
- Salt and pepper

Directions:

1. Cut 1 lemon in half, squeeze halves into container filled with 2 quarts water, then put in spent halves. Working with 1 artichoke at a time, trim stem to about ¾ inch and cut off top quarter of artichoke. Break off bottom 3 or 4 rows of tough outer leaves by pulling them downward. Use a paring knife to trim outer layer of stem and base, removing any dark green

parts. Cut artichoke into quarters and submerge in lemon water.
2. Bring 2 cups water and baking soda to boil in small saucepan. Put in beans and cook until edges begin to darken, 1 to 2 minutes. Drain and wash thoroughly with cold water.
3. Heat oil in 12-inch frying pan on moderate heat until it starts to shimmer. Put in leek, 1 tablespoon water, and 1 teaspoon salt and cook till they become tender, approximately three minutes. Mix in garlic and cook until aromatic, approximately half a minute.
4. Take artichokes out of lemon water, shaking off excess water, and put in to skillet. Mix in broth and bring to simmer. Decrease heat to moderate to low, cover, and cook until artichokes are almost tender, six to eight minutes. Mix in asparagus and peas, cover, and cook until crisp-tender, 5 to 7 minutes. Mix in beans and cook until heated through and artichokes are fully tender, approximately two minutes. Remove from the heat, mix in basil, mint, and lemon zest. Sprinkle with salt and pepper to taste and drizzle with extra oil. Serve instantly.

Flavourful Grilled Radicchio

Yield: 4 to 6 Servings

✒ This recipe can be made quickly ✒

Ⓥ This is a Vegetarian Recipe Ⓥ

Ingredients:

- 1 garlic clove, minced
- 1 teaspoon minced fresh rosemary
- 3 heads radicchio (10 ounces each), quartered
- 6 tablespoons extra-virgin olive oil
- Salt and pepper

Directions:

1. Microwave oil, garlic, and rosemary in a container until bubbling, approximately one minute; let mixture steep for about sixty seconds. Brush radicchio with ¼ cup oil mixture and sprinkle with salt and pepper.
2. **FOR A CHARCOAL GRILL**: Open bottom vent fully. Light large chimney starter half filled with charcoal briquettes (3 quarts). When top coals are partially covered with ash, pour uniformly over grill. Set cooking grate in place, cover, and open lid vent fully. Heat grill until hot, approximately five minutes. **FOR A GAS GRILL**: Turn all burners to high, cover, and heat grill until hot, about fifteen minutes. Turn all burners to medium.
3. Clean and oil cooking grate. Place radicchio on grill. Cook (covered if using gas), flipping as required, until radicchio becomes tender and mildly charred, 3 to 5 minutes. Move to serving platter and drizzle with remaining oil mixture. Serve.

Garlic-flavoured Braised Kale

Yield: 8 Servings

ⓥ This is a Vegetarian Recipe ⓥ

Ingredients:

- ¼ teaspoon red pepper flakes
- 1 cup water
- 1 large onion, chopped fine
- 1 tablespoon lemon juice, plus extra for seasoning
- 10 garlic cloves, minced
- 2 cups chicken or vegetable broth
- 4 pounds kale, stemmed and cut into 3-inch pieces
- 6 tablespoons extra-virgin olive oil
- Salt and pepper

Directions:

1. Heat 3 tablespoons oil in a Dutch oven on moderate heat until it starts to shimmer. Put in onion and cook till they become tender and lightly browned, 5 to 7 minutes. Mix in garlic and pepper flakes and cook until aromatic, approximately one minute. Mix in broth, water, and ½ teaspoon salt and bring to simmer.
2. Put in one-third of kale, cover, and cook, stirring intermittently, until wilted, 2 to 4 minutes. Replicate the process with the rest of the kale in 2 batches. Carry on cooking, covered, until kale is tender, 13 to fifteen minutes.
3. Remove lid and increase heat to medium-high. Cook, stirring intermittently, until most liquid has evaporated and greens begin to sizzle, 10 to 12 minutes. Remove from the heat, mix in remaining 3 tablespoons oil and lemon juice. Sprinkle with salt, pepper, and extra lemon juice to taste. Serve.

Greek Garlic-Lemon Potatoes Basic

Yield: 4 to 6 Servings

This recipe can be made quickly

Ⓥ *This is a Vegetarian Recipe* Ⓥ

Ingredients:

- 1½ pounds Yukon Gold potatoes, peeled and cut along the length into ¾-inch-thick wedges
- 1½ tablespoons minced fresh oregano
- 1½ tablespoons minced fresh parsley
- 2 teaspoons grated lemon zest plus 1½ tablespoons juice
- 3 garlic cloves, minced
- 3 tablespoons extra-virgin olive oil
- Salt and pepper

Directions:

1. Heat 2 tablespoons oil in 12-inch non-stick frying pan on moderate to high heat until it starts to shimmer. Put in potatoes cut side down in one layer and cook until golden brown on first side (frying pan should sizzle but not smoke), about 6 minutes. Using tongs, flip potatoes onto second cut side and cook until golden brown, approximately five minutes. Decrease heat to moderate to low, cover, and cook until potatoes are tender, 8 to 12 minutes.
2. In the meantime, beat remaining 1 tablespoon oil, oregano, garlic, lemon zest and juice, ½ teaspoon salt, and ½ teaspoon pepper together in a small-sized container. When potatoes are tender, gently mix in garlic mixture and cook, uncovered, until aromatic, approximately two minutes. Remove from the heat, gently mix in parsley and sprinkle with salt and pepper to taste. Serve.

Greek Garlic-Lemon Potatoes Mix 1

This recipe can be made quickly

Ⓥ This is a Vegetarian Recipe Ⓥ

Refer to the recipe "Greek Garlic-Lemon Potatoes Basic". Stir ½ cup crumbled feta cheese and 2 tablespoons chopped pitted kalamata olives into potatoes with parsley.

Greek Grilled Zucchini

Yield: 4 Servings

This recipe can be made quickly

Ⓥ This is a Vegetarian Recipe Ⓥ

Ingredients:

- ¼ teaspoon Dijon mustard
- 1 large red onion, peeled and sliced into ½-inch-thick rings
- 1 pound zucchini, sliced along the length into ¾-inch-thick planks
- 1 small garlic clove, minced
- 1 tablespoon chopped fresh basil
- 1 teaspoon grated lemon zest plus 1 tablespoon juice
- 6 tablespoons extra-virgin olive oil
- Salt and pepper

Directions:

1. Thread onion rounds from side to side onto two 12-inch metal skewers. Brush onion and zucchini with ¼ cup oil, drizzle with 1 teaspoon salt, and season with pepper. Beat remaining 2 tablespoons oil, lemon zest and juice, garlic, mustard, and ¼ teaspoon salt together in a container; set aside for serving.
2. **FOR A CHARCOAL GRILL**: Open bottom vent fully. Light large chimney starter half filled with charcoal briquettes (3 quarts). When top coals are partially covered with ash, pour uniformly over grill. Set cooking grate in place, cover, and open lid vent fully. Heat grill until hot, approximately five minutes. **FOR A GAS GRILL**: Turn all burners to high, cover, and heat grill until hot, about fifteen minutes. Turn all burners to medium.
3. Clean and oil cooking grate. Place vegetables cut side down on grill. Cook (covered if using gas), turning as required, until soft and caramelized, 18 to 22 minutes; move vegetables to serving platter as they finish cooking. Remove skewers from onion and discard any charred outer rings. Beat dressing to recombine, then drizzle over vegetables. Sprinkle with basil and serve.

Greek Marinated Eggplant

Yield: 4 to 6 Servings

ⓥ This is a Vegetarian Recipe ⓥ

Ingredients:

- ¼ cup extra-virgin olive oil
- ½ teaspoon grated lemon zest
- ½ teaspoon minced fresh oregano
- 1 garlic clove, minced
- 1 tablespoon capers, rinsed and minced
- 1½ pounds Italian eggplant, sliced into 1-inch-thick rounds
- 3 tablespoons minced fresh mint
- 4 teaspoons red wine vinegar
- Kosher salt and pepper

Directions:

1. Lay out eggplant on paper towel–lined baking sheet, drizzle both sides with ½ teaspoon salt, and allow to sit for 30 minutes.
2. Place oven rack 4 inches from broiler element and heat broiler. Comprehensively pat eggplant dry using paper towels, arrange on aluminium foil–lined rimmed baking sheet in one layer, and lightly brush both sides with 1 tablespoon oil. Broil eggplant until mahogany brown and mildly charred, six to eight minutes each side.
3. Beat remaining 3 tablespoons oil, vinegar, capers, garlic, lemon zest, oregano, and ¼ teaspoon pepper together in a big container. Put in eggplant and mint and gently toss to combine. Let eggplant cool to room temperature, about 1 hour. Season with pepper to taste and serve.

Greek Stewed Zucchini

Yield: 6 to 8 Servings

(V) This is a Vegetarian Recipe (V)

Ingredients:

- ¼ teaspoon red pepper flakes

- 1 (28-ounce) can whole peeled tomatoes
- 1 onion, chopped fine
- 1 teaspoon minced fresh oregano or ¼ teaspoon dried
- 2 tablespoons chopped pitted kalamata olives
- 2 tablespoons shredded fresh mint
- 3 garlic cloves, minced
- 3 tablespoons extra-virgin olive oil
- 5 zucchinis (8 ounces each), trimmed, quartered along the length, seeded, and cut into 2-inch lengths
- Salt and pepper

Directions:

1. Place oven rack to lower-middle position and pre-heat your oven to 325 degrees. Process tomatoes and their juice using a food processor until smoothened thoroughly, approximately one minute; set aside.
2. Heat 2 teaspoons oil in a Dutch oven on moderate to high heat until just smoking. Brown one-third of zucchini, approximately three minutes each side; move to a container. Repeat with 4 teaspoons oil and remaining zucchini in 2 batches.
3. Put in remaining 1 tablespoon oil, onion, and ¾ teaspoon salt to now-empty pot and cook, stirring intermittently, over moderate to low heat until onion is very soft and golden brown, 9 to 11 minutes. Mix in garlic, oregano, and pepper flakes and cook until aromatic, approximately half a minute. Mix in olives and tomatoes, bring to simmer, and cook, stirring intermittently, until sauce has thickened, approximately half an hour.
4. Mix in zucchini and any accumulated juice, cover, and move pot to oven. Bake until zucchini is very tender, 30 to 40 minutes. Mix in mint and adjust sauce consistency with hot water as required. Sprinkle with salt and pepper to taste. Serve.

Grilled Eggplant

Yield: **4 to 6 Servings**

(V) This is a Vegetarian Recipe (V)

Ingredients:

- ⅛ teaspoon red pepper flakes
- ½ cup plain whole-milk yogurt
- 1 teaspoon grated lemon zest plus 2 teaspoons juice
- 1 teaspoon ground cumin
- 2 pounds eggplant, sliced into ¼-inch-thick rounds
- 3 tablespoons chopped fresh mint
- 5 garlic cloves, minced
- 6 tablespoons extra-virgin olive oil
- Salt and pepper

Directions:

1. Mix oil, garlic, and pepper flakes in a container. Microwave until garlic is golden brown and crisp, approximately two minutes. Strain garlic oil through fine-mesh strainer into small-sized container. Reserve garlic oil and garlic separately.
2. Beat 1 tablespoon garlic oil, yogurt, mint, lemon zest and juice, cumin, and ¼ teaspoon salt together in different container; set aside for serving.
3. **FOR A CHARCOAL GRILL**: Open bottom vent fully. Light large chimney starter filled with charcoal briquettes (6 quarts). When top coals are partially covered with ash, pour uniformly over grill. Set cooking grate in place, cover, and open lid vent fully. Heat grill until hot, approximately five minutes. **FOR A GAS GRILL**: Turn all burners to high, cover, and heat grill until hot, about fifteen minutes. Turn all burners to medium-high.
4. Clean and oil cooking grate. Brush eggplant with remaining garlic oil and sprinkle with salt and pepper. Place half of eggplant on grill and cook (covered if using gas) until browned and tender, about 4 minutes each side; move to serving platter. Replicate the process with the rest of the eggplant; move to platter. Sprinkle yogurt sauce over eggplant and drizzle with garlic. Serve.

Grilled Portobello Mushrooms and Shallots

Yield: 4 to 6 Servings

✄ *This recipe can be made quickly* ✄

Ⓥ *This is a Vegetarian Recipe* Ⓥ

Ingredients:

- 1 small garlic clove, minced
- 1 teaspoon Dijon mustard
- 1 teaspoon minced fresh rosemary
- 2 teaspoons lemon juice
- 6 portobello mushroom caps (4 to 5 inches in diameter)
- 6 tablespoons extra-virgin olive oil
- 8 shallots, peeled
- Salt and pepper

Directions:

1. Beat 2 tablespoons oil, garlic, lemon juice, mustard, rosemary, and ¼ teaspoon salt together in a small-sized container. Sprinkle with salt and pepper to taste; set aside for serving.
2. Thread shallots through roots and stem ends onto two 12-inch metal skewers. Use a paring knife to cut ½-inch crosshatch pattern, ¼ inch deep, on tops of mushroom caps. Brush shallots and mushroom caps with remaining ¼ cup oil and sprinkle with salt and pepper.
3. FOR A CHARCOAL GRILL Open bottom vent fully. Light large chimney starter half filled with charcoal briquettes (3 quarts). When top coals are partially covered with ash, pour uniformly over grill. Set cooking grate in place, cover, and open lid vent fully. Heat grill until hot, approximately five minutes. 3B. FOR A

GAS GRILL Turn all burners to high, cover, and heat grill until hot, about fifteen minutes. Turn all burners to medium.
4. Clean and oil cooking grate. Place shallots and mushrooms, gill side up, on grill. Cook (covered if using gas) until mushrooms have released their liquid and vegetables are charred on first side, approximately eight minutes. Flip mushrooms and shallots and carry on cooking (covered if using gas) until vegetables are soft and charred on second side, approximately eight minutes. Move vegetables to serving platter. Remove skewers from shallots and discard any charred outer layers. Beat vinaigrette to recombine and drizzle over vegetables. Serve.

Hearty North-African Tagine

Yield: 4 to 6 Servings

ⓥ This is a Vegetarian Recipe ⓥ

Ingredients:

- ⅛ teaspoon cayenne pepper
- ¼ cup extra-virgin olive oil, plus extra for serving
- ¼ teaspoon ground cinnamon
- ¼ teaspoon ground coriander
- ¼ teaspoon ground ginger
- ½ cup golden raisins
- ½ cup minced fresh cilantro
- ½ cup pitted kalamata olives, halved
- ½ cup plain whole-milk Greek yogurt
- ½ teaspoon ground cumin
- 1 onion, halved and sliced ¼ inch thick
- 1 tablespoon paprika
- 2 (15-ounce) cans chickpeas, rinsed
- 2 tablespoons all-purpose flour
- 2 tablespoons honey

- 2 yellow or red bell peppers, stemmed, seeded, and cut into ½-inch-wide strips
- 3 cups jarred whole baby artichoke hearts packed in water, quartered, rinsed, and patted dry
- 3 cups vegetable broth
- 4 (2-inch) strips lemon zest plus 1 teaspoon grated zest (2 lemons)
- 8 garlic cloves, minced
- Salt and pepper

Directions:

1. Heat 1 tablespoon oil in a Dutch oven on moderate heat until it starts to shimmer. Put in artichokes and cook until golden brown, 5 to 7 minutes; move to a container.
2. Put in bell peppers, onion, lemon zest strips, and 1 tablespoon oil to now-empty pot and cook on moderate heat until vegetables are softened and lightly browned, 5 to 7 minutes. Mix in two-thirds of garlic, paprika, cumin, ginger, coriander, cinnamon, and cayenne and cook until aromatic, approximately half a minute. Mix in flour and cook for about sixty seconds.
3. Slowly beat in broth, scraping up any browned bits and smoothing out any lumps. Mix in artichoke hearts, chickpeas, olives, raisins, and honey and bring to simmer. Decrease heat to low, cover, and simmer gently until vegetables are tender, about fifteen minutes.
4. Remove from the heat, discard lemon zest strips. Mix ¼ cup hot liquid and yogurt in a container to temper, then stir yogurt mixture into pot. Mix in remaining 2 tablespoons oil, remaining garlic, cilantro, and grated lemon zest. Sprinkle with salt and pepper to taste. Serve, drizzling individual portions with extra oil.

Italian Broccoli Rabe Mix 1

Yield: 4 Servings

This recipe can be made quickly

This is a Vegetarian Recipe

Ingredients:

- ¼ teaspoon red pepper flakes
- 14 ounces broccoli rabe, trimmed and cut into 1-inch pieces
- 2 tablespoons extra-virgin olive oil
- 3 garlic cloves, minced
- Salt and pepper

Directions:

1. Bring 3 quarts water to boil in a big saucepan. Fill big container halfway with ice and water. Put in broccoli rabe and 2 teaspoons salt to boiling water and cook until wilted and tender, about 2½ minutes. Drain broccoli rabe, then move to ice water and allow to sit until chilled. Drain again and thoroughly pat dry.
2. Cook oil, garlic, and pepper flakes in 10-inch frying pan on moderate heat, stirring frequently, until garlic begins to sizzle, approximately two minutes. Increase heat to medium-high, put in broccoli rabe, and cook, stirring to coat with oil, until heated through, approximately one minute. Sprinkle with salt and pepper to taste and serve.

Italian Broccoli Rabe Mix 2

This recipe can be made quickly

This is a Vegetarian Recipe

Refer to Italian Broccoli Rabe Mix 1. Put in ¼ cup oil-packed sun-dried tomatoes, cut into thin strips, to frying pan with oil. Sprinkle broccoli rabe with 3 tablespoons toasted pine nuts before you serve.

Italian Broccoli Rabe Mix 3

This recipe can be made quickly

Ⓥ *This is a Vegetarian Recipe* Ⓥ

Refer to Italian Broccoli Rabe Mix 1. Substitute 1 teaspoon minced fresh oregano for pepper flakes. Put in 1 red bell pepper, stemmed, seeded, and cut into ½-inch pieces, to frying pan with oil and oregano. Put in ¼ cup chopped kalamata olives to frying pan with broccoli rabe. Sprinkle broccoli rabe with ¼ cup crumbled feta cheese before you serve.

Lamb-Stuffed Zucchini

Yield: 4 Servings

Ingredients:

- ¼ cup dried apricots, chopped fine
- ½ cup medium-grind bulgur, rinsed
- ⅔ cup chicken broth
- 1 onion, chopped fine
- 2 tablespoons minced fresh parsley
- 2 tablespoons pine nuts, toasted
- 2 tablespoons plus 1 teaspoon extra-virgin olive oil
- 2 teaspoons ras el hanout
- 4 garlic cloves, minced
- 4 zucchinis (8 ounces each), halved along the length and seeded
- 8 ounces ground lamb
- Salt and pepper

Directions:

1. Adjust oven racks to upper-middle and lowest positions, place rimmed baking sheet on lower rack, and pre-heat your oven to 400 degrees.

2. Brush cut sides of zucchini with 2 tablespoons oil and sprinkle with salt and pepper. Lay zucchini cut side down in hot sheet and roast until slightly softened and skins are wrinkled, eight to ten minutes. Remove zucchini from oven and flip cut side up on sheet; set aside.
3. In the meantime, heat remaining 1 teaspoon oil in a big saucepan on moderate to high heat until just smoking. Put in lamb, ½ teaspoon salt, and ¼ teaspoon pepper and cook, breaking up meat with wooden spoon, until browned, 3 to 5 minutes. Use a slotted spoon to move lamb to paper towel–lined plate.
4. Pour off all but 1 tablespoon fat from saucepan. Put in onion to fat left in saucepan and cook on moderate heat till they become tender, approximately five minutes. Mix in garlic and ras el hanout and cook until aromatic, approximately half a minute. Mix in broth, bulgur, and apricots and bring to simmer. Decrease heat to low, cover, and simmer gently until bulgur is tender, 16 to 18 minutes.
5. Remove from the heat, lay clean dish towel underneath lid and let pilaf sit for about ten minutes. Put in pine nuts and parsley to pilaf and gently fluff with fork to combine. Sprinkle with salt and pepper to taste.
6. Pack each zucchini half with bulgur mixture, about ½ cup per zucchini half, mounding excess. Place baking sheet on upper rack and bake zucchini until heated through, about 6 minutes. Serve.

Lemony Roasted Artichokes

Yield: 4 Servings

Ⓥ *This is a Vegetarian Recipe* Ⓥ

Ingredients:

- ½ teaspoon Dijon mustard
- ½ teaspoon garlic, minced to paste
- 2 teaspoons chopped fresh parsley
- 3 lemons
- 4 artichokes (8 to 10 ounces each)
- 9 tablespoons extra-virgin olive oil
- Salt and pepper

Directions:

1. Place oven rack to lower-middle position and pre-heat your oven to 475 degrees. Cut 1 lemon in half, squeeze halves into container filled with 2 quarts water, then put in spent halves.
2. Working with 1 artichoke at a time, trim stem to about ¾ inch and cut off top quarter of artichoke. Break off bottom 3 or 4 rows of tough outer leaves by pulling them downward. Use a paring knife to trim outer layer of stem and base, removing any dark green parts. Cut artichoke in half along the length, then remove fuzzy choke and any tiny inner purple-tinged leaves with the help of a small spoon. Immerse prepped artichokes in lemon water.
3. Coat bottom of 13 by 9-inch baking dish with 1 tablespoon oil. Take artichokes out of lemon water and shake off water, leaving some water still remaining on leaves. Toss artichokes with 2 tablespoons oil, ¾ teaspoon salt, and pinch pepper; gently rub oil and seasonings between leaves. Arrange artichokes cut side down in prepared dish. Trim ends off remaining 2 lemons, halve crosswise, and arrange cut side up next to artichokes. Cover tightly with aluminium foil and roast until cut sides of artichokes begin to brown and bases and leaves are soft when poked with tip of paring knife, about half an hour.
4. Move artichokes to serving platter. Let lemons cool slightly, then squeeze into fine-mesh strainer set over bowl, extracting as much juice and pulp as possible; press firmly on solids to yield 1½ tablespoons juice. Beat garlic, mustard, and ½ teaspoon salt into juice. Whisking continuously, slowly drizzle in remaining 6 tablespoons oil until completely blended. Beat in

parsley and sprinkle with salt and pepper to taste. Serve artichokes with dressing.

Ratatouille

Yield: 4 to 6 Servings

Ⓥ This is a Vegetarian Recipe Ⓥ

Ingredients:

- ¼ teaspoon red pepper flakes
- ⅓ cup plus 1 tablespoon extra-virgin olive oil
- 1 bay leaf
- 1 red bell pepper, stemmed, seeded, and cut into 1-inch pieces
- 1 tablespoon minced fresh parsley
- 1 tablespoon sherry vinegar
- 1 yellow bell pepper, stemmed, seeded, and cut into 1-inch pieces
- 1½ pounds eggplant, peeled and cut into 1-inch pieces
- 1½ teaspoons herbes de Provence
- 2 large onions, cut into 1-inch pieces
- 2 pounds plum tomatoes, peeled, cored, and chopped coarse
- 2 small zucchinis, halved along the length and cut into 1-inch pieces
- 2 tablespoons chopped fresh basil
- 8 large garlic cloves, peeled and smashed
- Salt and pepper

Directions:

1. Place the oven rack in the centre of the oven and pre-heat your oven to 400 degrees. Heat ⅓ cup oil in a Dutch oven on moderate to high heat until it starts to shimmer. Put in onions, garlic, 1 teaspoon salt, and ¼ teaspoon pepper and cook, stirring intermittently, until onions are translucent and starting to soften, about 10 minutes. Put in herbes de Provence, pepper

flakes, and bay leaf and cook, stirring often, for about sixty seconds. Mix in eggplant and tomatoes. Sprinkle with ½ teaspoon salt and ¼ teaspoon pepper and stir to combine. Move pot to oven and cook, uncovered, until vegetables are very soft and spotty brown, 40 to 45 minutes.

2. Remove pot from oven and, using potato masher or heavy wooden spoon, smash and stir eggplant mixture until broken down to sauce like consistency. Mix in zucchini, bell peppers, ¼ teaspoon salt, and ¼ teaspoon pepper and return to oven. Cook, uncovered, until zucchini and bell peppers are just tender, 20 minutes to half an hour.

3. Remove pot from oven, cover, and allow to sit until zucchini is translucent and easily pierced with tip of paring knife, 10 to fifteen minutes. Using wooden spoon, scrape any browned bits from sides of pot and stir back into ratatouille. Discard bay leaf. Mix in 1 tablespoon basil, parsley, and vinegar. Sprinkle with salt and pepper to taste. Move ratatouille to serving platter, drizzle with remaining 1 tablespoon oil, and drizzle with remaining 1 tablespoon basil. Serve.

Roasted Asparagus Basic

Yield: 4 to 6 Servings

This recipe can be made quickly

Ⓥ *This is a Vegetarian Recipe* Ⓥ

Ingredients:

- ¼ teaspoon pepper
- ½ teaspoon salt
- 2 pounds thick asparagus, trimmed
- 2 tablespoons plus 2 teaspoons extra-virgin olive oil

Directions:

1. Place oven rack to lowest position, place rimmed baking sheet on rack, and pre-heat your oven to 500 degrees. Peel bottom halves of asparagus spears until white flesh is exposed, then toss with 2 tablespoons oil, salt, and pepper.
2. Move asparagus to preheated sheet and spread into one layer. Roast, without moving asparagus, until undersides of spears become browned, tops are bright green, and tip of paring knife inserted at base of largest spear meets little resistance, eight to ten minutes. Move asparagus to serving platter and drizzle with remaining 2 teaspoons oil. Serve.

Roasted Asparagus Mix 1

This recipe can be made quickly

Ⓥ This is a Vegetarian Recipe Ⓥ

Mix 2 tablespoons minced fresh mint, 2 tablespoons minced fresh parsley, 2 teaspoons grated orange zest, 1 minced garlic clove, and pinch cayenne pepper in a container. Sprinkle gremolata over asparagus before you serve.

Roasted Asparagus Mix 2

This recipe can be made quickly

Ⓥ This is a Vegetarian Recipe Ⓥ

Mix 2 tablespoons minced fresh tarragon, 2 tablespoons minced fresh parsley, 2 teaspoons grated lemon zest, and 1 minced garlic clove in a container. Sprinkle gremolata over asparagus before you serve.

Roasted Carrot Cilantro Spice

Yield: 4 to 6 Servings

This recipe can be made quickly

Ⓥ This is a Vegetarian Recipe Ⓥ

Ingredients:

- ⅛ teaspoon ground cinnamon
- ¼ cup chopped fresh cilantro
- ¼ teaspoon ground cumin
- ½ teaspoon ground dried Aleppo pepper
- 1 tablespoon packed dark brown sugar
- 1½ pounds carrots, peeled
- 2 tablespoons extra-virgin olive oil
- 2 tablespoons orange juice
- Salt and pepper

Directions:

1. Place the oven rack in the centre of the oven and pre-heat your oven to 450 degrees. Beat oil, sugar, ½ teaspoon salt, and ½ teaspoon pepper together in a big container.
2. Cut carrots in half crosswise, then cut along the length into halves or quarters as required to create uniformly sized pieces. Put in carrots to oil mixture and toss to coat. Move to aluminium foil–lined rimmed baking sheet and spread into one layer.
3. Cover sheet tightly with foil and roast for 12 minutes. Remove foil and continue to roast until carrots are thoroughly browned and tender, 16 to 22 minutes, stirring halfway through roasting.
4. Beat orange juice, Aleppo, cumin, and cinnamon together in a big container. Put in carrots and cilantro and gently toss to combine. Sprinkle with salt and pepper to taste and serve.

Roasted Celery Root

Yield: 6 Servings

Ⓥ *This is a Vegetarian Recipe* Ⓥ

Ingredients:

- ¼ cup fresh cilantro leaves
- ¼ cup plain yogurt
- ¼ teaspoon dried thyme
- ¼ teaspoon grated lemon zest plus 1 teaspoon juice
- 1 teaspoon coriander seeds, toasted and crushed
- 1 teaspoon sesame seeds, toasted
- 3 celery roots (2½ pounds), peeled, halved, and sliced ½ inch thick
- 3 tablespoons extra-virgin olive oil
- Salt and pepper

Directions:

1. Place oven rack on the lowest position and pre-heat your oven to 425 degrees. Toss celery root with oil, ½ teaspoon salt, and ¼ teaspoon pepper and lay out on rimmed baking sheet in one layer. Roast celery root until sides touching sheet toward back of oven are well browned, about half an hour. Rotate sheet and continue to roast until sides touching sheet toward back of oven are well browned, 6 to 10 minutes.
2. Use metal spatula to flip each piece and continue to roast until celery root is very soft and sides touching sheet become browned, 10 to fifteen minutes.
3. Move celery root to serving platter. Beat yogurt, lemon zest and juice, and pinch salt together in a container. In a different container, combine sesame seeds, coriander seeds, thyme, and pinch salt. Sprinkle celery root with yogurt sauce and drizzle with seed mixture and cilantro. Serve.

Roasted Greek Winter Squash

Yield: 6 Servings

Ⓥ This is a Vegetarian Recipe Ⓥ

Ingredients:

- ¼ cup shelled pistachios, toasted and chopped fine
- 1 ounce feta cheese, crumbled (¼ cup)
- 1 tablespoon tahini
- 1 teaspoon honey
- 1½ teaspoons lemon juice
- 2 tablespoons chopped fresh mint
- 3 pounds butternut squash
- 3 tablespoons extra-virgin olive oil
- Salt and pepper

Directions:

1. Place oven rack on the lowest position and pre-heat your oven to 425 degrees. Using sharp vegetable peeler or chef's knife, remove squash skin and fibrous threads just below skin (squash should be completely orange with no white flesh). Halve squash along the length and scrape out seeds. Place squash cut side down on slicing board and slice crosswise into ½-inch-thick pieces.
2. Toss squash with 2 tablespoons oil, ½ teaspoon salt, and ½ teaspoon pepper and lay out on rimmed baking sheet in one layer. Roast squash until sides touching sheet toward back of oven are well browned, about half an hour. Rotate sheet and continue to roast until sides touching sheet toward back of oven are well browned, 6 to 10 minutes.
3. Use metal spatula to flip each piece and continue to roast until squash is very soft and sides touching sheet become browned, 10 to fifteen minutes.
4. Move squash to serving platter. Beat tahini, lemon juice, honey, remaining 1 tablespoon oil, and pinch salt together in a

container. Sprinkle squash with tahini dressing and drizzle with feta, pistachios, and mint. Serve.

Roasted Green Beans Mix 1

Yield: 4 to 6 Servings

This recipe can be made quickly

(V) This is a Vegetarian Recipe (V)

Ingredients:

- ¼ cup extra-virgin olive oil
- ¼ cup shredded Pecorino Romano cheese
- ¾ teaspoon sugar
- 1 teaspoon Dijon mustard
- 1 teaspoon grated lemon zest plus 1 tablespoon juice
- 1½ pounds green beans, trimmed
- 2 garlic cloves, minced
- 2 tablespoons chopped fresh basil
- 2 tablespoons pine nuts, toasted
- Salt and pepper

Directions:

1. Place oven rack on the lowest position and pre-heat your oven to 475 degrees. Toss green beans with 1 tablespoon oil, sugar, ¼ teaspoon salt, and ½ teaspoon pepper. Move to rimmed baking sheet and spread into one layer.
2. Cover sheet tightly with aluminium foil and roast for about ten minutes. Remove foil and continue to roast until green beans are spotty brown, about 10 minutes, stirring halfway through roasting.
3. In the meantime, combine garlic, lemon zest, and remaining 3 tablespoons oil in a moderate-sized container and microwave until bubbling, approximately one minute. Let mixture steep for

about sixty seconds, then beat in lemon juice, mustard, ⅛ teaspoon salt, and ¼ teaspoon pepper until combined.
4. Move green beans to a container with dressing, put in basil, and toss to combine. Sprinkle with salt and pepper to taste. Move green beans to serving platter and drizzle with Pecorino and pine nuts. Serve.

Roasted Green Beans Mix 2

This recipe can be made quickly

Ⓥ *This is a Vegetarian Recipe* Ⓥ

Refer to the recipe "Roasted Green Beans Mix 1. Omit Pecorino. Substitute 1 teaspoon lime zest and 1 tablespoon juice for lemon zest and juice, ¼ cup torn fresh mint leaves for basil, and 2 tablespoons toasted and chopped whole blanched almonds for pine nuts.

Roasted Mushrooms Mix 1

Yield: 4 Servings

Ⓥ *This is a Vegetarian Recipe* Ⓥ

Ingredients:

- 1 ounce Parmesan cheese, grated (½ cup)
- 1 pound shiitake mushrooms, stemmed, caps larger than 3 inches halved
- 1 teaspoon lemon juice
- 1½ pounds cremini mushrooms, trimmed and left whole if small, halved if medium, or quartered if large
- 2 tablespoons chopped fresh parsley
- 2 tablespoons pine nuts, toasted

- 3 tablespoons extra-virgin olive oil
- Salt and pepper

Directions:

1. Place oven rack on the lowest position and pre-heat your oven to 450 degrees. Dissolve 5 teaspoons salt in 2 quarts room-temperature water in large container. Put in cremini mushrooms and shiitake mushrooms, cover with plate or bowl to submerge, and soak at room temperature for about ten minutes.
2. Drain mushrooms and pat dry using paper towels. Toss mushrooms with 2 tablespoons oil, then spread into one layer in rimmed baking sheet. Roast until liquid from mushrooms has completely evaporated, 35 to 45 minutes.
3. Remove sheet from oven (be careful of escaping steam when opening oven) and, using metal spatula, carefully stir mushrooms. Return to oven and continue to roast until mushrooms are deeply browned, 5 to 10 minutes.
4. Beat residual 1 tablespoon oil and lemon juice together in a big container. Put in mushrooms and toss to coat. Mix in Parmesan, pine nuts, and parsley and sprinkle with salt and pepper to taste. Serve instantly.

Roasted Mushrooms Mix 2

Ⓥ This is a Vegetarian Recipe Ⓥ

Refer to the recipe "Roasted Mushrooms Mix 1". Use our homemade Harissa if you can, but you can substitute store-bought harissa if you wish, though spiciness can vary greatly by brand. Omit Parmesan and pine nuts and increase lemon juice to 2 teaspoons. Beat 1 minced garlic clove, 2 teaspoons harissa, ¼ teaspoon ground cumin, and ¼ teaspoon salt into oil mixture in step 4. Substitute 2 tablespoons mint for parsley.

Roasted Mushrooms Mix 3

(V) This is a Vegetarian Recipe (V)

Refer to the recipe "Roasted Mushrooms Mix 1". Omit Parmesan and pine nuts. Put in 3 unpeeled whole garlic cloves to sheet with mushrooms. Remove garlic from sheet in step 3 when stirring mushrooms. When garlic is cool enough to handle, peel and mash. Substitute 2 teaspoons sherry vinegar for lemon juice. Beat mashed garlic, ½ teaspoon smoked paprika, and ¼ teaspoon salt into oil mixture in step 4.

Roasted Tomatoes

Yield: 4 Servings

(V) This is a Vegetarian Recipe (V)

Ingredients:

- ¼ teaspoon dried oregano
- ¾ cup extra-virgin olive oil
- 2 garlic cloves, peeled and smashed
- 3 pounds large tomatoes, cored, bottom ⅛ inch trimmed, and sliced ¾ inch thick
- Kosher salt and pepper

Directions:

1. Place the oven rack in the centre of the oven and pre-heat your oven to 425 degrees. Line rimmed baking sheet with aluminium foil. Arrange tomatoes in a uniform layer in readied sheet, with larger slices around edge and smaller slices in center. Place garlic cloves on tomatoes. Sprinkle with oregano and ¼ teaspoon salt and season with pepper to taste. Sprinkle oil evenly over tomatoes.

2. Bake for 30 minutes, rotating sheet halfway through baking. Remove sheet from oven. Reduce oven temperature to 300 degrees and prop open door with wooden spoon to cool oven. Using thin spatula, flip tomatoes.
3. Return tomatoes to oven, close oven door, and carry on cooking until spotty brown, skins are blistered, and tomatoes have collapsed to ¼ to ½ inch thick, 1 to 2 hours. Remove from oven and allow to cool completely, approximately half an hour. Discard garlic and move tomatoes and oil to airtight container. (Tomatoes will keep safely in a fridge for maximum 5 days or frozen for maximum 2 months.)

Sautéed Cabbage Mix 1

Yield: 4 to 6 Servings

This recipe can be made quickly

Ⓥ This is a Vegetarian Recipe Ⓥ

Ingredients:

- ¼ cup chopped fresh parsley
- 1 onion, halved and sliced thin
- 1 small head green cabbage (1¼ pounds), cored and sliced thin
- 1½ teaspoons lemon juice
- 2 tablespoons extra-virgin olive oil
- Salt and pepper

Directions:

1. Place cabbage in a big container and cover with cold water. Allow to sit for about three minutes; drain well.
2. Heat 1 tablespoon oil in 12-inch non-stick frying pan on moderate to high heat until it starts to shimmer. Put in onion and ¼ teaspoon salt and cook till they become tender and lightly browned, 5 to 7 minutes; move to a container.

3. Heat residual 1 tablespoon oil in now-empty frying pan on moderate to high heat until it starts to shimmer. Put in cabbage and drizzle with ½ teaspoon salt and ¼ teaspoon pepper. Cover and cook, without stirring, until cabbage is wilted and lightly browned on bottom, approximately three minutes. Stir and continue to cook, uncovered, until cabbage is crisp-tender and lightly browned in places, about 4 minutes, stirring once halfway through cooking. Remove from the heat, mix in onion, parsley, and lemon juice. Sprinkle with salt and pepper to taste and serve.

Sautéed Cabbage Mix 2

This recipe can be made quickly

Ⓥ This is a Vegetarian Recipe Ⓥ

Refer the previous recipe. Omit pepper. Substitute 1 small head savoy cabbage for green cabbage and 1 fennel bulb, fronds minced, stalks discarded, bulb halved, cored, and sliced thin, for onion. Cook fennel till they become tender, eight to ten minutes, then put in 2 minced garlic cloves and ¼ teaspoon red pepper flakes and cook until aromatic, approximately half a minute. Substitute fennel fronds for parsley and increase lemon juice to 2 teaspoons. Sprinkle cabbage with extra 1 tablespoon oil and drizzle with 2 tablespoons grated Parmesan cheese before you serve.

Sautéed Cherry Tomatoes Basic

Yield: 4 to 6 Servings

This recipe can be made quickly

Ⓥ This is a Vegetarian Recipe Ⓥ

Ingredients:

- 1 garlic clove, minced
- 1 tablespoon extra-virgin olive oil
- 1½ pounds cherry tomatoes, halved
- 2 tablespoons chopped fresh basil
- 2 teaspoons sugar, or to taste
- Salt and pepper

Directions:

1. Heat oil in 12-inch frying pan on moderate to high heat until it starts to shimmer. Toss tomatoes with sugar and ¼ teaspoon salt, then put in to frying pan and cook, stirring frequently, for about sixty seconds. Mix in garlic and cook until aromatic, approximately half a minute.
2. Remove from the heat, mix in basil and sprinkle with salt and pepper to taste. Serve.

Sautéed Cherry Tomatoes Mix 1

✰ This recipe can be made quickly ✰

Refer to the recipe "Sautéed Cherry Tomatoes Basic". Heat 2 anchovy fillets, rinsed and minced, with oil until starting to sizzle, approximately two minutes. Increase garlic to 2 cloves and put in 2 tablespoons rinsed capers to tomatoes with garlic. Substitute 2 tablespoons minced fresh parsley for basil.

Sautéed Swiss Chard Mix 1

Yield: 4 Servings

✰ This recipe can be made quickly ✰

Ⓥ This is a Vegetarian Recipe Ⓥ

Ingredients:

- 1½ pounds Swiss chard, stems sliced ¼ inch thick on bias, leaves sliced into ½-inch-wide strips
- 2 tablespoons extra-virgin olive oil
- 2 teaspoons lemon juice
- 3 garlic cloves, sliced thin
- Salt and pepper

Directions:

1. Heat oil in 12-inch non-stick frying pan on moderate to high heat until it barely starts shimmering. Put in garlic and cook, stirring continuously, until lightly browned, 30 to 60 seconds. Put in chard stems and ⅛ teaspoon salt and cook, stirring intermittently, until spotty brown and crisp-tender, about 6 minutes.
2. Put in two-thirds of chard leaves and cook, tossing with tongs, until just starting to wilt, 30 to 60 seconds. Put in remaining chard leaves and continue to cook, stirring often, until leaves are tender, approximately three minutes. Remove from the heat, mix in lemon juice and sprinkle with salt and pepper to taste. Serve.

Sautéed Swiss Chard Mix 2

This recipe can be made quickly

Refer to the recipe "Sautéed Swiss Chard Mix 1". Omit garlic. Heat 1 tablespoon of oil in 12-inch non-stick frying pan on moderate heat until it starts to shimmer. Put in 3 thinly sliced shallots and cook, stirring often, until thoroughly browned and softened, 10 to 12 minutes. Move shallots to a container and wipe frying pan clean using paper towels. Cook 2 ounces pancetta, cut into ¼-inch pieces, and residual 1 tablespoon oil in now-empty frying pan on moderate to high heat, stirring intermittently, until rendered and crisp, six to eight minutes. Use a slotted spoon to move pancetta to paper towel–lined plate. Pour off all but 2 tablespoons fat from frying pan and return to medium-high heat. Proceed with recipe, adding ⅛ teaspoon red pepper flakes to frying pan with chard stems. Substitute 1 tablespoon balsamic vinegar for lemon juice and stir pancetta and shallots into chard with vinegar.

Sautéed Swiss Chard Mix 3

This recipe can be made quickly

Ⓥ This is a Vegetarian Recipe Ⓥ

Refer to the recipe "Sautéed Swiss Chard Mix 1". Reduce garlic to 1 minced clove and put in ¼ teaspoon ground cumin to frying pan with garlic. Substitute 2 teaspoons sherry vinegar for lemon juice and stir 3 tablespoons dried currants and 3 tablespoons toasted pine nuts into chard with vinegar.

Sautéed Zucchini Ribbons Basic

Yield: 4 to 6 Servings

This recipe can be made quickly

Ⓥ This is a Vegetarian Recipe Ⓥ

Ingredients:

- 1 small garlic clove, minced
- 1 teaspoon grated lemon zest plus 1 tablespoon juice
- 1½ tablespoons chopped fresh parsley
- 2 tablespoons plus 1 teaspoon extra-virgin olive oil
- 4 (6- to 8-ounce) zucchini or yellow summer squash, trimmed
- Salt and pepper

Directions:

1. Mix garlic and lemon juice in a big container and set aside for minimum 10 minutes. Take a vegetable peeler and use it to shave off 3 ribbons from 1 side of summer squash, then turn

squash 90 degrees and shave off 3 more ribbons. Continue to turn and shave ribbons until you reach seeds; discard core. Replicate the process with the rest of the squash.
2. Beat 2 tablespoons oil, ¼ teaspoon salt, ⅛ teaspoon pepper, and lemon zest into garlic–lemon juice mixture.
3. Heat remaining 1 teaspoon oil in 12-inch non-stick frying pan on moderate to high heat until just smoking. Put in summer squash and cook, tossing occasionally with tongs, until squash has softened and is translucent, three to five minutes. Move squash to a container with dressing, put in parsley, and gently toss to coat. Sprinkle with salt and pepper to taste. Serve.

Sautéed Zucchini Ribbons Mix

This recipe can be made quickly

Ⓥ *This is a Vegetarian Recipe* Ⓥ

Refer to the previous recipe. Omit lemon zest and substitute 1½ teaspoons cider vinegar for lemon juice. Substitute ⅓ cup chopped fresh mint for parsley and drizzle squash with 2 tablespoons toasted and chopped pistachios before you serve.

Simmered Braised Green Beans

Yield: 6 Servings

Ⓥ *This is a Vegetarian Recipe* Ⓥ

Ingredients:

- ½ teaspoon baking soda
- 1 (14.5-ounce) can diced tomatoes, drained with juice reserved, chopped
- 1 onion, chopped fine
- 1 pound Yukon Gold potatoes, peeled and cut into 1-inch pieces

- 1 tablespoon tomato paste
- 1½ cups water
- 1½ pounds green beans, trimmed and cut into 2-inch lengths
- 2 tablespoons minced fresh oregano or 2 teaspoons dried
- 3 tablespoons chopped fresh basil
- 4 garlic cloves, minced
- 5 tablespoons extra-virgin olive oil
- Lemon juice
- Salt and pepper

Directions:

1. Place oven rack to lower-middle position and pre-heat your oven to 275 degrees. Heat 3 tablespoons oil in a Dutch oven on moderate heat until it starts to shimmer. Put in onion and cook till they become tender, approximately five minutes. Mix in oregano and garlic and cook until aromatic, approximately half a minute. Mix in water, green beans, potatoes, and baking soda, bring to simmer, and cook, stirring intermittently, for about ten minutes.
2. Mix in tomatoes and their juice, tomato paste, 2 teaspoons salt, and ¼ teaspoon pepper. Cover, move pot to oven, and cook until sauce is slightly thickened and green beans can be cut easily with side of fork, forty to fifty minutes.
3. Mix in basil and season with salt, pepper, and lemon juice to taste. Move green beans to serving bowl and drizzle with remaining 2 tablespoons oil. Serve.

Skillet-Roasted Cauliflower Basic

Yield: 4 to 6 Servings

✎ This recipe can be made quickly ✎

Ⓥ This is a Vegetarian Recipe Ⓥ

Ingredients:

- ¼ cup chopped fresh parsley
- 1 garlic clove, minced
- 1 head cauliflower (2 pounds)
- 1 slice hearty white sandwich bread, torn into 1-inch pieces
- 1 teaspoon grated lemon zest, plus lemon wedges for serving
- 5 tablespoons extra-virgin olive oil
- Salt and pepper

Directions:

1. Trim outer leaves of cauliflower and cut stem flush with bottom of head. Turn head so stem is facing down and cut head into ¾-inch-thick slices. Cut around core to remove florets; discard core. Cut large florets into 1½-inch pieces. Move florets to a container, including any small pieces that may have been created during trimming, and set aside.
2. Pulse bread using a food processor to coarse crumbs, approximately ten pulses. Heat bread crumbs, 1 tablespoon oil, pinch salt, and pinch pepper in 12-inch non-stick frying pan on moderate heat, stirring often, until bread crumbs start to look golden brown, 3 to 5 minutes. Move crumbs to a container and wipe frying pan clean using paper towels.
3. Mix 2 tablespoons oil and cauliflower florets in now-empty frying pan and drizzle with 1 teaspoon salt and ½ teaspoon pepper. Cover frying pan and cook on moderate to high heat until florets start to brown and edges just start to become translucent (do not lift lid), approximately five minutes. Remove lid and continue to cook, stirring every 2 minutes, until florets turn golden brown in many spots, about 12 minutes.
4. Push cauliflower to sides of skillet. Put in remaining 2 tablespoons oil, garlic, and lemon zest to center and cook, stirring using a rubber spatula, until aromatic, approximately half a minute. Stir garlic mixture into cauliflower and continue to cook, stirring intermittently, until cauliflower becomes soft but still firm, approximately three minutes. Remove from the heat, mix in parsley and sprinkle with salt and pepper to taste.

Move cauliflower to serving platter and drizzle with bread crumbs. Serve with lemon wedges.

Skillet-Roasted Cauliflower Mix 1

This recipe can be made quickly

Ⓥ This is a Vegetarian Recipe Ⓥ

Refer to the recipe "Skillet-Roasted Cauliflower Basic". Omit bread and reduce oil to ¼ cup. Reduce salt in step 3 to ¾ teaspoon. Substitute 2 tablespoons capers, rinsed and minced, for garlic. Substitute 2 tablespoons minced fresh chives for parsley, and stir ¼ cup toasted pine nuts into cauliflower with chives.

Skillet-Roasted Cauliflower Spicy Mix

This recipe can be made quickly

Ⓥ This is a Vegetarian Recipe Ⓥ

Refer to the recipe "Skillet-Roasted Cauliflower Basic". Omit bread and reduce oil to ¼ cup. Heat 1 teaspoon cumin seeds and 1 teaspoon coriander seeds in 12-inch non-stick frying pan on moderate heat, stirring often, until lightly toasted and aromatic, approximately two minutes. Move to spice grinder or mortar and pestle and coarsely grind. Wipe frying pan clean using paper towels. Substitute ground cumin-coriander mixture, ½ teaspoon paprika, and pinch cayenne pepper for garlic, 1 teaspoon grated lime zest for lemon zest, and 3 tablespoons chopped fresh mint for parsley. Sprinkle cauliflower with ¼ cup pistachios, toasted and chopped, before you serve with lime wedges.

Slow Cooked Braised Fennel

Yield: 6 Servings

Ⓥ This is a Vegetarian Recipe Ⓥ

Ingredients:

- ¼ cup water
- ½ cup dry white wine
- ½ teaspoon grated lemon zest plus 2 teaspoons juice
- 1 head radicchio (10 ounces), cored and sliced thin
- 2 tablespoons pine nuts, toasted and chopped
- 2 teaspoons honey
- 3 fennel bulbs (12 ounces each), 2 tablespoons fronds minced, stalks discarded, bulbs cut vertically into ½-inch-thick slabs
- 3 tablespoons extra-virgin olive oil
- Salt and pepper
- Shaved Parmesan cheese

Directions:

1. Heat oil in 12-inch frying pan on moderate heat until it starts to shimmer. Put in fennel pieces, lemon zest, ½ teaspoon salt, and ¼ teaspoon pepper, then pour wine over fennel. (Skillet will be slightly crowded at first, but fennel will fit into one layer as it cooks.) Cover, decrease the heat to moderate to low, and cook until fennel is just tender, approximately twenty minutes.
2. Increase heat to medium, flip fennel pieces, and continue to cook, uncovered, until fennel is thoroughly browned on first side and liquid is almost completely evaporated, five to ten minutes. Flip fennel pieces and carry on cooking until thoroughly browned on second side, 2 to 4 minutes. Move fennel to serving platter and tent loosely with aluminium foil.
3. Put in radicchio, water, honey, and pinch salt to now-empty frying pan and cook on low heat, scraping up any browned bits, until wilted, 3 to 5 minutes. Remove from the heat, mix in lemon juice and sprinkle with salt and pepper to taste. Arrange

radicchio over fennel and drizzle with pine nuts, minced fennel fronds, and shaved Parmesan. Serve.

Slow-Cooked Whole Carrots Basic

Yield: 4 to 6 Servings

(V) This is a Vegetarian Recipe (V)

Ingredients:

- ½ teaspoon salt
- 1 tablespoon extra-virgin olive oil
- 1½ pounds carrots, peeled

Directions:

1. Cut parchment paper into 11-inch circle, then cut 1-inch hole in center, folding paper as required.
2. Bring 3 cups water, oil, and salt to simmer in 12-inch frying pan on high heat. Remove from the heat, put in carrots, top with parchment, cover skillet, and allow to sit for 20 minutes.
3. Uncover, leaving parchment in place, and bring to simmer on high heat. Decrease heat to moderate to low and cook until most of water has evaporated and carrots are very tender, about 45 minutes.
4. Discard parchment, increase heat to medium-high, and cook carrots, shaking frying pan often, until lightly glazed and no water remains, 2 to 4 minutes. Serve.

Slow-Cooked Whole Carrots Mix 1

(V) This is a Vegetarian Recipe (V)

Refer to the recipe "Slow Cooked Whole Carrots Basic". Microwave ⅓ cup raisins and 1 tablespoon water in a moderate-sized container until hot, approximately one minute; allow to sit for about five minutes. Mix in ½ cup chopped green olives, 1 minced shallot, 2 tablespoons extra-virgin olive oil, 1 tablespoon red wine vinegar, 1 tablespoon minced fresh parsley, ½ teaspoon ground fennel, and ¼ teaspoon salt. Spoon relish over carrots before you serve.

Slow-Cooked Whole Carrots Mix 2

Ⓥ This is a Vegetarian Recipe Ⓥ

Refer to the recipe "Slow Cooked Whole Carrots Basic". Mix ⅓ cup toasted pine nuts, 1 minced shallot, 1 tablespoon sherry vinegar, 1 tablespoon minced fresh parsley, 1 teaspoon honey, ½ teaspoon minced fresh rosemary, ¼ teaspoon smoked paprika, ¼ teaspoon salt, and pinch cayenne pepper in a container. Spoon relish over carrots before you serve.

Slow-Cooked Whole Carrots Mix 3

Ⓥ This is a Vegetarian Recipe Ⓥ

Refer to the recipe "Slow Cooked Whole Carrots Basic". Heat 3 tablespoons extra-virgin olive oil in moderate-sized saucepan on moderate heat until it starts to shimmer. Put in 1 thinly sliceped red onion and ¼ teaspoon salt and cook until soft and well browned, about fifteen minutes. Mix in 2 minced garlic cloves and cook until aromatic, approximately half a minute. Mix in 2 tablespoons balsamic vinegar and cook for about sixty seconds. Allow it to cool for about fifteen minutes. Mix in 2 tablespoons minced fresh mint. Spoon relish over carrots before you serve.

Stuffed Bell Peppers Beef Mix

Yield: 4 Servings

Ingredients:

- ¼ cup currants
- ¼ cup slivered almonds, toasted and chopped
- ¼ teaspoon ground cinnamon
- ½ cup long-grain white rice
- ½ teaspoon red pepper flakes
- ¾ teaspoon ground cardamom
- 1 (14.5-ounce) can diced tomatoes, drained with 2 tablespoons juice reserved
- 1 onion, chopped fine
- 1 tablespoon extra-virgin olive oil, plus extra for serving
- 10 ounces 90 percent lean ground beef
- 2 ounces feta cheese, crumbled (½ cup)
- 2 teaspoons chopped fresh oregano or ½ teaspoon dried
- 2 teaspoons grated fresh ginger
- 2 teaspoons ground cumin
- 3 garlic cloves, minced
- 4 red, yellow, or orange bell peppers, ½ inch trimmed off tops, cores and seeds discarded
- Salt and pepper

Directions:

1. Bring 4 quarts water to boil in large pot. Put in bell peppers and 1 tablespoon salt and cook until just starting to soften, 3 to 5 minutes. Using tongs, remove peppers from pot, drain excess water, and place peppers cut side up on paper towels. Return water to boil, put in rice, and cook until tender, about 13 minutes. Drain rice and move to big container; set aside.
2. Place the oven rack in the centre of the oven and pre-heat your oven to 350 degrees. Heat oil in 12-inch frying pan on moderate to high heat until it starts to shimmer. Put in onion and ¼ teaspoon salt and cook till they become tender and lightly browned, 5 to 7 minutes. Mix in garlic, ginger, cumin, cardamom, pepper flakes, and cinnamon and cook until aromatic, approximately half a minute. Put in ground beef and

cook, breaking up meat with wooden spoon, until no longer pink, about 4 minutes. Remove from the heat, mix in tomatoes and reserved juice, currants, and oregano, scraping up any browned bits. Move mixture to a container with rice. Put in ¼ cup feta and almonds and gently toss to combine. Sprinkle with salt and pepper to taste.
3. Place peppers cut side up in 8-inch square baking dish. Pack each pepper with rice mixture, mounding filling on top. Bake until filling is heated through, approximately half an hour. Sprinkle remaining ¼ cup feta over peppers and drizzle with extra oil. Serve.

Stuffed Bell Peppers Lamb Mix

Refer to the previous recipe. Substitute 10 ounces ground lamb for ground beef. Increase ginger to 1 tablespoon, cumin to 1 tablespoon, cardamom to 1 teaspoon, and cinnamon to ½ teaspoon.

Stuffed Tomato Mix 1

Yield: 6 Servings

Ⓥ This is a Vegetarian Recipe Ⓥ

Ingredients:

- ⅛ teaspoon red pepper flakes
- ¼ cup panko bread crumbs
- ¼ cup pitted kalamata olives, chopped
- ½ teaspoon grated orange zest
- 1 cup couscous
- 1 onion, halved and sliced thin
- 1 tablespoon red wine vinegar
- 1 tablespoon sugar
- 2 garlic cloves, minced

- 3 ounces Manchego cheese, shredded (¾ cup)
- 4½ tablespoons extra-virgin olive oil
- 6 large ripe tomatoes (8 to 10 ounces each)
- 8 ounces (8 cups) baby spinach, chopped coarse
- Kosher salt and pepper

Directions:

1. Place the oven rack in the centre of the oven and pre-heat your oven to 375 degrees. Cut top ½ inch off stem end of tomatoes and set aside. Using melon baller or teaspoon measure, scoop out tomato pulp and move to fine-mesh strainer set over bowl. Press on pulp with wooden spoon to extract juice; set aside juice and discard pulp. (You should have about ⅔ cup tomato juice; if not, put in water as required to equal ⅔ cup.)
2. Mix sugar and 1 tablespoon salt in a container. Sprinkle each tomato cavity with 1 teaspoon sugar mixture, then turn tomatoes upside down on plate to drain for 30 minutes.
3. Mix 1½ teaspoons oil and panko in 10-inch frying pan and toast on moderate to high heat, stirring often, until golden brown, approximately three minutes. Move to a container and allow to cool for about ten minutes. Mix in ¼ cup Manchego.
4. Heat 2 tablespoons oil in now-empty frying pan on moderate heat until it starts to shimmer. Put in onion and ½ teaspoon salt and cook till they become tender, approximately five minutes. Mix in garlic and pepper flakes and cook until aromatic, approximately half a minute. Put in spinach, 1 handful at a time, and cook until wilted, approximately three minutes. Mix in couscous, orange zest, and reserved tomato juice. Cover, remove frying pan from heat, and allow to sit until couscous is tender, approximately seven minutes. Put in olives and remaining ½ cup Manchego to couscous and gently fluff with fork to combine. Sprinkle with salt and pepper to taste.
5. Coat bottom of 13 by 9-inch baking dish with remaining 2 tablespoons oil. Blot tomato cavities dry using paper towels and sprinkle with salt and pepper. Pack each tomato with couscous mixture, about ½ cup per tomato, mounding excess. Top stuffed

tomatoes with 1 heaping tablespoon panko mixture. Place tomatoes in prepared dish. Season reserved tops with salt and pepper and place in empty spaces in dish.
6. Bake, uncovered, until tomatoes have softened but still hold their shape, approximately twenty minutes. Use a slotted spoon to move to serving platter. Beat vinegar into oil remaining in dish, then drizzle over tomatoes. Place tops on tomatoes and serve.

Stuffed Tomato Mix 2

Ⓥ This is a Vegetarian Recipe Ⓥ

Refer to the recipe "Stuffed Tomato Mix 1". Substitute ¾ cup shredded mozzarella cheese for Manchego. Stir 2 tablespoons rinsed capers and 2 tablespoons toasted pine nuts into cooked couscous mixture with mozzarella.

Stuffed Tomatoes Mix 3

Ⓥ This is a Vegetarian Recipe Ⓥ

Refer to the recipe "Stuffed Tomato Mix 1". Substitute ¾ cup crumbled feta cheese for Manchego. Stir 2 tablespoons dried currants and 2 tablespoons chopped pistachios into cooked couscous mixture with feta.

Tangy & Tender Sautéed Spinach

Yield: 4 Servings

This recipe can be made quickly

Ⓥ This is a Vegetarian Recipe Ⓥ

Ingredients:

- ¼ cup dukkah
- ½ cup plain yogurt
- 1½ teaspoons lemon zest plus 1 teaspoon juice
- 2 garlic cloves, minced
- 20 ounces curly-leaf spinach, stemmed
- 3 tablespoons extra-virgin olive oil
- Salt and pepper

Directions:

1. Mix yogurt and lemon zest and juice in a container; set aside for serving. Heat 1 tablespoon oil in a Dutch oven on high heat until it starts to shimmer. Put in spinach, 1 handful at a time, stirring and tossing each handful to wilt slightly before adding more. Cook spinach, stirring continuously, until uniformly wilted, approximately one minute. Move spinach to colander and squeeze between tongs to release excess liquid.
2. Wipe pot dry using paper towels. Put in remaining 2 tablespoons oil and garlic to now-empty pot and cook on moderate heat until aromatic, approximately half a minute. Put in spinach and toss to coat, gently separating leaves to evenly coat with garlic oil. Remove from the heat, sprinkle with salt and pepper to taste. Move spinach to serving platter, drizzle with yogurt sauce, and drizzle with dukkah. Serve.

Tangy Grilled Vegetable Kebabs

Yield: 4 to 6 Servings

✓ This recipe can be made quickly ✓

Ⓥ This is a Vegetarian Recipe Ⓥ

Ingredients:

- ¼ cup extra-virgin olive oil
- 1 garlic clove, minced
- 1 teaspoon Dijon mustard
- 1 teaspoon minced fresh rosemary
- 2 lemons, quartered
- 2 red bell peppers, stemmed, seeded, and cut into 1½-inch pieces
- 2 zucchini, halved along the length and sliced ¾ inch thick
- 6 portobello mushroom caps (4 to 5 inches in diameter), quartered
- Salt and pepper

Directions:

1. Beat oil, mustard, rosemary, garlic, ½ teaspoon salt, and ¼ teaspoon pepper together in a big container. Measure out and reserve half of oil mixture for serving. Toss mushrooms, zucchini, and bell peppers with remaining oil mixture, then thread in alternating order onto eight 12-inch metal skewers.
2. **FOR A CHARCOAL GRILL:** Open bottom vent fully. Light large chimney starter half filled with charcoal briquettes (3 quarts). When top coals are partially covered with ash, pour uniformly over grill. Set cooking grate in place, cover, and open lid vent fully. Heat grill until hot, approximately five minutes. **FOR A GAS GRILL:** Turn all burners to high, cover, and heat grill until hot, about fifteen minutes. Turn all burners to medium.
3. Clean and oil cooking grate. Place kebabs and lemons on grill. Cook (covered if using gas), turning as required, until vegetables are soft and thoroughly browned and lemons are juicy and mildly charred, 16 to 18 minutes.
4. Move kebabs and lemons to serving platter and remove skewers. Juice 2 lemon quarters and beat juice into reserved oil mixture. Sprinkle vegetables with dressing and serve with remaining lemon quarters.

Tomato-Thyme Braised Artichokes

Yield: 4 to 6 Servings

Ingredients:

- ½ cup dry white wine
- 1 cup chicken broth
- 1 lemon
- 1 onion, chopped fine
- 1 teaspoon minced fresh thyme or ¼ teaspoon dried
- 2 anchovy fillets, rinsed, patted dry, and minced
- 2 tablespoons chopped fresh parsley
- 2 tablespoons extra-virgin olive oil
- 3 garlic cloves, minced
- 4 artichokes (8 to 10 ounces each)
- 6 ounces cherry tomatoes, halved
- Salt and pepper

Directions:

1. Cut lemon in half, squeeze halves into container filled with 2 quarts water, then put in spent halves. Working with 1 artichoke at a time, trim stem to about ¾ inch and cut off top quarter of artichoke. Break off bottom 3 or 4 rows of tough outer leaves by pulling them downward. Use a paring knife to trim outer layer of stem and base, removing any dark green parts. Cut artichoke in half along the length, remove fuzzy choke and any tiny inner purple-tinged leaves with the help of a small spoon, then cut each half into 1-inch-thick wedges. Immerse prepped artichokes in lemon water.
2. Heat oil in 12-inch frying pan on moderate heat until it starts to shimmer. Put in onion, ¾ teaspoon salt, and ¼ teaspoon pepper and cook till they become tender and lightly browned, 5 to 7 minutes. Mix in garlic, anchovies, and thyme and cook until aromatic, approximately half a minute. Mix in wine and cook until almost evaporated, approximately one minute. Mix in broth and bring to simmer.

3. Take artichokes out of lemon water, shaking off excess water, and put in to skillet. Cover, decrease the heat to moderate to low, and simmer until artichokes are tender, 20 minutes to half an hour.
4. Mix in tomatoes, bring to simmer, and cook until tomatoes start to break down, 3 to 5 minutes. Remove from the heat, mix in parsley and sprinkle with salt and pepper to taste. Serve.

Tunisian Mechouia

Yield: 4 to 6 Servings

(V) This is a Vegetarian Recipe (V)

Ingredients:

DRESSING

- ⅛ teaspoon cayenne pepper
- ¼ cup chopped fresh cilantro
- ¼ cup chopped fresh parsley
- ½ teaspoon paprika
- 1 teaspoon cumin seeds
- 1 teaspoon grated lemon zest plus 2 tablespoons juice
- 1½ teaspoons caraway seeds
- 2 tablespoons chopped fresh mint
- 2 teaspoons coriander seeds
- 3 garlic cloves, minced
- 5 tablespoons extra-virgin olive oil
- Salt

VEGETABLES

- 1 small eggplant, halved along the length and scored on cut side
- 1 zucchini (8 to 10 ounces), halved along the length and scored on cut side

- 2 red or green bell peppers, tops and bottoms trimmed, stemmed and seeded, and peppers flattened
- 2 shallots, unpeeled
- 4 plum tomatoes, cored and halved along the length
- Salt and pepper

Directions:

1. **FOR THE DRESSING** Grind coriander seeds, caraway seeds, and cumin seeds in spice grinder until finely ground. Beat ground spices, oil, paprika, and cayenne together in a container. Reserve 3 tablespoons oil mixture for brushing vegetables before grilling. Heat remaining oil mixture and garlic in 8-inch frying pan on low heat, stirring intermittently, until aromatic and small bubbles appear, eight to ten minutes. Move to big container, allow to cool for about ten minutes, then beat in parsley, cilantro, mint, and lemon zest and juice and sprinkle with salt to taste; set aside for serving.
2. **FOR THE VEGETABLES** Brush interior of bell peppers and cut sides of eggplant, zucchini, and tomatoes with reserved oil mixture and season with salt.
3. **FOR A CHARCOAL GRILL:** Open bottom vent fully. Light large chimney starter three-quarters filled with charcoal briquettes (4½ quarts). When top coals are partially covered with ash, pour uniformly over grill. Set cooking grate in place, cover, and open lid vent fully. Heat grill until hot, approximately five minutes. **FOR A GAS GRILL:** Turn all burners to high, cover, and heat grill until hot, about fifteen minutes. Turn all burners to medium-high.
4. Clean and oil cooking grate. Place bell peppers, eggplant, zucchini, tomatoes, and shallots cut side down on grill. Cook (covered if using gas), turning as required, until soft and mildly charred, 8 to 16 minutes. Move eggplant, zucchini, tomatoes, and shallots to baking sheet as they finish cooking; place bell peppers in a container, cover up using plastic wrap, and let steam to loosen skins.
5. Let vegetables cool slightly. Peel bell peppers, tomatoes, and shallots. Chop all vegetables into ½-inch pieces, then toss gently

with dressing in a container. Sprinkle with salt and pepper to taste. Serve warm or at room temperature.

Turkish Stuffed Eggplant

Yield: 4 Servings

Ⓥ This is a Vegetarian Recipe Ⓥ

Ingredients:

- ¼ cup water
- ¼ teaspoon ground cinnamon
- ½ cup medium-grind bulgur, rinsed
- 1 onion, chopped fine
- 1 pound plum tomatoes, cored, seeded, and chopped
- 2 ounces Pecorino Romano cheese, grated (1 cup)
- 2 tablespoons extra-virgin olive oil
- 2 tablespoons minced fresh parsley
- 2 tablespoons pine nuts, toasted
- 2 teaspoons minced fresh oregano or ½ teaspoon dried
- 2 teaspoons red wine vinegar
- 3 garlic cloves, minced
- 4 (10-ounce) Italian eggplants, halved along the length
- Pinch cayenne pepper
- Salt and pepper

Directions:

1. Adjust oven racks to upper-middle and lowest positions, place parchment paper–lined rimmed baking sheet on lowest rack, and pre-heat your oven to 400 degrees.
2. Score flesh of each eggplant half in 1-inch diamond pattern, about 1 inch deep. Brush scored sides of eggplant with 1 tablespoon oil and sprinkle with salt and pepper. Lay eggplant cut side down on hot sheet and roast until flesh is tender, forty

to fifty minutes. Move eggplant cut side down to paper towel–lined baking sheet and let drain.
3. Toss bulgur with water in a container and allow to sit until grains are softened and liquid is fully absorbed, 20 to 40 minutes.
4. Heat residual 1 tablespoon oil in 12-inch frying pan on moderate heat until it starts to shimmer. Put in onion and cook till they become tender, 5 minutes. Mix in garlic, oregano, ½ teaspoon salt, cinnamon, and cayenne and cook until aromatic, approximately half a minute. Remove from the heat, mix in bulgur, tomatoes, ¾ cup Pecorino, pine nuts, and vinegar and allow to sit until heated through, approximately one minute. Sprinkle with salt and pepper to taste.
5. Return eggplant cut side up to rimmed baking sheet. Using 2 forks, gently push eggplant flesh to sides to make room for filling. Mound bulgur mixture into eggplant halves and pack lightly with back of spoon. Sprinkle with remaining ¼ cup Pecorino. Bake on upper rack until cheese is melted, 5 to 10 minutes. Sprinkle with parsley and serve.

Zesty Roasted Radicchio, Fennel, and Parsnips

Ⓥ This is a Vegetarian Recipe Ⓥ

Refer to the precious recipe. Substitute 2 fennel bulbs, halved, cored, and sliced into ½-inch wedges, 8 ounces parsnips, peeled and cut into 2-inch pieces, and 1 head radicchio, cored and cut into 2-inch wedges, for Brussels sprouts and carrots. Arrange radicchio in center of baking sheet before roasting. Omit capers and parsley and put in 2 tablespoons chopped fresh basil and 2 tablespoons minced fresh chives to oil mixture in step 3.

Zesty Roasted Root Vegetables

Yield: 4 to 6 Servings

(V) This is a Vegetarian Recipe (V)

Ingredients:

- 1 pound Brussels sprouts, trimmed and halved
- 1 pound red potatoes, unpeeled, cut into 1-inch pieces
- 1 tablespoon lemon juice, plus extra for seasoning
- 1 teaspoon minced fresh rosemary
- 1 teaspoon sugar
- 1½ tablespoons capers, rinsed and minced
- 2 tablespoons minced fresh parsley
- 2 teaspoons minced fresh thyme
- 3 tablespoons extra-virgin olive oil
- 4 carrots, peeled and cut into 2-inch lengths, thick ends halved along the length
- 6 garlic cloves, peeled
- 8 shallots, peeled and halved
- Salt and pepper

Directions:

1. Place the oven rack in the centre of the oven and pre-heat your oven to 450 degrees. Toss Brussels sprouts, potatoes, shallots, and carrots with garlic, 1 tablespoon oil, thyme, rosemary, sugar, ¾ teaspoon salt, and ¼ teaspoon pepper.
2. Lay out vegetables into one layer in rimmed baking sheet, arranging Brussels sprouts cut side down in center of sheet. Roast until vegetables are soft and golden brown, 30 to 35 minutes, rotating sheet halfway through roasting.
3. Beat parsley, capers, lemon juice, and remaining 2 tablespoons oil together in a big container. Put in roasted vegetables and toss to combine. Sprinkle with salt, pepper, and extra lemon juice to taste. Serve.

Zucchini-Feta Fritters

Yield: 4 to 6 Servings

(V) This is a Vegetarian Recipe (V)

Ingredients:

- ¼ cup all-purpose flour
- 1 garlic clove, minced
- 1 pound zucchini, shredded
- 2 large eggs, lightly beaten
- 2 scallions, minced
- 2 tablespoons minced fresh dill
- 4 ounces feta cheese, crumbled (1 cup)
- 6 tablespoons extra-virgin olive oil
- Lemon wedges
- Salt and pepper

Directions:

1. Place the oven rack in the centre of the oven and pre-heat your oven to 200 degrees. Toss zucchini with 1 teaspoon salt and allow to drain using a fine-mesh strainer for about ten minutes.
2. Wrap zucchini in clean dish towel, squeeze out excess liquid, and move to big container. Mix in feta, scallions, eggs, dill, garlic, and ¼ teaspoon pepper. Sprinkle flour over mixture and stir to incorporate.
3. Heat 3 tablespoons oil in 12-inch non-stick frying pan on moderate heat until it starts to shimmer. Drop 2-tablespoon-size portions of batter into frying pan and use back of spoon to press batter into 2-inch-wide fritter (you should fit about 6 fritters in frying pan at a time). Fry until golden brown, approximately three minutes each side.
4. Move fritters to paper towel–lined baking sheet and keep warm in oven. Wipe frying pan clean using paper towels and repeat with remaining 3 tablespoons oil and remaining batter. Serve with lemon wedges.

Vegetable Sauces

Cucumber-Yogurt Sauce

Yield: Approximately 2½ cups

This recipe can be made quickly

Ⓥ *This is a Vegetarian Recipe* Ⓥ

Ingredients:

- 1 cucumber, peeled, halved along the length, seeded, and shredded
- 1 cup plain Greek yogurt
- 1 garlic clove, minced
- 2 tablespoons extra-virgin olive oil
- 2 tablespoons minced fresh dill
- Cilantro, mint, parsley, or tarragon can be substituted for the dill if desired.
- Salt and pepper

Directions:

1. Beat yogurt, oil, dill, and garlic together in a moderate-sized container until combined.
2. Mix in cucumber and sprinkle with salt and pepper to taste. (Sauce will keep safely in a fridge for maximum 1 day.)

Garlic Aïoli

Yield: Approximately 1¼ cups

This recipe can be made quickly

(V) This is a Vegetarian Recipe (V)

Ingredients:

- ¼ cup extra-virgin olive oil
- ¾ cup vegetable oil
- 1 garlic clove, minced
- 1 tablespoon water
- 2 large egg yolks
- 2 teaspoons Dijon mustard
- 2 teaspoons lemon juice
- A combination of vegetable oil and extra-virgin olive oil is crucial to the flavor of the aïoli.
- Salt and pepper

Directions:

1. Process egg yolks, mustard, lemon juice, and garlic using a food processor until combined, about 10 seconds. While your food processor runs slowly drizzle in vegetable oil, approximately one minute. Move mixture to medium bowl and beat in water, ½ teaspoon salt, and ¼ teaspoon pepper.
2. Whisking continuously, slowly drizzle in olive oil until completely blended. (Aïoli will keep safely in a fridge for maximum 4 days.)

Lemon-Yogurt Sauce

Yield: Approximately 1 cup

This recipe can be made quickly

(V) This is a Vegetarian Recipe (V)

Ingredients:

- 1 cup plain yogurt
- 1 garlic clove, minced
- 1 tablespoon minced fresh mint
- 1 teaspoon grated lemon zest plus 2 tablespoons juice
- Salt and pepper

Directions:

1. Beat yogurt, mint, lemon zest and juice, and garlic together in a container until combined.
2. Sprinkle with salt and pepper to taste. Allow to sit until flavours blend, approximately half an hour. (Sauce will keep safely in a fridge for maximum 2 days.)

Tahini Sauce

Yield: Approximately 1¼ cups

✐ *This recipe can be made quickly* ✐

Ⓥ *This is a Vegetarian Recipe* Ⓥ

Ingredients:

- ¼ cup lemon juice (2 lemons)
- ½ cup tahini
- ½ cup water
- 2 garlic cloves, minced
- Salt and pepper

Directions:

1. Beat tahini, water, lemon juice, and garlic together in a container until combined.

2. Sprinkle with salt and pepper to taste. Allow to sit until flavours blend, approximately half an hour. (Sauce will keep safely in a fridge for maximum 4 days.)

Tahini-Yogurt Sauce

Yield: Approximately 1 cup

⚡ This recipe can be made quickly ⚡

Ⓥ This is a Vegetarian Recipe Ⓥ

Ingredients:

- ¼ cup water
- ⅓ cup plain Greek yogurt
- ⅓ cup tahini
- 1 garlic clove, minced
- 3 tablespoons lemon juice
- Salt and pepper

Directions:

1. Beat tahini, yogurt, water, lemon juice, garlic, and ¾ teaspoon salt together in a container until combined.
2. Sprinkle with salt and pepper to taste. Allow to sit until flavours blend, approximately half an hour. (Sauce will keep safely in a fridge for maximum 4 days.)

Yogurt-Herb Sauce

Yield: Approximately 1 cup

⚡ This recipe can be made quickly ⚡

Ⓥ This is a Vegetarian Recipe Ⓥ

Ingredients:

- 1 cup plain yogurt
- 1 garlic clove, minced
- 2 tablespoons minced fresh cilantro
- 2 tablespoons minced fresh mint
- Salt and pepper

Directions:

1. Beat yogurt, cilantro, mint, and garlic together in a container until combined.
2. Sprinkle with salt and pepper to taste. Allow to sit until flavours blend, approximately half an hour. (Sauce will keep safely in a fridge for maximum 2 days.)

Seafood

Seafood is a vital part of the Mediterranean diet, and should be consumed at least twice a week. Make sure the seafood ingredients you use in the recipes are fresh! Feel free to substitute one kind of fish for another in a recipe if you cannot find a particular type of ingredient. Everything works!

Fish

Aromatic Grilled Swordfish Skewers

Yield: 4 to 6 Servings

This recipe can be made quickly

Ingredients:

- ⅛ teaspoon ground nutmeg
- ¼ cup extra-virgin olive oil
- ¼ cup pitted kalamata olives, chopped
- ¼ teaspoon ground cinnamon
- 1 small eggplant (12 ounces), cut crosswise on bias into ½-inch-thick ovals
- 1 tablespoon grated lemon zest, plus 2 lemons, halved
- 1 teaspoon ground cumin
- 1½ pounds skinless swordfish steaks, 1¼ to 1½ inches thick, cut into 1¼-inch pieces
- 1½ tablespoons honey
- 12 ounces cherry tomatoes
- 2 garlic cloves, minced
- 2 tablespoons minced fresh basil
- 5 teaspoons ground coriander
- 6 scallions, trimmed

- Salt and pepper

Directions:

1. Pat swordfish dry using paper towels, rub with 1 tablespoon coriander, and sprinkle with salt and pepper. Thread fish onto three 12-inch metal skewers. Thread tomatoes onto three 12-inch metal skewers. Brush swordfish, tomatoes, eggplant, and scallions with 2 tablespoons oil.
2. **FOR A CHARCOAL GRILL:** Open bottom vent fully. Light large chimney starter filled with charcoal briquettes (6 quarts). When top coals are partly covered with ash, pour uniformly over grill. Set cooking grate in place, cover, and open lid vent fully. Heat grill until hot, approximately five minutes. **FOR A GAS GRILL:** Turn all burners to high, cover, and heat grill until hot, about fifteen minutes. Leave all burners on high.
3. Clean cooking grate, then repetitively brush grate with thoroughly oiled paper towels until black and glossy, 5 to 10 times. Place swordfish, tomatoes, eggplant, scallions, and lemon halves on grill. Cook (covered if using gas), turning as required, until swordfish flakes apart when softly poked using paring knife and registers 140 degrees and tomatoes, eggplant, scallions, and lemon halves are softened and mildly charred, 5 to fifteen minutes. Move items to serving platter as they finish grilling and tent loosely with aluminium foil. Let swordfish rest while finishing caponata.
4. Beat remaining 2 teaspoons coriander, remaining 2 tablespoons oil, lemon zest, honey, garlic, cumin, ¾ teaspoon salt, ¼ teaspoon pepper, cinnamon, and nutmeg together in a big container. Microwave, stirring intermittently, until aromatic, approximately one minute. Once lemons are cool enough to handle, squeeze into fine-mesh strainer set over bowl with oil-honey mixture, extracting as much juice as possible; beat to combine. Mix in olives.
5. Using tongs, slide tomatoes off skewers onto slicing board. Coarsely chop tomatoes, eggplant, and scallions, move to a container with dressing, and gently toss to combine. Sprinkle

with salt and pepper to taste. Remove swordfish from skewers, drizzle with basil, and serve with caponata.

Aromatic Provençal Braised Hake

Yield: 4 Servings

Ingredients:

- ½ cup dry white wine
- 1 (14.5-ounce) can diced tomatoes, drained
- 1 fennel bulb, stalks discarded, bulb halved, cored, and sliced thin
- 1 onion, halved and sliced thin
- 1 teaspoon minced fresh thyme or ¼ teaspoon dried
- 2 tablespoons extra-virgin olive oil, plus extra for serving
- 2 tablespoons minced fresh parsley
- 4 (4- to 6-ounce) skinless hake fillets, 1 to 1½ inches thick
- 4 garlic cloves, minced
- Salt and pepper

Directions:

1. Heat oil in 12-inch frying pan on moderate heat until it starts to shimmer. Put in onion, fennel, and ½ teaspoon salt and cook till they become tender, approximately five minutes. Mix in garlic and thyme and cook until aromatic, approximately half a minute. Mix in tomatoes and wine and bring to simmer.
2. Pat hake dry using paper towels and sprinkle with salt and pepper. Nestle hake skinned side down into skillet, spoon some sauce over top, and bring to simmer. Decrease heat to moderate to low, cover, and cook until hake flakes apart when softly poked using paring knife and registers 140 degrees, 10 to 12 minutes.
3. Cautiously move hake to individual shallow bowls. Stir parsley into sauce and sprinkle with salt and pepper to taste. Spoon sauce over hake and drizzle with extra oil. Serve.

Aromatic Sicilian Fish Stew

Yield: 4 to 6 Servings

Ingredients:

- ¼ cup chopped fresh mint
- ¼ cup golden raisins
- ¼ cup pine nuts, toasted
- ½ cup dry white wine
- 1 (28-ounce) can whole peeled tomatoes, drained with juice reserved, chopped coarse
- 1 celery rib, minced
- 1 teaspoon grated orange zest
- 1 teaspoon minced fresh thyme or ¼ teaspoon dried
- 1½ pounds skinless swordfish steaks, 1 to 1 ½ inches thick, cut into 1-inch pieces
- 2 (8-ounce) bottles clam juice
- 2 onions, chopped fine
- 2 tablespoons capers, rinsed
- 2 tablespoons extra-virgin olive oil
- 4 garlic cloves, minced
- Pinch red pepper flakes
- Salt and pepper

Directions:

1. Mix pine nuts, mint, one-quarter of garlic, and orange zest in a container; set aside for serving. Heat oil in a Dutch oven on moderate heat until it starts to shimmer. Put in onions, celery, ½ teaspoon salt, and ¼ teaspoon pepper and cook till they become tender, approximately five minutes. Mix in thyme, pepper flakes, and remaining garlic and cook until aromatic, approximately half a minute.
2. Mix in wine and reserved tomato juice, bring to simmer, and cook until reduced by half, about 4 minutes. Mix in tomatoes,

clam juice, raisins, and capers, bring to simmer, and cook until flavours blend, about fifteen minutes.
3. Pat swordfish dry using paper towels and sprinkle with salt and pepper. Nestle swordfish into pot and spoon some cooking liquid over top. Bring to simmer and cook for 4 minutes. Remove from the heat, cover and allow to sit until swordfish flakes apart when softly poked using paring knife, approximately three minutes. Sprinkle with salt and pepper to taste. Serve, sprinkling individual bowls with pine nut mixture.

Braised Halibut

Yield: 4 Servings

Use Sea Bass if you can't find halibut.

Ingredients:

- ¼ cup extra-virgin olive oil, plus extra for serving
- ¾ cup dry white wine
- 1 pound leeks, white and light green parts only, halved along the length, sliced thin, and washed thoroughly
- 1 tablespoon minced fresh parsley
- 1 teaspoon Dijon mustard
- 4 (4- to 6-ounce) skinless halibut fillets, ¾ to 1 inch thick
- Lemon wedges
- Salt and pepper

Directions:

1. Pat halibut dry using paper towels and drizzle with ½ teaspoon salt. Heat oil in 12-inch frying pan on moderate heat until warm, approximately fifteen seconds. Place halibut skinned side up in frying pan and cook until bottom half of halibut begins to turn opaque (halibut should not brown), about 4 minutes. Cautiously move halibut raw side down to large plate.

2. Put in leeks, mustard, and ¼ teaspoon salt to oil left in frying pan and cook on moderate heat, stirring often, till they become tender, 10 to 12 minutes. Mix in wine and bring to simmer. Place halibut raw side down on top of leeks. Decrease heat to moderate to low, cover, and simmer gently until halibut flakes apart when softly poked using paring knife and registers 140 degrees, 6 to 10 minutes. Cautiously move halibut to serving platter, tent loosely with aluminium foil, and allow to rest while finishing leeks.
3. Return leeks to high heat and simmer briskly until mixture becomes thick slightly, 2 to 4 minutes. Sprinkle with salt and pepper to taste. Arrange leek mixture around halibut, drizzle with extra oil, and drizzle with parsley. Serve with lemon wedges.

Broiled Grouper Wrap

Yield: 4 Servings

If you can't find the Grouper, feel free to use Snapper or sea bass instead.

Ingredients:

- ½ cup Tahini-Lemon Dressing
- ½ teaspoon pepper
- ½ teaspoon salt
- 1 (16-ounce) jar grape leaves
- 1 tablespoon capers, rinsed and minced
- 1 teaspoon grated lemon zest
- 2 tablespoons minced fresh parsley
- 3 tablespoons extra-virgin olive oil, plus extra for brushing
- 4 (4- to 6-ounce) skinless grouper fillets, ¾ to 1 inch thick

Directions:

1. Beat oil, parsley, capers, lemon zest, salt, and pepper together in medium bowl. Put in grouper and gently turn to coat. Cover and put in the fridge while preparing grape leaves.
2. Reserve 24 undamaged grape leaves, approximately 6 inches in diameter; save for later rest of the leaves for another use. Bring 8 cups water to boil in a big saucepan. Put in grape leaves and cook for about five minutes. Gently drain leaves and move to a container of cold water to cool, approximately five minutes. Drain again thoroughly.
3. Place oven rack 8 inches from broiler element and heat broiler. Set wire rack in rimmed baking sheet and spray using vegetable oil spray. Shingle 5 leaves smooth side down on counter into 9-inch circle with stems pointing toward center of circle, then place 1 leaf smooth side down over opening in center. Place 1 fillet in center of leaf circle and spoon portion of remaining marinade on top. Fold sides of leaf circle over grouper, then fold up bottom of circle and continue to roll tightly into packet. Move packet seam side down to prepared rack. Replicate the process with the rest of the grape leaves, fillets, and marinade.
4. Pat tops of grouper packets dry using paper towels and brush with extra oil. Broil until grape leaves are crisp and mildly charred and grouper registers 140 degrees, 12 to 18 minutes, rotating sheet halfway through broiling. Serve with Tahini-Lemon Dressing.

Charred Whole Sardines

Yield: 4 to 6 Servings

✦ This recipe can be made quickly ✦

Ingredients:

- ½ teaspoon honey
- 12 (2- to 3-ounce) whole sardines, scaled, gutted, fins snipped off with scissors
- 2 tablespoons mayonnaise

- Lemon wedges
- Pepper

Directions:

1. Wash each sardine under cold running water and pat dry using paper towels inside and out. Open cavity of each sardine and season flesh with pepper. Mix mayonnaise and honey, then brush mixture uniformly exterior of each fish.
2. **FOR A CHARCOAL GRILL**: Open bottom vent fully. Light large chimney starter filled with charcoal briquettes (6 quarts). When top coals are partly covered with ash, pour uniformly over grill. Set cooking grate in place, cover, and open lid vent fully. Heat grill until hot, approximately five minutes. **FOR A GAS GRILL**: Turn all burners to high, cover, and heat grill until hot, about fifteen minutes. Leave all burners on high.
3. Clean cooking grate, then repetitively brush grate with thoroughly oiled paper towels until grate is black and glossy, 5 to 10 times. Place sardines on grill and cook (covered if using gas) until skin is browned and starting to blister, 2 to 4 minutes. Gently flip sardines using spatula and carry on cooking until second side is browned and starting to blister, 2 to 4 minutes. Serve with lemon wedges.

Classic Provençal Bouillabaisse

Yield: 6 to 8 Servings

Ingredients:

- ⅛ teaspoon red pepper flakes
- ¼ cup extra-virgin olive oil
- ¼ teaspoon saffron threads, crumbled
- ¾ cup dry white wine or dry vermouth
- 1 (14.5-ounce) can whole peeled tomatoes, drained with juice reserved, chopped
- 1 onion, chopped fine

- 1 pound large sea scallops, tendons removed
- 1 pound skinless halibut fillets, ¾ to 1 inch thick, cut into 3- to 4-inch pieces
- 1 small fennel bulb, stalks discarded, bulb halved, cored, and chopped fine
- 1 teaspoon minced fresh thyme or ¼ teaspoon dried
- 12 ounces mussels, scrubbed and debearded
- 2 (8-ounce) bottles clam juice
- 2 bay leaves
- 2 tablespoons minced fresh tarragon
- 8 garlic cloves, minced
- 8 ounces medium-large shrimp (31 to 40 per pound), peeled and deveined
- Salt and pepper

Directions:

1. Heat oil in a Dutch oven on moderate to high heat until it starts to shimmer. Put in fennel and onion and cook till they become tender, approximately five minutes. Mix in garlic, thyme, saffron, and pepper flakes and cook until aromatic, approximately half a minute. Mix in wine and cook until slightly reduced, approximately half a minute.
2. Mix in clam juice, tomatoes with their juice, and bay leaves. Bring to simmer and cook until liquid has reduced by about half, seven to nine minutes.
3. Pat halibut dry using paper towels and sprinkle with salt and pepper. Nestle halibut into pot, spoon some cooking liquid over top, and bring to simmer. Decrease heat to moderate to low, cover, and simmer slowly for 2 minutes. Nestle mussels and scallops into pot, cover, and carry on cooking until halibut is almost cooked through, approximately three minutes.
4. Arrange shrimp uniformly over stew, cover, and carry on cooking until halibut flakes apart when softly poked using paring knife, shrimp and scallops are firm and opaque in center, and mussels have opened, approximately two minutes.

5. Remove from the heat, discard bay leaves and any mussels that refuse to open. Gently mix in tarragon and sprinkle with salt and pepper to taste. Serve in wide, shallow bowls.

Easy-Roasted Halibut with Chermoula

Yield: 8 Servings

✒ This recipe can be made quickly ✒

Ingredients:

CHERMOULA

- ⅛ teaspoon cayenne pepper
- ¼ cup extra-virgin olive oil
- ¼ teaspoon salt
- ½ teaspoon ground cumin
- ½ teaspoon paprika
- ¾ cup fresh cilantro leaves
- 2 tablespoons lemon juice
- 4 garlic cloves, minced

FISH

- 2 (1¼-pound) skin-on full halibut steaks, 1 to 1½ inches thick and 10 to 12 inches long, trimmed
- 2 tablespoons extra-virgin olive oil
- Salt and pepper

Directions:

1. **FOR THE CHERMOULA**: Process all ingredients using a food processor until smooth, approximately one minute, scraping down sides of the container as required; set aside for serving.
2. **FOR THE FISH**: Place the oven rack in the centre of the oven and pre-heat your oven to 325 degrees. Pat halibut dry using paper towels and sprinkle with salt and pepper. Heat oil in 12-inch

oven-safe non-stick frying pan on moderate to high heat until just smoking. Place halibut in frying pan and cook until thoroughly browned on first side, approximately five minutes.
3. Gently flip halibut using 2 spatulas and move frying pan to oven. Roast until halibut flakes apart when softly poked using paring knife and registers 140 degrees, 6 to 9 minutes.
4. Cautiously move halibut to slicing board, tent loosely with aluminium foil, and allow to rest for about five minutes. Remove skin from steaks and separate each quadrant of meat from bones by slipping knife or spatula between them. Serve with chermoula.

Easy-Roasted Monkfish

Yield: 4 Servings

This recipe can be made quickly

Ingredients:

- ¼ cup extra-virgin olive oil
- ¼ cup pitted kalamata olives, minced
- ½ teaspoon sugar
- 1 small shallot, minced
- 1 teaspoon Dijon mustard
- 2 tablespoons minced fresh oregano
- 2 tablespoons red wine vinegar
- 4 (4- to 6-ounce) skinless monkfish fillets, 1 to 1½ inches thick, trimmed
- Salt and pepper

Directions:

1. Mix 2 tablespoons oil and oregano in a moderate-sized container and microwave until bubbling, approximately half a minute. Let mixture steep for about five minutes, then beat in

vinegar, shallot, mustard, and ¼ teaspoon pepper. Mix in olives and set aside for serving.
2. Place the oven rack in the centre of the oven and pre-heat your oven to 425 degrees. Pat monkfish dry using paper towels, sprinkle with salt and pepper, and drizzle evenly with sugar.
3. Heat remaining 2 tablespoons oil in 12-inch oven-safe frying pan on moderate to high heat until just smoking. Place monkfish in frying pan and press lightly to ensure even contact with skillet. Cook until browned on first side, approximately two minutes. Gently flip monkfish using 2 spatulas and cook until browned on second side, approximately two minutes. Move frying pan to oven and roast until monkfish is opaque in center and registers 160 degrees, 8 to 12 minutes. Cautiously move monkfish to serving platter, tent loosely with aluminium foil, and allow to rest for about five minutes. Serve with relish.

French Swordfish en Cocotte

Yield: 4 Servings

Ingredients:

- ¼ cup fresh parsley leaves
- ¼ teaspoon cayenne pepper
- ¾ cup fresh mint leaves
- 1 cucumber, peeled, seeded, and sliced thin
- 1 teaspoon ground cumin
- 2 tablespoons lemon juice
- 3 shallots, sliced thin
- 4 (4- to 6-ounce) skin-on swordfish steaks, 1 to 1½ inches thick
- 4 garlic cloves, minced
- 5 tablespoons extra-virgin olive oil
- Salt and pepper

Directions:

1. Place oven rack on the lowest position and pre-heat your oven to 250 degrees. Process mint, parsley, 3 tablespoons oil, lemon juice, garlic, cumin, cayenne, and ¼ teaspoon salt using a food processor until smooth, approximately half a minute, scraping down sides of the container as required.
2. Heat remaining 2 tablespoons oil in a Dutch oven over moderate to low heat until it starts to shimmer. Put in shallots, cover, and cook, stirring intermittently, till they become tender, approximately five minutes. Remove from the heat, mix in processed mint mixture and cucumber.
3. Pat swordfish dry using paper towels and sprinkle with salt and pepper. Place swordfish on top of cucumber-mint mixture. Place large sheet of aluminium foil over pot and press to seal, then cover firmly with lid. Move pot to oven and cook until swordfish flakes apart when softly poked using paring knife and registers 140 degrees, 35 to 40 minutes.
4. Cautiously move swordfish to serving platter. Season cucumber-mint mixture with salt and pepper to taste, then spoon over swordfish. Serve.

Grilled Swordfish Salad

Yield: 4 Servings

This recipe can be made quickly

Ingredients:

- ⅛ teaspoon ground cinnamon
- ¼ teaspoon cayenne pepper
- ½ red onion, chopped coarse
- 1 (15-ounce) can chickpeas, rinsed
- 1 cup fresh cilantro leaves
- 1 large eggplant, sliced into ½-inch-thick rounds
- 1 teaspoon ground cumin
- 1 teaspoon paprika

- 3 tablespoons lemon juice
- 4 (4- to 6-ounce) skin-on swordfish steaks, 1 to 1½ inches thick
- 4 garlic cloves, chopped
- 6 ounces cherry tomatoes, halved
- 6 tablespoons extra-virgin olive oil
- Salt and pepper

Directions:

1. Process cilantro, onion, 3 tablespoons oil, lemon juice, garlic, cumin, paprika, cayenne, cinnamon, and ½ teaspoon salt using a food processor until smooth, approximately two minutes, scraping down sides of the container as required. Measure out and reserve ½ cup cilantro mixture. Move remaining cilantro mixture to big container and set aside.
2. Brush swordfish with reserved ½ cup cilantro mixture. Brush eggplant with remaining 3 tablespoons oil and sprinkle with salt and pepper.
3. **FOR A CHARCOAL GRILL:** Open bottom vent fully. Light large chimney starter filled with charcoal briquettes (6 quarts). When top coals are partly covered with ash, pour two-thirds uniformly over half of grill, then pour remaining coals over other half of grill. Set cooking grate in place, cover, and open lid vent fully. Heat grill until hot, approximately five minutes. **FOR A GAS GRILL:** Turn all burners to high, cover, and heat grill until hot, about fifteen minutes. Leave primary burner on high and turn other burner(s) to moderate to high.
4. Clean cooking grate, then repetitively brush grate with thoroughly oiled paper towels until black and glossy, 5 to 10 times. Place swordfish and eggplant on hotter part of grill. Cook swordfish, uncovered, until dark grill marks appear, 6 to 9 minutes, gently flipping steaks using 2 spatulas halfway through cooking. Cook eggplant, flipping as required, till they become tender and mildly charred, approximately eight minutes; move to serving platter and tent loosely with aluminium foil.
5. Gently move swordfish to cooler part of grill and continue to cook, uncovered, until fish flakes apart when softly poked using

paring knife and registers 140 degrees, 1 to 3 minutes each side; move to platter and tent loosely with foil. Let swordfish rest while finishing salad.
6. Coarsely chop eggplant and put in to a container with cilantro mixture along with tomatoes and chickpeas. Gently toss to combine and sprinkle with salt and pepper to taste. Serve.

Grilled Swordfish with Italian Salsa Verde

Yield: 4 Servings

✎This recipe can be made quickly✎

Ingredients:

- ½ cup Italian Salsa Verde
- 2 tablespoons extra-virgin olive oil
- 4 (4- to 6-ounce) skin-on swordfish steaks, 1 to 1½ inches thick
- Salt and pepper

Directions:

1. Pat swordfish dry using paper towels, rub with oil, and sprinkle with salt and pepper.
2. **FOR A CHARCOAL GRILL:** Open bottom vent fully. Light large chimney starter filled with charcoal briquettes (6 quarts). When top coals are partly covered with ash, pour two-thirds uniformly over half of grill, then pour remaining coals over other half of grill. Set cooking grate in place, cover, and open lid vent fully. Heat grill until hot, approximately five minutes. **FOR A GAS GRILL:** Turn all burners to high, cover, and heat grill until hot, about fifteen minutes. Leave primary burner on high and turn other burner(s) to moderate to high.
3. Clean cooking grate, then repetitively brush grate with thoroughly oiled paper towels until black and glossy, 5 to 10

times. Place swordfish on hotter part of grill and cook, uncovered, until dark grill marks appear, 6 to 9 minutes, gently flipping steaks using 2 spatulas halfway through cooking.
4. Gently move swordfish to cooler part of grill and continue to cook, uncovered, until fish flakes apart when softly poked using paring knife and registers 140 degrees, 1 to 3 minutes each side. Serve with Italian Salsa Verde.

Grilled Tuna Steaks

Yield: 4 Servings

✒ This recipe can be made quickly ✒

Ingredients:

- ⅛ teaspoon cayenne pepper
- ¼ cup extra-virgin olive oil
- 1 cup jarred roasted red peppers, rinsed, patted dry, and chopped coarse
- 1 garlic clove, minced
- 1 plum tomato, cored, seeded, and chopped
- 1 slice hearty white sandwich bread, crusts removed, bread lightly toasted and cut into ½-inch pieces (½ cup)
- 1 teaspoon water
- 1½ tablespoons slivered almonds, toasted
- 2 (8- to 12-ounce) skinless tuna steaks, 1 inch thick, halved crosswise
- 2 teaspoons honey
- 2¼ teaspoons sherry vinegar
- Salt and pepper

Directions:

1. Process bread and almonds using a food processor until nuts are finely ground, 10 to 15 seconds. Put in red peppers, tomato, 1 tablespoon oil, vinegar, garlic, cayenne, and ½ teaspoon salt.

Process until smooth and mixture has texture similar to mayonnaise, 20 to 30 seconds, scraping down sides of the container as required. Sprinkle with salt to taste; set aside for serving.
2. Beat remaining 3 tablespoons oil, honey, water, ½ teaspoon salt, and pinch pepper together in a container. Pat tuna dry using paper towels and heavily brush with oil mixture.
3. FOR A CHARCOAL GRILL Open bottom vent fully. Light large chimney starter filled with charcoal briquettes (6 quarts). When top coals are partly covered with ash, pour uniformly over half of grill. Set cooking grate in place, cover, and open lid vent fully. Heat grill until hot, approximately five minutes. FOR A GAS GRILL Turn all burners to high, cover, and heat grill until hot, about fifteen minutes. Leave all burners on high.
4. Clean cooking grate, then repetitively brush grate with thoroughly oiled paper towels until grate is black and glossy, 5 to 10 times. Place tuna on grill (on hotter side if using charcoal) and cook (covered if using gas) until opaque and streaked with dark grill marks on first side, 1 to 3 minutes. Gently flip tuna using 2 spatulas and carry on cooking until opaque at perimeter and translucent red at center when checked with tip of paring knife and registers 110 degrees (for rare), about 1½ minutes, or until opaque at perimeter and reddish pink at center when checked with tip of paring knife and registers 125 degrees (for medium-rare), approximately three minutes. Serve with sauce.

Grilled Whole Mackerel Variation 1

This recipe can be made quickly

Substitute 1 teaspoon ground fennel seeds for marjoram and 1 teaspoon grated orange zest for lemon zest.

Grilled Whole Mackerel Variation 2

This recipe can be made quickly

Substitute 1 teaspoon ground coriander for marjoram and 1 teaspoon grated lime zest and wedges for lemon zest and wedges.

Grilled Whole Mackerel with Lemon and Marjoram

Yield: 4 Servings

This recipe can be made quickly

Ingredients:

- ½ teaspoon honey
- 1 (13 by 9-inch) disposable aluminium roasting pan (if using charcoal)
- 1 teaspoon grated lemon zest, plus lemon wedges for serving
- 2 tablespoons mayonnaise
- 2 teaspoons chopped fresh marjoram
- 4 (8- to 10-ounce) whole mackerel, gutted, fins snipped off with scissors
- Salt and pepper

Directions:

1. Place marjoram, lemon zest, and 1 teaspoon salt on slicing board and chop until finely minced and thoroughly mixed. Wash each mackerel under cold running water and pat dry using paper towels inside and out. Open cavity of each mackerel, season flesh with pepper, and drizzle evenly with marjoram mixture; allow to sit for about ten minutes. Mix mayonnaise and honey, then brush mixture uniformly exterior of each fish.

2. **FOR A CHARCOAL GRILL:** Using kitchen shears, poke twelve ½-inch holes in bottom of disposable pan. Open bottom vent completely and place prepared pan in center of grill. Light large chimney starter two-thirds filled with charcoal briquettes (4 quarts). When top coals are partly covered with ash, pour into even layer in pan. Set cooking grate over coals with bars parallel to long side of pan, cover, and open lid vent fully. Heat grill until hot, approximately five minutes. **FOR A GAS GRILL:** Turn all burners to high, cover, and heat grill until hot, about fifteen minutes. Leave all burners on high.
3. Clean cooking grate, then repetitively brush grate with thoroughly oiled paper towels until grate is black and glossy, 5 to 10 times. Place mackerel on grill (directly over coals if using charcoal) and cook (covered if using gas) until skin is browned and starting to blister on first side, 2 to 4 minutes. Using spatula, lift bottom of thick backbone edge of mackerel from cooking grate just enough to slide second spatula under fish. Remove first spatula, then use it to support raw side of mackerel as you use second spatula to flip fish over. Cook until second side is browned and starting to blister and thickest part of mackerel registers 130 to 135 degrees, 2 to 4 minutes. Cautiously move mackerel to serving platter and allow to rest for about five minutes. Serve with lemon wedges.

Italian Grilled Whole Sea Bass

Yield: 4 Servings

✒ This recipe can be made quickly ✒

Ingredients:

SALMORIGLIO SAUCE

- ⅛ teaspoon pepper
- ⅛ teaspoon salt
- ¼ cup extra-virgin olive oil

- 1 small garlic clove, minced
- 1 tablespoon lemon juice
- 1½ tablespoons minced fresh oregano

FISH

- 2 (1½- to 2-pound) whole sea bass, scaled, gutted, fins snipped off with scissors
- 3 tablespoons extra-virgin olive oil
- Salt and pepper

Directions:

1. **FOR THE SALMORIGLIO SAUCE:** Beat all ingredients together in a container until combined; cover and set aside for serving.
2. **FOR A CHARCOAL GRILL:** Open bottom vent fully. Light large chimney starter filled with charcoal briquettes (6 quarts). When top coals are partly covered with ash, pour uniformly over grill. Set cooking grate in place, cover, and open lid vent fully. Heat grill until hot, approximately five minutes. **FOR A GAS GRILL:** Turn all burners to high, cover, and heat grill until hot, about fifteen minutes. Leave all burners on high.
3. Wash each sea bass under cold running water and pat dry using paper towels inside and out. Using sharp knife, make 3 or 4 shallow slashes, about 2 inches apart, on both sides of sea bass. Rub sea bass with oil and season heavily with salt and pepper inside and outside.
4. Clean cooking grate, then repetitively brush grate with thoroughly oiled paper towels until black and glossy, 5 to 10 times. Place sea bass on grill and cook (covered if using gas) until skin is browned and starting to blister on first side, six to eight minutes. Using spatula, lift bottom of thick backbone edge of sea bass from cooking grate just enough to slide second spatula under fish. Remove first spatula, then use it to support raw side of sea bass as you use second spatula to flip fish over. Cook (covered if using gas) until second side is browned, starting to blister, and sea bass registers 140 degrees, six to eight minutes.

5. Cautiously move sea bass to carving board and allow to rest for about five minutes. Fillet sea bass by making vertical cut just behind head from top of fish to belly. Make another cut on top of sea bass from head to tail. Use spatula to lift meat from bones, starting at head end and running spatula over bones to lift out fillet. Repeat on other side of sea bass. Discard head and skeleton. Serve with sauce.

Poached Snapper

Yield: 4 Servings

Ingredients:

FISH

- ½ onion, peeled
- ¾ cup extra-virgin olive oil
- 1 cup jarred whole baby artichokes packed in water, quartered, rinsed, and patted dry
- 1 tablespoon cornstarch
- 3 garlic cloves, minced
- 4 (4- to 6-ounce) skinless red snapper fillets, about 1 inch thick
- Salt

VINAIGRETTE

- ½ small shallot, peeled
- 1 tablespoon minced fresh parsley
- 4 teaspoons sherry vinegar
- 6 ounces cherry tomatoes (2 ounces cut into ⅛-inch-thick rounds)
- Salt and pepper

Directions:

1. **FOR THE FISH:** Adjust oven racks to middle and lower-middle positions and pre-heat your oven to 250 degrees. Pat snapper

dry using paper towels and season each fillet with ⅛ teaspoon salt. Allow to sit at room temperature for 20 minutes.

2. In the meantime, toss artichokes with cornstarch in a container to coat. Heat ½ cup oil in 10-inch oven-safe non-stick frying pan on moderate heat until it starts to shimmer. Shake excess cornstarch from artichokes and put in to skillet. Cook, stirring intermittently, until crisp and golden, 2 to 4 minutes. Put in garlic and carry on cooking until garlic is golden, 30 to 60 seconds. Strain oil through fine-mesh strainer into a container. Move artichokes and garlic to oven-safe plate coated using paper towels and season with salt. Do not wash strainer.

3. Return strained oil to now-empty frying pan and put in remaining ¼ cup oil. Place onion half in center of skillet. Let oil cool until it registers about 180 degrees, five to ten minutes. Arrange fillets skinned side up around onion (oil should come approximately halfway up fillets) and spoon some oil over each fillet. Cover, move frying pan to upper rack, and cook for about fifteen minutes.

4. Using potholders, remove frying pan from oven. Being careful of hot frying pan handle, gently flip fillets using 2 spatulas. Cover, return frying pan to upper rack, and place plate with artichokes and garlic on lower rack. Continue to bake snapper until it registers 130 to 135 degrees, 9 to 14 minutes. Cautiously move snapper to serving platter, reserving ½ cup oil, and tent loosely with aluminium foil. Turn off oven, leaving plate of artichokes in oven.

5. **FOR THE VINAIGRETTE**: Process reserved ½ cup fish cooking oil, whole tomatoes, shallot, vinegar, ½ teaspoon pepper, and ¼ teaspoon salt using a blender until smooth, approximately two minutes, scraping down sides of the container as required. Put in any accumulated fish juices, sprinkle with salt to taste, and blend for 10 seconds. Strain sauce through fine-mesh strainer into a container; discard solids. To serve, spoon vinaigrette around fish. Garnish each fillet with warmed crisped artichokes and garlic, parsley, and tomato rounds. Serve.

Quick-Roasted Sea Bass

Yield: 4 Servings

✎This recipe can be made quickly ✎

Ingredients:

- ½ teaspoon sugar
- 1 tablespoon extra-virgin olive oil
- 4 (4- to 6-ounce) skinless sea bass fillets, 1 to 1½ inches thick
- Lemon wedges
- Salt and pepper

Directions:

1. Place the oven rack in the centre of the oven and pre-heat your oven to 425 degrees. Pat sea bass dry using paper towels, sprinkle with salt and pepper, and drizzle sugar uniformly 1 side of each fillet.
2. Heat oil in 12-inch oven-safe frying pan on moderate to high heat until just smoking. Place sea bass sugared side down in frying pan and press lightly to ensure even contact with skillet. Cook until browned on first side, approximately two minutes. Gently flip sea bass using 2 spatulas, move frying pan to oven, and roast until fish flakes apart when softly poked using paring knife and registers 140 degrees, 7 to 10 minutes. Serve with lemon wedges.

Quick-Roasted Sea Bass with Orange Relish

✎This recipe can be made quickly ✎

Pulse ½ cup toasted slivered almonds, ½ cup pitted brine-cured green olives, chopped coarse, 1 small minced garlic clove, and 1 teaspoon grated orange zest using a food processor until thinly sliceped, 10 to 12 pulses. Move to a container and mix in ¼ cup orange juice, ¼ cup extra-virgin olive oil, ¼ cup minced fresh mint, and 2 teaspoons white wine vinegar. Sprinkle with salt and cayenne to taste. Serve with fish.

Quick-Roasted Sea Bass with Thyme Relish

This recipe can be made quickly

Pulse ½ cup toasted and skinned hazelnuts, ½ cup jarred roasted red peppers, rinsed, patted dry, and chopped coarse, 1 minced garlic clove, and ½ teaspoon grated lemon zest using a food processor until thinly sliceped, 10 to 12 pulses. Move to a container and mix in ¼ cup extra-virgin olive oil, 2 tablespoons chopped fresh parsley, 4 teaspoons lemon juice, 1 teaspoon minced fresh thyme, and ¼ teaspoon smoked paprika. Sprinkle with salt and pepper to taste. Serve with fish.

Quick-Roasted Sea Bass with Wild Mushrooms

Yield: 4 Servings

Ingredients:

- ¼ cup extra virgin olive oil, plus extra for serving
- ⅓ ounce dried porcini mushrooms
- ½ cup water
- 1 pound cremini mushrooms, trimmed and halved if small or quartered if large
- 1 red onion, halved and sliced thin
- 1 sprig fresh rosemary

- 1 tablespoon minced fresh parsley
- 12 ounces portobello mushroom caps, halved and sliced ½ inch thick
- 2 garlic cloves, minced
- 4 (4- to 6-ounce) skinless sea bass fillets, 1 to 1½ inches thick
- Lemon wedges
- Salt and pepper

Directions:

1. Microwave water and porcini mushrooms in covered bowl until steaming, approximately one minute. Allow to sit till they become tender, approximately five minutes. Drain mushrooms using a fine-mesh strainer lined with coffee filter, reserve porcini liquid, and mince mushrooms.
2. Place oven rack to lower-middle position and pre-heat your oven to 475 degrees. Pat sea bass dry using paper towels, rub with 2 tablespoons oil, and sprinkle with salt and pepper.
3. Heat remaining 2 tablespoons oil and rosemary in 12-inch oven-safe frying pan on moderate to high heat until it starts to shimmer. Put in onion, portobello mushrooms, cremini mushrooms, and ½ teaspoon salt. Cook, stirring intermittently, until mushrooms have released their liquid and are starting to brown, eight to ten minutes. Mix in garlic and porcini mushrooms and cook until aromatic, approximately half a minute.
4. Remove from the heat, mix in reserved porcini liquid. Nestle sea bass skinned side down into skillet, move to oven, and roast until fish flakes apart when softly poked using paring knife and registers 140 degrees, 10 to 12 minutes. Sprinkle with parsley and drizzle with extra oil. Serve with lemon wedges.

Sautéed Sole

Yield: 4 Servings

✏This recipe can be made quickly✏

Ingredients:

- ¼ cup extra-virgin olive oil
- ½ cup all-purpose flour
- 8 (2- to 3-ounce) skinless sole fillets, ¼ to ½ inch thick
- Lemon wedges
- Salt and pepper

Directions:

1. Place flour in shallow dish. Pat sole dry using paper towels and sprinkle with salt and pepper. Working with 1 fillet at a time, dredge in flour to coat, shaking off any excess.
2. Heat 2 tablespoons oil in 12-inch non-stick frying pan on moderate to high heat until it starts to shimmer. Place half of sole in frying pan and cook until lightly browned on first side, 2 to 3 minutes. Gently flip sole using 2 spatulas and carry on cooking until fish flakes apart when softly poked using paring knife, 30 to 60 seconds.
3. Cautiously move sole to serving platter and tent loosely with aluminium foil. Wipe frying pan clean using paper towels and repeat with remaining 2 tablespoons oil and fillets. Serve with lemon wedges.

Tomato Relish

✏This recipe can be made quickly✏

This relish is a great accompaniment to simple seafood dishes.

Mix 2 ripe tomatoes, cored, seeded, and cut into ¼-inch pieces, 1 small minced shallot, 2 tablespoons chopped fresh basil, 1 tablespoon extra-virgin olive oil, 1 small minced garlic clove, and 1 teaspoon red wine vinegar in a container. Allow to sit for about fifteen minutes. Sprinkle with salt and pepper to taste. Serve over sole.

Grapefruit and Basil Relish

This recipe can be made quickly

This relish is a great accompaniment to simple seafood dishes.

Cut away peel and pith from 2 red grapefruits. Cut each grapefruit into 8 wedges, then slice wedges crosswise into ½-inch-thick pieces. Place grapefruit in strainer set over bowl and allow to drain for about fifteen minutes; reserve 1 tablespoon drained juice. Mix reserved juice, 2 tablespoons chopped fresh basil, 1 small minced shallot, 2 teaspoons lemon juice, and 2 teaspoons extra-virgin olive oil in a container. Mix in drained grapefruits and allow to sit for about fifteen minutes. Sprinkle with salt, pepper, and sugar to taste. Serve over sole.

Spanish Smokey Hake

Yield: 4 Servings

Ingredients:

- ¼ teaspoon saffron threads, crumbled
- ½ cup dry white wine
- ¾ cup water
- 1 (8-ounce) bottle clam juice
- 1 bay leaf
- 1 onion, chopped fine
- 1 tablespoon extra-virgin olive oil, plus extra for serving
- 1 teaspoon lemon juice
- 2 tablespoons minced fresh parsley
- 3 ounces Spanish-style chorizo sausage, sliced ¼ inch thick
- 4 (4- to 6-ounce) skinless hake fillets, 1 to 1½ inches thick
- 4 garlic cloves, minced
- 4 ounces small red potatoes, unpeeled, sliced ¼ inch thick
- Salt and pepper

Directions:

1. Heat oil in 12-inch frying pan on moderate heat until it starts to shimmer. Put in onion and chorizo and cook until onion becomes tender and lightly browned, 5 to 7 minutes. Mix in garlic and saffron and cook until aromatic, approximately half a minute. Mix in clam juice, water, wine, potatoes, and bay leaf and bring to simmer. Decrease heat to moderate to low, cover, and cook until potatoes are almost tender, about 10 minutes.
2. Pat hake dry using paper towels and sprinkle with salt and pepper. Nestle hake skinned side down into frying pan and spoon some broth over top. Bring to simmer, cover, and cook until potatoes are fully soft and hake flakes apart when softly poked using paring knife and registers 140 degrees, 10 to 12 minutes.
3. Cautiously move hake to individual shallow bowls. Use a slotted spoon to divide potatoes and chorizo evenly among bowls. Discard bay leaf. Stir lemon juice into broth and sprinkle with salt and pepper to taste. Spoon broth over hake, drizzle with parsley, and drizzle with extra oil. Serve.

Tangy Baked Stuffed Mackerel

Yield: 4 Servings

Ingredients:

- ⅓ cup pitted brine-cured green olives, chopped
- ½ preserved lemon, pulp and white pith removed, rind rinsed and minced (2 tablespoons)
- 1 red bell pepper, stemmed, seeded, and chopped fine
- 1 red onion, chopped fine
- 1 tablespoon minced fresh parsley
- 3 tablespoons extra-virgin olive oil
- 4 (8- to 10-ounce) whole mackerel, gutted, fins snipped off with scissors
- Lemon wedges
- Salt and pepper

Directions:

1. Place the oven rack in the centre of the oven and pre-heat your oven to 500 degrees. Heat 2 tablespoons oil in 12-inch frying pan on moderate to high heat until it starts to shimmer. Put in bell pepper and onion and cook until vegetables are softened and well browned, eight to ten minutes. Mix in preserved lemon and cook until aromatic, approximately half a minute. Remove from the heat, mix in olives and parsley and sprinkle with salt and pepper to taste.
2. Grease rimmed baking sheet with remaining 1 tablespoon oil. Wash each mackerel under cold running water and pat dry using paper towels inside and out. Open cavity of each mackerel, season flesh with salt and pepper, and spoon one-quarter of filling into opening. Place mackerel on readied sheet, spaced at least 2 inches apart. Bake until thickest part of mackerel registers 130 to 135 degrees, 10 to 12 minutes. Cautiously move mackerel to serving platter and allow to rest for about five minutes. Serve with lemon wedges.

Tangy Broiled Bluefish

Yield: 4 Servings

This recipe can be made quickly

Ingredients:

- ¼ cup Green Zhoug
- ¼ cup mayonnaise
- ¼ preserved lemon, pulp and white pith removed, rind rinsed and minced (1 tablespoon)
- ¼ teaspoon sugar
- 1 garlic clove, minced
- 4 (4- to 6-ounce) skinless bluefish fillets, 1 to 1½ inches thick

- Lemon wedges
- Salt and pepper

Directions:

1. Place oven rack 4 inches from broiler element and heat broiler. Pat bluefish dry using paper towels, sprinkle with salt and pepper, and place skinned side down in greased rimmed baking sheet.
2. Mix mayonnaise, preserved lemon, garlic, and sugar in a container, then spread mixture uniformly tops of fillets. Broil until bluefish flakes apart when softly poked using paring knife and registers 140 degrees, approximately five minutes. Serve with Green Zhoug and lemon wedges.

Tangy Grilled Sea Bass

Yield: 4 Servings

This recipe can be made quickly

Ingredients:

- ¼ cup pitted kalamata olives, chopped
- ½ teaspoon ground cumin
- ½ teaspoon paprika
- 1 red grapefruit
- 2 oranges
- 2 tablespoons extra-virgin olive oil
- 2 tablespoons minced fresh parsley
- 4 (4- to 6-ounce) skinless sea bass fillets, 1 to 1½ inches thick
- Pinch cayenne pepper
- Salt and pepper

Directions:

1. Cut away peel and pith from oranges and grapefruit. Quarter oranges, then slice crosswise into ½-inch-thick pieces. Cut

grapefruit into 8 wedges, then slice wedges crosswise into ½-inch-thick pieces. Mix oranges, grapefruit, olives, parsley, cumin, paprika, and cayenne in a container. Sprinkle with salt to taste, cover, and set aside for serving.
2. Pat sea bass dry using paper towels, rub with oil, and sprinkle with salt and pepper.
3. **FOR A CHARCOAL:** GRILL Open bottom vent fully. Light large chimney starter filled with charcoal briquettes (6 quarts). When top coals are partly covered with ash, pour uniformly over half of grill. Set cooking grate in place, cover, and open lid vent fully. Heat grill until hot, approximately five minutes. **FOR A GAS GRILL:** Turn all burners to high, cover, and heat grill until hot, about fifteen minutes. Leave primary burner on high and turn other burner(s) to moderate to low.
4. Clean cooking grate, then repetitively brush grate with thoroughly oiled paper towels until grate is black and glossy, 5 to 10 times. Place sea bass on hotter part of grill and cook, uncovered, until well browned, about 10 minutes, gently flipping fillets using 2 spatulas halfway through cooking.
5. Slowly move sea bass to cooler part of grill and cook, uncovered, until fish flakes apart when softly poked using paring knife and registers 140 degrees, 3 to 6 minutes. Serve with salad.

Tangy Whole Roasted Snapper

Yield: 4 Servings

This recipe can be made quickly

Ingredients:

- ⅛ teaspoon red pepper flakes
- ¼ cup minced fresh cilantro
- 1 small shallot, minced

- 2 (1½- to 2-pound) whole red snapper, scaled, gutted, fins snipped off with scissors
- 2 teaspoons grated lime zest plus 2 tablespoons juice
- 2 teaspoons grated orange zest plus 2 tablespoons juice
- 6 tablespoons extra-virgin olive oil
- Salt and pepper

Directions:

1. Place the oven rack in the centre of the oven and pre-heat your oven to 500 degrees. Line rimmed baking sheet with parchment paper and grease parchment. Beat ¼ cup oil, cilantro, lime juice, orange juice, shallot, and pepper flakes together in a container. Sprinkle with salt and pepper to taste; set aside for serving.
2. In a different container, combine lime zest, orange zest, 1½ teaspoons salt, and ½ teaspoon pepper. Wash each snapper under cold running water and pat dry using paper towels inside and out. Using sharp knife, make 3 or 4 shallow slashes, about 2 inches apart, on both sides of snapper. Open cavity of each snapper and drizzle 1 teaspoon salt mixture on flesh. Brush 1 tablespoon oil on outside of each snapper and season with remaining salt mixture; move to readied sheet and allow to sit for about ten minutes.
3. Roast until snapper flakes apart when softly poked using paring knife and registers 140 degrees, fifteen to twenty minutes. (To check for doneness, peek into slashed flesh or into interior through opened bottom area of each fish.)
4. Cautiously move snapper to carving board and allow to rest for about five minutes. Fillet snapper by making vertical cut just behind head from top of fish to belly. Make another cut along top of snapper from head to tail. Use spatula to lift meat from bones, starting at head end and running spatula over bones to lift out fillet. Repeat on other side of snapper. Discard head and skeleton. Beat dressing to recombine and serve with snapper.

Traditional North African Monkfish Tagine

Yield: 4 to 6 Servings

Ingredients:

- ¼ cup pitted oil-cured black olives, quartered
- ¼ teaspoon saffron threads, crumbled
- ½ teaspoon dried mint
- 1 (8-ounce) bottle clam juice
- 1 large onion, halved and sliced ¼ inch thick
- 1 tablespoon tomato paste
- 1 teaspoon ground cumin
- 1 teaspoon sherry vinegar
- 1¼ teaspoons paprika
- 1½ pounds skinless monkfish fillets, 1 to 1½ inches thick, trimmed and cut into 3-inch pieces
- 2 tablespoons extra-virgin olive oil
- 2 tablespoons minced fresh mint
- 3 (2-inch) strips orange zest
- 3 carrots, peeled, halved along the length, and sliced ¼ inch thick
- 5 garlic cloves, minced
- Salt and pepper

Directions:

1. Mince 1 strip orange zest and combine with 1 teaspoon garlic in a container; set aside.
2. Heat oil in a Dutch oven on moderate heat until it starts to shimmer. Put in onion, carrots, ¼ teaspoon salt, and remaining 2 strips orange zest and cook until vegetables are softened and lightly browned, 10 to 12 minutes. Mix in remaining garlic, tomato paste, paprika, cumin, dried mint, and saffron and cook until aromatic, approximately half a minute. Mix in clam juice, scraping up any browned bits.

3. Pat monkfish dry using paper towels and sprinkle with salt and pepper. Nestle monkfish into pot, spoon some cooking liquid over top, and bring to simmer. Decrease heat to moderate to low, cover, and simmer gently until monkfish is opaque in center and registers 160 degrees, 8 to 12 minutes.
4. Discard orange zest. Gently mix in olives, fresh mint, vinegar, and garlic–orange zest mixture. Sprinkle with salt and pepper to taste. Serve.

Zesty Hake Fillets

Yield: 4 Servings

This recipe can be made quickly

If you can't find Hake, feel free to use Haddock or cod instead.

Ingredients:

- ¼ cup extra-virgin olive oil
- 1 lemon, sliced thin
- 1½ pounds russet potatoes, unpeeled, sliced into ¼-inch-thick rounds
- 3 garlic cloves, minced
- 4 (4- to 6-ounce) skinless hake fillets, 1 to 1½ inches thick
- 4 sprigs fresh thyme
- Salt and pepper

Directions:

1. Place oven rack to lower-middle position and pre-heat your oven to 425 degrees. Toss potatoes with 2 tablespoons oil and garlic in a container and sprinkle with salt and pepper. Microwave, uncovered, until potatoes are just tender, 12 to 14 minutes, stirring halfway through microwaving.
2. Move potatoes to 13 by 9-inch baking dish and press gently into even layer. Pat hake dry using paper towels, sprinkle with salt and pepper, and arrange skinned side down on top of potatoes.

Sprinkle hake with remaining 2 tablespoons oil, then place thyme sprigs and lemon slices on top. Bake until hake flakes apart when softly poked using paring knife and registers 140 degrees, fifteen to twenty minutes. Slide spatula underneath potatoes and hake and carefully move to individual plates. Serve.

Shellfish

Citric Seared Scallops

Yield: 4 to 6 Servings

This recipe can be made quickly

Ingredients:

- ⅛ teaspoon red pepper flakes
- 1 small shallot, minced
- 1 tablespoon minced fresh cilantro
- 1½ pounds large sea scallops, tendons removed
- 2 tablespoons lime juice
- 2 tablespoons orange juice
- 6 tablespoons extra-virgin olive oil
- Salt and pepper

Directions:

1. Place scallops in rimmed baking sheet lined with clean kitchen towel. Place second clean kitchen towel on top of scallops and press gently on towel to blot liquid. Let scallops sit at room temperature, covered with towel, for about ten minutes.
2. Beat ¼ cup oil, orange juice, lime juice, shallot, cilantro, and pepper flakes together in a container. Sprinkle with salt to taste and set aside for serving.

3. Heat 1 tablespoon oil in 12-inch non-stick frying pan on moderate to high heat until just smoking. Put in half of scallops to frying pan in one layer and cook, without moving them, until thoroughly browned on first side, about 1½ minutes. Flip scallops and continue to cook, without moving them, until thoroughly browned on second side, about 1½ minutes. Move scallops to serving platter and tent loosely with aluminium foil. Repeat with residual 1 tablespoon oil and remaining scallops. Beat dressing to recombine and serve with scallops.

Greek-Style Shrimp

Yield: 4 to 6 Servings

Ingredients:

- ¼ cup dry white wine
- ¼ cup extra-virgin olive oil
- ½ teaspoon red pepper flakes
- 1 (28-ounce) can diced tomatoes, drained with ⅓ cup juice reserved
- 1 red or green bell pepper, stemmed, seeded, and chopped
- 1 small onion, chopped
- 1 teaspoon grated lemon zest
- 1½ pounds extra-large shrimp (21 to 25 per pound), peeled and deveined
- 2 tablespoons chopped fresh dill
- 2 tablespoons coarsely chopped fresh parsley
- 3 tablespoons ouzo
- 5 garlic cloves, minced
- 6 ounces feta cheese, crumbled (1½ cups)
- Salt and pepper

Directions:

1. Toss shrimp in a container with 1 tablespoon oil, 1 tablespoon ouzo, 1 teaspoon garlic, lemon zest, ¼ teaspoon salt, and ⅛ teaspoon pepper; set aside.
2. Heat 2 tablespoons oil in 12-inch frying pan on moderate heat until it starts to shimmer. Put in onion, bell pepper, and ¼ teaspoon salt, cover, and cook, stirring intermittently, until vegetables release their liquid, 3 to 5 minutes. Uncover and continue to cook, stirring intermittently, until liquid evaporates and vegetables are softened, approximately five minutes. Mix in remaining garlic and pepper flakes and cook until aromatic, approximately one minute.
3. Mix in tomatoes and reserved juice, wine, and remaining 2 tablespoons ouzo. Bring to simmer and cook, stirring intermittently, until flavours blend and sauce is slightly thickened (sauce should not be completely dry), five to ten minutes. Mix in parsley and sprinkle with salt and pepper to taste.
4. Decrease heat to moderate to low and put in shrimp along with any accumulated juices; stir to coat and distribute evenly. Cover and cook, stirring intermittently, until shrimp are opaque throughout, 6 to 9 minutes, adjusting heat as required to maintain bare simmer. Remove from the heat, drizzle with feta and dill and drizzle with remaining 1 tablespoon oil. Serve.

Grilled Scallop-Zucchini Skewers

Yield: 4 to 6 Servings

Ingredients:

- ½ cup extra-virgin olive oil
- ¾ cup fresh basil leaves
- 1 (13 by 9-inch) disposable aluminium roasting pan (if using charcoal)
- 1 tablespoon all-purpose flour
- 1 tablespoon white wine vinegar

- 1 teaspoon cornstarch
- 1½ pounds large sea scallops, tendons removed
- 1¾ teaspoons sugar
- 2 garlic cloves, minced
- 2 tablespoons minced fresh chives
- 2 zucchini, halved along the length and sliced ¾ inch thick
- Salt and pepper

Directions:

1. Place scallops in rimmed baking sheet lined with clean kitchen towel. Place second clean kitchen towel on top of scallops and press gently on towel to blot liquid. Let scallops sit at room temperature, covered with towel, for about ten minutes.
2. In the meantime, pulse basil, chives, vinegar, garlic, ¾ teaspoon sugar, ¾ teaspoon salt, and ¼ teaspoon pepper using a food processor until approximately chopped, about 5 pulses. While your food processor runs slowly drizzle in 6 tablespoons oil and process until completely blended, approximately half a minute, scraping down sides of the container as necessary. Measure out and reserve 2 tablespoons vinaigrette in a big container. Set aside remaining vinaigrette for serving. Toss zucchini with reserved 2 tablespoons vinaigrette, then thread onto two 12-inch metal skewers.
3. With scallops on flat work surface, thread onto doubled skewers so that flat sides will directly touch grill grate, 4 to 6 scallops per doubled skewer (3 doubled skewers total). Return skewered scallops to towel-lined sheet and refrigerate, covered with second towel, while preparing grill.
4. **FOR A CHARCOAL GRILL:** Using kitchen shears, poke twelve ½-inch holes in bottom of disposable pan. Open bottom vent completely and place prepared pan in center of grill. Light large chimney starter mounded with charcoal briquettes (7 quarts). When top coals are partly covered with ash, pour into even layer in pan. Set cooking grate over coals with bars parallel to long side of pan, cover, and open lid vent fully. Heat grill until hot, approximately five minutes. **FOR A GAS GRILL:** Turn all

burners to high, cover, and heat grill until hot, about fifteen minutes. Leave all burners on high.
5. Beat remaining 2 tablespoons oil, remaining 1 teaspoon sugar, flour, and cornstarch together in a small-sized container. Remove towels from scallops. Brush both sides of scallops with oil mixture and sprinkle with salt and pepper.
6. Clean cooking grate, then repetitively brush grate with thoroughly oiled paper towels until grate is black and glossy, 5 to 10 times. Place scallops and zucchini on grill (directly over coals if using charcoal). Cook (covered if using gas), without moving them, until lightly browned on first side, 2½ to 4 minutes. Gently flip skewers and continue to cook, without moving them, until zucchini becomes soft and lightly browned and scallop sides are firm and centers are opaque, 2 to 4 minutes. Using tongs, slide zucchini and scallops off skewers onto serving platter. Serve with remaining vinaigrette.

Italian Shrimp & White Beans

Yield: 4 Servings

This recipe can be made quickly

Ingredients:

- ¼ teaspoon red pepper flakes
- 1 pound extra-large shrimp (21 to 25 per pound), peeled and deveined
- 1 red bell pepper, stemmed, seeded, and chopped fine
- 1 small red onion, chopped fine
- 2 (15-ounce) cans cannellini beans, rinsed
- 2 garlic cloves, minced
- 2 ounces (2 cups) baby arugula, chopped coarse
- 2 tablespoons lemon juice
- 5 tablespoons extra-virgin olive oil
- Pinch sugar

- Salt and pepper

Directions:

1. Pat shrimp dry using paper towels and season with sugar, salt, and pepper. Heat 1 tablespoon oil in 12-inch non-stick frying pan on high heat until just smoking. Put in shrimp to frying pan in one layer and cook, without stirring, until spotty brown and edges turn pink on first side, approximately one minute.
2. Remove from the heat, flip shrimp and allow to sit until opaque throughout, approximately half a minute. Move shrimp to a container and cover to keep warm.
3. Heat remaining ¼ cup oil in now-empty frying pan on moderate heat until it starts to shimmer. Put in bell pepper, onion, and ½ teaspoon salt and cook till they become tender, approximately five minutes. Mix in garlic and pepper flakes and cook until aromatic, approximately half a minute. Mix in beans and cook until heated through, approximately five minutes.
4. Put in arugula and shrimp along with any accumulated juices and gently toss until arugula is wilted, approximately one minute. Mix in lemon juice and sprinkle with salt and pepper to taste. Serve.

Moroccan Grilled Marinated Shrimp Skewers

Yield: 4 to 6 Servings

Ingredients:

MARINADE

- ¼ teaspoon cayenne pepper
- ½ teaspoon ground cumin
- ½ teaspoon ground ginger
- ½ teaspoon salt
- ½ teaspoon smoked paprika

- 1 teaspoon grated lime zest
- 3 tablespoons extra-virgin olive oil
- 6 garlic cloves, minced

SHRIMP

- ½ Teaspoon Sugar
- 1 Tablespoon Minced Fresh Cilantro
- 1½ pounds extra-large shrimp (21 to 25 per pound), peeled and deveined
- Lime Wedges

Directions:

1. **FOR THE MARINADE:** Beat all ingredients together in medium bowl.
2. **FOR THE SHRIMP:** Pat shrimp dry using paper towels. Using sharp paring knife, make shallow cut down outside curve of shrimp. Put in shrimp to a container with marinade and toss to coat. Cover and put in the fridge for minimum half an hour or maximum 1 hour.
3. **FOR A CHARCOAL:** GRILL Open bottom vent fully. Light large chimney starter filled with charcoal briquettes (6 quarts). When top coals are partly covered with ash, pour uniformly over half of grill. Set cooking grate in place, cover, and open lid vent fully. Heat grill until hot, approximately five minutes. FOR A GAS GRILL Turn all burners to high, cover, and heat grill until hot, about fifteen minutes. Leave all burners on high.
4. Clean and oil cooking grate. Thread shrimp tightly onto four 12-inch metal skewers (about 12 shrimp per skewer), alternating direction of heads and tails. Sprinkle 1 side of skewered shrimp with sugar. Place shrimp skewers sugared side down on grill (on hotter side if using charcoal). Cook (covered if using gas), without moving them, until mildly charred on first side, three to five minutes. Flip skewers and move to cooler side of grill (if using charcoal) or turn all burners off (if using gas) and cook, covered, until shrimp are opaque throughout, 1 to 2 minutes. Using tongs, slide shrimp off skewers onto serving platter and

sprinkle with salt and pepper to taste. Sprinkle with cilantro and serve with lime wedges.

Oven-Steamed Mussels

Yield: 4 to 6 Servings

✓ This recipe can be made quickly ✓

Ingredients:

- ¼ teaspoon salt
- 1 cup dry white wine
- 2 bay leaves
- 2 tablespoons minced fresh parsley
- 3 garlic cloves, minced
- 3 sprigs fresh thyme
- 3 tablespoons extra-virgin olive oil
- 4 pounds mussels, scrubbed and debearded
- Pinch red pepper flakes

Directions:

1. Place oven rack on the lowest position and pre-heat your oven to 500 degrees. Heat 1 tablespoon oil, garlic, and pepper flakes in large roasting pan on moderate heat and cook, stirring continuously, until aromatic, approximately half a minute. Mix in wine, thyme sprigs, and bay leaves, bring to boil, and cook until wine is slightly reduced, approximately one minute.
2. Mix in mussels and salt. Cover pan tightly with aluminium foil and move to oven. Cook until most mussels have opened (a few may remain closed), fifteen to twenty minutes.
3. Remove pan from oven. Discard thyme sprigs, bay leaves, and any mussels that refuse to open. Sprinkle with remaining 2 tablespoons oil, drizzle with parsley, and toss to combine. Serve.

Oven-Steamed Mussels Variation

This recipe can be made quickly

Omit pepper flakes and thyme sprigs. Put in 1 pound leeks, white and light green parts only, halved along the length, sliced thin, and washed comprehensively, to pan with garlic and cook until leeks are wilted, approximately three minutes. Substitute ½ cup Pernod and ¼ cup water for wine. After removing pan from oven in step 3, push mussels to sides of pan. Put in ¼ cup crème fraîche and oil to center and beat until combined. Substitute 2 tablespoons chives for parsley.

Roasted Garlic Shrimp

Yield: 4 to 6 Servings

This recipe can be made quickly

Ingredients:

- ¼ cup extra-virgin olive oil
- ¼ cup salt
- ¼ teaspoon pepper
- ½ teaspoon red pepper flakes
- 1 teaspoon anise seeds
- 2 pounds shell-on jumbo shrimp (16 to 20 per pound)
- 2 tablespoons minced fresh parsley
- 6 garlic cloves, minced
- Lemon wedges

Directions:

1. Dissolve salt in 4 cups cold water in large container. Using kitchen shears or sharp paring knife, cut through shell of shrimp and devein but do not remove shell. Use a paring knife to continue to cut shrimp ½ inch deep, taking care not to cut in

half fully. Immerse shrimp in brine, cover, put inside your fridge for about fifteen minutes.
2. Place oven rack 4 inches from broiler element and heat broiler. Mix oil, garlic, anise seeds, pepper flakes, and pepper in a big container. Remove shrimp from brine and pat dry using paper towels. Put in shrimp and parsley to oil mixture and toss well, making sure oil mixture gets into interior of shrimp. Arrange shrimp in one layer on wire rack set in rimmed baking sheet.
3. Broil shrimp until opaque and shells are starting to brown, 2 to 4 minutes, rotating sheet halfway through broiling. Flip shrimp and continue to broil until second side is opaque and shells are starting to brown, 2 to 4 minutes, rotating sheet halfway through broiling. Serve with lemon wedges.

Spanish Clams Mix

Yield: 4 to 6 Servings

This recipe can be made quickly

Ingredients:

- ½ cup minced fresh parsley
- 1 cup dry vermouth or dry white wine
- 1 tablespoon minced fresh thyme or 1 teaspoon dried
- 1½ pounds leeks, white and light green parts only, halved along the length, sliced thin, and washed thoroughly
- 2 cups pearl couscous
- 2 tablespoons extra-virgin olive oil
- 3 garlic cloves, minced
- 3 tomatoes, cored, seeded, and chopped
- 4 pounds littleneck clams, scrubbed
- 6 ounces Spanish-style chorizo sausage, halved along the length and sliced thin
- Salt and pepper

Directions:

1. Bring 2 quarts water to boil in moderate-sized saucepan. Mix in couscous and 2 teaspoons salt and cook until al dente, approximately eight minutes; drain.
2. In the meantime, heat oil in a Dutch oven on moderate heat. Put in leeks and chorizo and cook until leeks are tender, about 4 minutes. Mix in garlic and thyme and cook until aromatic, approximately half a minute. Mix in vermouth and cook until slightly reduced, approximately one minute. Mix in tomatoes and clams, cover, and cook until clams open, 8 to 12 minutes.
3. Use slotted spoon to move clams to large serving bowl, discarding any that refuse to open. Stir couscous and parsley into cooking liquid and sprinkle with salt and pepper to taste. Portion couscous mixture into individual bowls, top with clams, and serve.

Spanish Shellfish Stew

Yield: 4 to 6 Servings

Ingredients:

- ⅛ teaspoon red pepper flakes
- ¼ cup extra-virgin olive oil
- ¼ teaspoon saffron threads, crumbled
- 1 (28-ounce) can whole peeled tomatoes, drained with juice reserved, chopped
- 1 onion, chopped fine
- 1 recipe Picada
- 1 red bell pepper, stemmed, seeded, and chopped fine
- 1 tablespoon minced fresh parsley
- 1 teaspoon paprika
- 1½ cups dry white wine or dry vermouth
- 1½ pounds littleneck clams, scrubbed
- 12 ounces large sea scallops, tendons removed
- 2 bay leaves
- 2 tablespoons brandy

- 3 garlic cloves, minced
- 8 ounces medium-large shrimp (31 to 40 per pound), peeled and deveined, shells reserved
- 8 ounces mussels, scrubbed and debearded
- Lemon wedges
- Salt and pepper

Directions:

1. Heat 1 tablespoon oil in moderate-sized saucepan on moderate heat until it starts to shimmer. Put in shrimp shells and cook, stirring often, until they begin to turn spotty brown and pot starts to brown, 2 to 4 minutes. Remove from the heat, mix in wine, cover, and allow to steep until ready to use.
2. Heat remaining 3 tablespoons oil in large Dutch oven on moderate to high heat until it starts to shimmer. Put in onion and bell pepper and cook till they become tender and lightly browned, 5 to 7 minutes. Mix in garlic, paprika, saffron, and pepper flakes and cook until aromatic, approximately half a minute. Mix in brandy, scraping up any browned bits. Mix in tomatoes and their juice and bay leaves and cook until slightly thickened, 5 to 7 minutes.
3. Strain wine mixture into Dutch oven, pressing on solids to extract as much liquid as possible; discard solids. Bring to simmer and cook until flavours blend, 3 to 5 minutes.
4. Nestle clams into pot, cover, and cook for 4 minutes. Nestle mussels and scallops into pot, cover, and carry on cooking until most clams have opened, approximately three minutes. Arrange shrimp uniformly over stew, cover, and carry on cooking until shrimp are opaque throughout, scallops are firm and opaque in center, and clams and mussels have opened, 1 to 2 minutes.
5. Remove from the heat, discard bay leaves and any clams and mussels that refuse to open. Mix in picada and parsley and sprinkle with salt and pepper to taste. Serve in wide, shallow bowls with lemon wedges.

White Wine Steamed Clams

Yield: 4 to 6 Servings

✎This recipe can be made quickly✎

Ingredients:

- 1 bay leaf
- 1½ cups dry white wine
- 2 tablespoons minced fresh parsley
- 3 shallots, minced
- 3 tablespoons extra-virgin olive oil
- 4 garlic cloves, minced
- 4 pounds littleneck clams, scrubbed
- Lemon wedges

Directions:

1. Bring wine, shallots, garlic, and bay leaf to simmer in a Dutch oven on high heat and cook for about three minutes. Put in clams, cover, and cook, stirring twice, until clams open, about four to eight minutes. Use a slotted spoon to move clams to serving bowl, discarding any that refuse to open.
2. Remove from the heat, beat oil into cooking liquid until combined. Pour sauce over clams and drizzle with parsley. Serve with lemon wedges.

Squid and Octopus

Classic Calamari Stew

Yield: 4 to 6 Servings

Ingredients:

- ¼ cup extra-virgin olive oil, plus extra for serving
- ¼ teaspoon red pepper flakes
- ⅓ cup pitted brine-cured green olives, chopped coarse
- ½ cup dry white wine or dry vermouth
- 1 tablespoon capers, rinsed
- 2 celery ribs, sliced thin
- 2 onions, chopped fine
- 2 pounds small squid, bodies sliced crosswise into 1-inch-thick rings, tentacles halved
- 3 (28-ounce) cans whole peeled tomatoes, drained and chopped coarse
- 3 tablespoons minced fresh parsley
- 8 garlic cloves, minced
- Salt and pepper

Directions:

1. Heat oil in a Dutch oven on moderate to high heat until it starts to shimmer. Put in onions and celery and cook till they become tender, approximately five minutes. Mix in garlic and pepper flakes and cook until aromatic, approximately half a minute. Mix in wine, scraping up any browned bits, and cook until nearly evaporated, approximately one minute.
2. Pat squid dry using paper towels and sprinkle with salt and pepper. Stir squid into pot. Decrease heat to moderate to low, cover, and simmer gently until squid has released its liquid, about fifteen minutes. Mix in tomatoes, olives, and capers, cover, and carry on cooking until squid is very tender, 30 to 35 minutes.
3. Remove from the heat, mix in parsley and sprinkle with salt and pepper to taste. Serve, drizzling individual portions with extra oil.

Greek Stuffed Squid

Yield: 4 Servings

Ingredients:

- ¼ cup golden raisins
- ¼ cup pine nuts, toasted
- ½ cup dry white wine
- ½ cup plain dried bread crumbs
- 1 (15-ounce) can tomato sauce
- 1 garlic clove, minced
- 1 tablespoon dried mint
- 16 medium squid bodies, plus 6 ounces tentacles, chopped (¾ cup)
- 2 tablespoons extra-virgin olive oil
- 3 onions, chopped fine
- 4 anchovy fillets, rinsed and minced
- 5 tablespoons minced fresh parsley
- Salt and pepper

Directions:

1. Heat 1 tablespoon oil in 12-inch non-stick frying pan on moderate to high heat until it starts to shimmer. Put in two-thirds of onions and cook till they become tender, approximately five minutes. Mix in squid tentacles and cook until no longer translucent, 1 to 2 minutes. Mix in pine nuts, mint, and ¼ teaspoon pepper and cook until aromatic, approximately one minute. Move mixture to big container and mix in bread crumbs, ¼ cup parsley, raisins, and anchovies. Sprinkle with salt and pepper to taste and allow to cool slightly.
2. Using small soup spoon, portion 2 tablespoons filling into each squid body, pressing on filling gently to create 1-inch space at top. Thread toothpick through opening of each squid to secure closed.
3. Heat residual 1 tablespoon oil in now-empty frying pan on moderate to high heat until it starts to shimmer. Put in remaining onions and cook till they become tender, approximately five minutes. Mix in garlic, ¼ teaspoon salt, and ¼ teaspoon pepper and cook until aromatic, approximately half a minute. Mix in wine and tomato sauce and bring to simmer.

4. Nestle squid into sauce. Decrease heat to low, cover, and simmer gently until sauce has thickened slightly and squid is easily pierced with paring knife, about 1 hour, turning squid halfway through cooking. Season sauce with salt and pepper to taste. Remove toothpicks from squid and drizzle with remaining 1 tablespoon parsley. Serve.

Greek Tangy Grilled Squid

Yield: 4 Servings

Ingredients:

- 1 garlic clove, minced
- 1 pound small squid
- 1 tablespoon lemon juice, plus lemon wedges for serving
- 2 tablespoons baking soda
- 2 teaspoons minced fresh parsley
- 5 tablespoons extra-virgin olive oil
- Salt and pepper

Directions:

1. Mix 3 tablespoons oil, lemon juice, parsley, garlic, and ¼ teaspoon pepper in a big container; set aside for serving.
2. Using kitchen shears, cut squid bodies along the length down one side. Open squid bodies and flatten into planks. Dissolve baking soda and 2 tablespoons salt in 3 cups cold water in large container. Immerse squid bodies and tentacles in brine, cover, put inside your fridge for about fifteen minutes. Remove squid from brine and spread in a uniform layer in rimmed baking sheet lined with clean kitchen towel. Place second clean kitchen towel on top of squid and press gently on towel to blot liquid. Let squid sit at room temperature, covered with towel, for about ten minutes.
3. Toss squid with remaining 2 tablespoons oil and season with pepper. Thread tentacles onto two 12-inch metal skewers.

4. **FOR A CHARCOAL GRILL:** Open bottom vent fully. Light large chimney starter mounded with charcoal briquettes (7 quarts). When top coals are partly covered with ash, pour uniformly over half of grill. Set cooking grate in place, cover, and open lid vent fully. Heat grill until hot, approximately five minutes. **FOR A GAS GRILL:** Turn all burners to high, cover, and heat grill until hot, about fifteen minutes. Leave all burners on high.
5. Clean cooking grate, then repetitively brush grate with thoroughly oiled paper towels until black and glossy, 5 to 10 times. Place squid bodies and tentacles on grill (directly over coals if using charcoal), draping long tentacles over skewers to stop them from falling through grates. Cook (covered if using gas) until squid is opaque and mildly charred, approximately five minutes, flipping halfway through cooking. Move bodies to plate and tent loosely with aluminium foil. Continue to grill tentacles until ends become browned and crisp, approximately three minutes; move to plate with bodies.
6. Using tongs, remove tentacles from skewers. Move bodies to slicing board and slice into ½-inch-thick strips. Put in tentacles and bodies to a container with oil mixture and toss to coat. Serve with lemon wedges.

Greek-Style Octopus Braised in Red Wine

Yield: 4 Servings

Ingredients:

- 1 (4-pound) octopus, rinsed
- 1 cup dry red wine
- 1 sprig fresh rosemary
- 1 tablespoon extra-virgin olive oil
- 2 bay leaves
- 2 tablespoons red wine vinegar

- 2 tablespoons tomato paste
- 2 tablespoons unflavored gelatin
- 2 teaspoons chopped fresh parsley
- 4 garlic cloves, peeled and smashed
- Pepper
- Pinch ground cinnamon
- Pinch ground nutmeg

Directions:

1. Using sharp knife, separate octopus mantle (large sac) and body (lower section with tentacles) from head (midsection containing eyes); discard head. Place octopus in large pot, cover with water by 2 inches, and bring to simmer on high heat. Decrease heat to low, cover, and simmer gently, flipping octopus occasionally, until skin between tentacle joints tears easily when pulled, 45 minutes to 1¼ hours.
2. Move octopus to slicing board and allow to cool slightly. Measure out and reserve 3 cups octopus cooking liquid; discard remaining liquid and wipe pot dry using paper towels.
3. While octopus is still warm, use paring knife to cut mantle into quarters, then trim and scrape away skin and interior fibers; move to a container. Using your fingers, remove skin from body, being careful not to remove suction cups from tentacles. Cut tentacles from around core of body in three sections; discard core. Separate tentacles and cut into 2-inch lengths; move to a container.
4. Heat oil in now-empty pot on moderate to high heat until it starts to shimmer. Put in tomato paste and cook, stirring continuously, until starting to darken, approximately one minute. Mix in garlic, rosemary sprig, bay leaves, ½ teaspoon pepper, cinnamon, and nutmeg and cook until aromatic, approximately half a minute. Mix in reserved octopus cooking liquid, wine, vinegar, and gelatin, scraping up any browned bits. Bring to boil and cook, stirring intermittently, for 20 minutes.
5. Mix in octopus and any accumulated juices and bring to simmer. Cook, stirring intermittently, until octopus becomes

soft and sauce has thickened slightly and coats back of spoon, 20 minutes to half an hour. Remove from the heat, discard rosemary sprig and bay leaves. Mix in parsley and season with pepper to taste. Serve.

Spanish Grilled Octopus Salad

Yield: 4 to 6 Servings

Ingredients:

- ½ cup pitted brine-cured green olives, halved
- 1 (4-pound) octopus, rinsed
- 1 large orange
- 1 red bell pepper, stemmed, seeded, and cut into 2-inch-long matchsticks
- 1 teaspoon grated lemon zest plus ⅓ cup juice (2 lemons)
- 1 teaspoon sugar
- 2 bay leaves
- 2 celery ribs, sliced thin on bias
- 2 cups dry white wine
- 2 tablespoons chopped fresh parsley
- 2 teaspoons smoked paprika
- 3 tablespoons sherry vinegar
- 6 garlic cloves (4 peeled and smashed, 2 minced)
- 7 tablespoons extra-virgin olive oil
- Salt and pepper

Directions:

1. Using sharp knife, separate octopus mantle (large sac) and body (lower section with tentacles) from head (midsection containing eyes); discard head. Place octopus, wine, smashed garlic, and bay leaves in large pot, put in water to cover octopus by 2 inches, and bring to simmer on high heat. Decrease heat to low, cover, and simmer gently, flipping octopus occasionally, until

skin between tentacle joints tears easily when pulled, 45 minutes to 1¼ hours.
2. Move octopus to slicing board and allow to cool slightly; discard cooking liquid. Use a paring knife to cut mantle in half, then trim and scrape away skin and interior fibers; move to a container. Using your fingers, remove skin from body, being careful not to remove suction cups from tentacles. Cut tentacles from around core of body in three sections; discard core. Separate tentacles and move to a container.
3. Beat lemon juice and zest, 6 tablespoons oil, vinegar, paprika, minced garlic, sugar, ¼ teaspoon salt, and ¼ teaspoon pepper together in a container; move to 1-gallon zipper-lock bag and set aside.
4. **FOR A CHARCOAL GRILL**: Open bottom vent fully. Light large chimney starter filled with charcoal briquettes (6 quarts). When top coals are partly covered with ash, pour uniformly over half of grill. Set cooking grate in place, cover, and open lid vent fully. Heat grill until hot, approximately five minutes. **FOR A GAS GRILL:** Turn all burners to high, cover, and heat grill until hot, about fifteen minutes. Leave all burners on high.
5. Toss octopus with remaining 1 tablespoon oil. Clean cooking grate, then repetitively brush grate with thoroughly oiled paper towels until black and glossy, 5 to 10 times. Place octopus on grill (directly over coals if using charcoal). Cook (covered if using gas) until octopus is streaked with dark grill marks and mildly charred at tips of tentacles, eight to ten minutes, flipping halfway through grilling; move to slicing board.
6. While octopus is still warm, slice ¼ inch thick on bias, then move to zipper-lock bag with oil-lemon mixture and toss to coat. Press out as much air from bag as possible and seal bag. Refrigerate for minimum 2 hours or for maximum 24 hours, flipping bag occasionally.
7. Move octopus and marinade to big container and let come to room temperature, about 2 hours. Cut away peel and pith from orange. Holding fruit over bowl with octopus, use paring knife to slice between membranes to release segments. Put in celery,

bell pepper, olives, and parsley and gently toss to coat. Sprinkle with salt and pepper to taste. Serve.

Spanish Grilled Octopus Variation

To get a Greek-style salad instead of a Spanish one, omit orange. Substitute 1 tablespoon dried oregano for paprika, 1 fennel bulb, stalks discarded, bulb halved, cored, and sliced thin, for bell pepper, and 2 tablespoons chopped fresh dill for parsley.

Poultry and Meat

Although not a staple in the Mediterranean diet, poultry and meat recipes can still be enjoyed once or twice a month as long as the amount of meat in the recipes is moderate to small.

Beef Recipes

Beefy Grilled Flank Steak

Yield: 4 to 6 Servings

Ingredients:

- ½ cup Italian 1 pound eggplant, sliced along the length into ¾-inch-thick planks
- 1 red onion, sliced into ½-inch-thick rounds
- 1½ pounds flank steak, trimmed
- 2 tablespoons extra-virgin olive oil
- 2 zucchini, sliced along the length into ¾-inch-thick planks
- 8 ounces cherry tomatoes
- Salt and pepper
- Salsa Verde

Directions:

1. Thread onion rounds from side to side onto two 12-inch metal skewers. Thread cherry tomatoes onto two 12-inch metal skewers. Brush onion rounds, tomatoes, zucchini, and eggplant with oil and sprinkle with salt and pepper. Pat steak dry using paper towels and sprinkle with salt and pepper.
2. **For a Charcoal Grill:** Open bottom grill vent fully. Light large chimney starter filled with charcoal briquettes (6 quarts). When top coals are partly covered with ash, pour uniformly over grill. Set cooking grate in place, cover, and open lid vent fully. Heat

grill until hot, approximately five minutes. **For a Gas Grill:** Turn all burners to high, cover, and heat grill until hot, about fifteen minutes. Leave all burners on high.
3. Clean and oil cooking grate. Place steak, onion and tomato skewers, zucchini, and eggplant on grill. Cook (covered if using gas), flipping steak and turning vegetables as required, until steak is thoroughly browned and registers 120 to 125 degrees (for medium-rare) and vegetables are mildly charred and tender, 7 to 12 minutes. Move steak and vegetables to carving board as they finish grilling and tent loosely with aluminium foil. Let steak rest for about ten minutes.
4. In the meantime, slide tomatoes and onions off skewers using tongs. Cut onion rounds, zucchini, and eggplant into 2- to 3-inch pieces. Arrange vegetables on serving platter and sprinkle with salt and pepper to taste. Slice steak thin against grain on bias and arrange on platter with vegetables. Sprinkle steak with ¼ cup Salsa Verde. Serve, passing remaining sauce separately.

ITALIAN SALSA VERDE

Yield: 1 cup

◢This recipe can be made quickly◣

Ingredients:

- ⅛ teaspoon ½ cup extra-virgin olive oil
- 1 cup fresh mint leaves
- 1 garlic clove, minced
- 2 tablespoons capers, rinsed
- 3 anchovy fillets, rinsed
- 3 cups fresh parsley leaves
- 3 tablespoons white wine vinegar
- salt

Directions:

1. Pulse all ingredients using a food processor until mixture is thinly sliced (mixture should not be smooth), approximately ten pulses, scraping down sides of the container as required.
2. Move mixture to a container and serve. (Sauce will keep safely in a fridge for maximum 2 days; bring to room temperature before you serve.)

Braised Beef Short Ribs

Yield: 6 to 8 Servings

Make your own Ras el Hanout if you can.

Ingredients:

- ¾ cup prunes, halved
- 1 carrot, peeled and chopped fine
- 1 cup water
- 1 onion, chopped fine
- 1 tablespoon red wine vinegar
- 2 tablespoons chopped 2 tablespoons extra-virgin olive oil
- 2 tablespoons ras el hanout
- 2 tablespoons toasted sesame seeds
- 4 cups unsweetened pomegranate juice
- 4 garlic cloves, minced
- 4 pounds bone-in English-style short ribs, trimmed
- Salt and pepper
- fresh cilantro

Directions:

1. Place oven rack to lower-middle position and pre-heat your oven to 450 degrees. Pat short ribs dry using paper towels and sprinkle with salt and pepper. Arrange ribs bone side down in one layer in large roasting pan and roast until meat begins to brown, about 45 minutes.

2. Discard any accumulated fat and juices in pan and continue to roast until meat is well browned, fifteen to twenty minutes. Move ribs to a container and tent loosely with aluminium foil; set aside. Stir pomegranate juice and water into pan, scraping up any browned bits; set aside.
3. Reduce oven temperature to 300 degrees. Heat oil in a Dutch oven on moderate heat until it starts to shimmer. Put in onion, carrot, and ¼ teaspoon salt and cook till they become tender, approximately five minutes. Mix in ras el hanout and garlic and cook until aromatic, approximately half a minute.
4. Mix in pomegranate mixture from roasting pan and half of prunes and bring to simmer. Nestle short ribs bone side up into pot and bring to simmer. Cover, move pot to oven, and cook until ribs are soft and fork slips easily in and out of meat, about 2½ hours.
5. Move short ribs to a container, discard any loose bones, and tent loosely with aluminium foil. Strain braising liquid through fine-mesh strainer into fat separator; move solids to blender. Let braising liquid settle for about five minutes, then pour defatted liquid into blender with solids and process until smooth, approximately one minute.
6. Move sauce to now-empty pot and mix in vinegar and remaining prunes. Return short ribs and any accumulated juices to pot, bring to mild simmer on moderate heat, and cook, spooning sauce over ribs occasionally, until heated through, approximately five minutes. Sprinkle with salt and pepper to taste. Move short ribs to serving platter, spoon 1 cup sauce over top, and drizzle with sesame seeds and cilantro. Serve, passing remaining sauce separately.

Braised Oxtails

Yield: 6 to 8 Servings

Ingredients:

- 1 (15-ounce) can navy beans, rinsed
- 1 (28-ounce) can whole peeled tomatoes
- 1 carrot, peeled and chopped fine
- 1 onion, chopped fine
- 1 tablespoon 1 tablespoon minced fresh oregano
- 2 tablespoons extra-virgin olive oil
- 2 tablespoons ground dried Aleppo pepper
- 2 tablespoons tomato paste
- 4 cups chicken broth
- 4 pounds oxtails, trimmed
- 6 garlic cloves, minced
- Salt and pepper
- sherry vinegar

Directions:

1. Place oven rack to lower-middle position and pre-heat your oven to 450 degrees. Pat oxtails dry using paper towels and sprinkle with salt and pepper. Arrange oxtails cut side down in one layer in large roasting pan and roast until meat begins to brown, about 45 minutes.
2. Discard any accumulated fat and juices in pan and continue to roast until meat is well browned, fifteen to twenty minutes. Move oxtails to a container and tent loosely with aluminium foil; set aside. Stir chicken broth into pan, scraping up any browned bits; set aside.
3. Reduce oven temperature to 300 degrees. Heat oil in a Dutch oven on moderate heat until it starts to shimmer. Put in onion and carrot and cook till they become tender, approximately five minutes. Mix in garlic, tomato paste, Aleppo, and 1 teaspoon oregano and cook until aromatic, approximately half a minute.
4. Mix in broth mixture from roasting pan and tomatoes and their juice and bring to simmer. Nestle oxtails into pot and bring to simmer. Cover, move pot to oven, and cook until oxtails are soft and fork slips easily in and out of meat, about three hours.
5. Move oxtails to a container and tent loosely with aluminium foil. Strain braising liquid through fine-mesh strainer into fat

separator; return solids to now-empty pot. Let braising liquid settle for about five minutes, then pour defatted liquid into pot with solids.
6. Mix in beans, vinegar, and remaining 2 teaspoons oregano. Return oxtails and any accumulated juices to pot, bring to mild simmer on moderate heat, and cook until oxtails and beans are heated through, approximately five minutes. Sprinkle with salt and pepper to taste. Move oxtails to serving platter and spoon 1 cup sauce over top. Serve, passing remaining sauce separately.

Italian Flank Steak Peperonata

Yield: 4 to 6 Servings

Peperonata is an Italian combination of sweet peppers, onion, tomato, and garlic cooked in fruity olive oil.

Ingredients:

- ⅛ teaspoon red pepper flakes
- ⅓ cup plus 1 tablespoon extra-virgin olive oil, plus extra for serving
- ½ cup chopped 1 (1½-pound) flank steak, trimmed
- 1 (14.5-ounce) can diced tomatoes
- 1 onion, quartered through root end and sliced crosswise into ¼-inch-wide strips
- 2 tablespoons capers plus 4 teaspoons caper brine
- 2 teaspoons dried oregano
- 4 red or yellow bell peppers, quartered, stemmed, seeded, and cut crosswise into ¼-inch-wide strips
- 6 garlic cloves, lightly crushed and peeled
- Salt and pepper
- fresh basil

Directions:

1. Mix oregano and 1 teaspoon salt in a container. Cut steak with grain into 3 equivalent pieces. Sprinkle steak with oregano mixture, wrap tightly in plastic wrap, put inside your fridge for minimum half an hour or maximum 24 hours.
2. Heat ⅓ cup oil in 12-inch non-stick frying pan on moderate to high heat until just smoking. Put in bell peppers, onion, garlic, and ½ teaspoon salt. Cover and cook, stirring intermittently, until vegetables are soft, about 10 minutes.
3. Mix in tomatoes and their juice, capers and brine, and pepper flakes and cook, uncovered, until slightly thickened, approximately five minutes. Sprinkle with salt and pepper to taste. Move peperonata to a container, cover, and keep warm.
4. Wipe frying pan clean using paper towels. Pat steaks dry using paper towels and season with pepper. Heat residual 1 tablespoon oil in now-empty frying pan on moderate to high heat until just smoking. Cook steaks until thoroughly browned and meat registers 120 to 125 degrees (for medium-rare), 5 to 7 minutes each side. Move steaks to carving board, tent loosely with aluminium foil, and allow to rest for about ten minutes.
5. Stir basil into peperonata. Slice steaks thin against grain on bias. Season steak slices with salt and pepper and drizzle with extra oil. Serve steak with peperonata.

Kibbeh

Yield: 16

A popular Lebanese and Syrian Beef cuisine.

Ingredients:

DOUGH

- ¼ teaspoon ½ teaspoon ground cinnamon
- ½ teaspoon salt
- 1 cup medium-grind bulgur, rinsed
- 1 cup water

- 1 small onion, chopped
- 8 ounces ground lamb
- pepper

FILLING

- ⅛ teaspoon ground allspice
- ½ cup pine nuts, toasted
- ½ teaspoon ground cinnamon
- 1 small onion, chopped fine
- 1 tablespoon pomegranate molasses
- 1 teaspoon extra-virgin olive oil
- 2 cups vegeta8 ounces ground lamb
- Salt and pepper
- Vegetable oil

Directions:

1. **FOR THE DOUGH:** Mix bulgur and water in a container and allow to sit until grains start to become tender, 30 to 40 minutes. Drain bulgur well and move to a container of food processor. Put in lamb, onion, cinnamon, salt, and pepper and process to smooth paste, approximately one minute, scraping down sides of the container as required. Move dough to a container, cover, put inside your fridge until chilled, approximately half an hour.
2. **FOR THE FILLING:** Heat oil in 12-inch frying pan on moderate to high heat until just smoking. Put in lamb, ½ teaspoon salt, and ¼ teaspoon pepper and cook, breaking up meat with wooden spoon, until browned, 3 to 5 minutes. Use a slotted spoon to move meat to paper towel–lined plate. Pour off all but 1 tablespoon fat from skillet.
3. Put in onion to fat left in frying pan and cook on moderate heat till they become tender, approximately five minutes. Mix in pine nuts, cinnamon, and allspice and cook until aromatic, approximately half a minute. Remove from the heat, mix in lamb and pomegranate molasses and sprinkle with salt and pepper to taste.

4. Line rimmed baking sheet with parchment paper and grease parchment. Pinch off and roll dough into 2-inch balls (16 balls total). Working with 1 dough ball at a time, use your lightly oiled hands to press and stretch dough into rough cup with ¼-inch-thick sides. Spoon 1 tablespoon filling into cup, pressing gently to pack filling, and pinch seam closed. Gently form kibbeh into 3 by 1½-inch torpedo shape with tapered ends and move to readied sheet. Cover and put in the fridge kibbeh until firm, minimum half an hour or maximum 24 hours.
5. Place the oven rack in the centre of the oven and pre-heat your oven to 200 degrees. Set wire rack in second rimmed baking sheet and line with triple layer of paper towels. Heat oil in clean 12-inch frying pan on moderate to high heat to 375 degrees. Fry half of kibbeh until deep golden brown, 2 to 3 minutes each side. Adjust burner, if needed, to maintain oil temperature of 375 degrees. Use a slotted spoon to move kibbeh to prepared rack and keep warm in oven. Return oil to 375 degrees and repeat with remaining kibbeh. Serve.

Tangy Grilled Beef Kebabs

Yield: 4 to 6 Servings

Ingredients:

MARINADE

- ⅓ cup beef broth
- ⅓ cup extra-virgin olive oil
- ¾ teaspoon 1 onion, chopped
- 1½ teaspoons sugar
- 2 tablespoons chopped fresh rosemary
- 2 teaspoons grated lemon zest
- 2 teaspoons salt
- 3 tablespoons tomato paste
- 6 garlic cloves, chopped

- pepper

BEEF AND VEGETABLES

- 1½ pounds sirloin steak tips, trimmed and cut into 2-inch pieces
- 2 red onions, cut into 2 red or green bell peppers, stemmed, seeded, and cut into 1½-inch pieces
- 2 zucchini or yellow summer squash, halved along the length and sliced 1 inch thick
- 1-inch pieces, 3 layers thick

Directions:

1. **FOR THE MARINADE:** Process all ingredients using a blender until smooth, approximately fifty seconds, scraping down sides of blender jar as required. Move ¾ cup marinade to big container and set aside.
2. **FOR THE BEEF AND VEGETABLES:** Place remaining marinade and beef in 1-gallon zipper-lock bag and toss to coat. Press out as much air as possible and seal bag. Refrigerate for minimum sixty minutes or maximum 2 hours, flipping bag every half an hour.
3. Put in zucchini, bell peppers, and onions to a container with reserved marinade and toss to coat. Cover and allow to sit at room temperature for minimum half an hour.
4. Remove beef from bag and pat dry using paper towels. Thread beef tightly onto two 12-inch metal skewers. In alternating pattern of zucchini, bell pepper, and onion, thread vegetables onto four 12-inch metal skewers.
5. **For a Charcoal Grill:** Open bottom vent fully. Light large chimney starter mounded with charcoal briquettes (7 quarts). When top coals are partly covered with ash, pour uniformly over center of grill, leaving 2-inch gap between grill wall and charcoal. Set cooking grate in place, cover, and open lid vent fully. Heat grill until hot, approximately five minutes. **For a Gas Grill:** Turn all burners to high, cover, and heat grill until hot, about fifteen minutes. Leave primary burner on high and turn other burner(s) to moderate to low.

6. Clean and oil cooking grate. Place beef skewers on grill (directly over coals if using charcoal or over hotter side of grill if using gas). Place vegetable skewers on grill (near edge of coals but still over coals if using charcoal or on cooler side of grill if using gas). Cook (covered if using gas), turning skewers every three to five minutes, until beef is thoroughly browned and registers 120 to 125 degrees (for medium-rare), 12 to 16 minutes. Move beef skewers to serving platter, tent loosely with aluminium foil, and allow to rest while finishing vegetables.
7. Carry on cooking vegetable skewers until soft and mildly charred, approximately five minutes; move to platter. Using tongs, slide beef and vegetables off skewers onto platter. Serve.

Poultry

Sautéed Chicken Cutlets Alongside Romesco Sauce

Yield: 4 Servings

This recipe can be made quickly

Ingredients:

SAUCE

- ¼ cup hazelnuts, toasted and skinned
- ½ slice hearty white sandwich bread, cut into ½ inch pieces
- ½ teaspoon salt
- ½ teaspoon smoked paprika
- 1 cup jarred roasted red peppers, rinsed and patted dry
- 1 teaspoon honey
- 1½ tablespoons sherry vinegar
- 2 garlic cloves, sliced thin

- 2 tablespoons extra-virgin olive oil
- Pinch cayenne pepper

CHICKEN

- 4 (4- to 6-ounce) boneless, skinless chicken breasts, trimmed
- 4 teaspoons Salt and pepper
- extra-virgin olive oil

Directions:

1. **FOR THE SAUCE:** Cook bread, hazelnuts, and 1 tablespoon oil in 12-inch frying pan on moderate heat, stirring continuously, until bread and hazelnuts are lightly toasted, approximately three minutes. Put in garlic and cook, stirring continuously, until aromatic, approximately half a minute. Move mixture to your food processor and pulse until coarsely chopped, about 5 pulses. Put in red peppers, vinegar, honey, paprika, salt, cayenne, and residual 1 tablespoon oil to processor. Pulse until thinly sliced, 5 to 8 pulses. Move sauce to a container and set aside for serving. (Sauce will keep safely in a fridge for maximum 2 days.)
2. **FOR THE CHICKEN:** Cut chicken horizontally into 2 thin cutlets, then cover up using plastic wrap and pound to uniform ¼-inch thickness. Pat cutlets dry using paper towels and sprinkle with salt and pepper. Heat 2 teaspoons oil in 12-inch frying pan on moderate to high heat until just smoking. Place 4 cutlets in frying pan and cook, without moving, until browned on first side, approximately two minutes. Flip cutlets and carry on cooking until opaque on second side, approximately half a minute. Move chicken to serving platter and tent loosely with aluminium foil. Replicate the process with the rest of the 4 cutlets and remaining 2 teaspoons oil. Serve with sauce.

Sautéed Chicken Cutlets Variation 1

✒ This recipe can be made quickly ✒

Omit honey, smoked paprika, and cayenne. Substitute ¼ cup pine nuts for hazelnuts, 1 small tomato, cored and cut into ½-inch pieces, and ½ cup oil-packed sun-dried tomatoes for red peppers, and 2 tablespoons balsamic vinegar for sherry vinegar. Put in 2 tablespoons chopped fresh basil to your food processor with tomato.

Sautéed Chicken Cutlets Variation 2

This recipe can be made quickly

Omit smoked paprika and cayenne. Cut away peel and pith from 1 orange. Quarter orange, then slice crosswise into ½-inch-thick pieces. Substitute ¼ cup slivered almonds for hazelnuts, orange pieces and ¾ cup pitted kalamata olives for red peppers, and 1½ tablespoons red wine vinegar for sherry vinegar. Put in ¼ teaspoon fennel seeds to frying pan with garlic and 2 tablespoons chopped fresh mint to your food processor with orange.

Sautéed Chicken Breasts Veggie Blast

Yield: 4 Servings

This recipe can be made quickly

Ingredients:

- ¼ cup shredded ½ cup all-purpose flour
- 1 teaspoon herbes de Provence
- 12 ounces cherry tomatoes, halved
- 2 garlic cloves, minced
- 2 tablespoons capers, rinsed
- 2 yellow summer squash, quartered along the length and sliced ½ inch thick
- 2 zucchini, quartered along the length and sliced ½ inch thick
- 3 tablespoons plus 2 teaspoons extra-virgin olive oil
- 4 (4- to 6-ounce) boneless, skinless chicken breasts, trimmed
- Salt and pepper

- fresh basil or mint

Directions:

1. Lay out flour in shallow dish. Pound thicker ends of chicken breasts between 2 sheets of plastic wrap to uniform ½-inch thickness. Pat chicken dry using paper towels, drizzle with herbes de Provence, and sprinkle with salt and pepper. Working with 1 chicken breast at a time, dredge in flour to coat, shaking off any excess.
2. Heat 2 tablespoons oil in 12-inch non-stick frying pan on moderate to high heat until just smoking. Place chicken in frying pan and cook, turning as required, until golden brown on both sides and chicken registers 160 degrees, about 10 minutes. Move chicken to plate, tent loosely with aluminium foil, and allow to rest while preparing vegetables.
3. Heat 2 teaspoons oil in now-empty frying pan on moderate to high heat until it starts to shimmer. Put in zucchini and squash and cook until well browned, about 10 minutes. Mix in garlic and cook until aromatic, approximately half a minute. Mix in tomatoes and capers and cook until tomatoes are just softened, approximately two minutes. Remove from the heat, mix in basil and remaining 1 tablespoon oil. Sprinkle with salt and pepper to taste. Serve chicken with vegetables.

Tangy Pan-Seared Chicken Breasts Salad

Yield: 4 Servings

✐This recipe can be made quickly✐

Ingredients:

- ¼ cup chopped fresh mint
- ¼ cup lemon juice (2 lemons)
- ½ cup all-purpose flour
- ½ red onion, sliced thin

- ½ teaspoon ground cumin
- 1 teaspoon honey
- 1 teaspoon smoked paprika
- 2 (15-ounce) cans chickpeas, rinsed
- 4 (4- to 6-ounce) boneless6 tablespoons extra-virgin olive oil
- Salt and pepper
- , skinless chicken breasts, trimmed

Directions:

1. Beat ¼ cup oil, lemon juice, honey, paprika, cumin, ½ teaspoon salt, and ½ teaspoon pepper together in a big container until combined. Reserve 3 tablespoons dressing for serving. Put in chickpeas, onion, and mint to remaining dressing and toss to combine. Sprinkle with salt and pepper to taste and set aside for serving.
2. Lay out flour in shallow dish. Pound thicker ends of chicken breasts between 2 sheets of plastic wrap to uniform ½-inch thickness. Pat chicken dry using paper towels and sprinkle with salt and pepper. Working with 1 chicken breast at a time, dredge in flour to coat, shaking off any excess.
3. Heat remaining 2 tablespoons oil in 12-inch frying pan on moderate to high heat until just smoking. Place chicken in frying pan and cook, turning as required, until golden brown on both sides and chicken registers 160 degrees, about 10 minutes. Move chicken to serving platter, tent loosely with aluminium foil, and allow to rest for about five minutes. Sprinkle reserved dressing over chicken and serve with salad.

Circassian Chicken

Yield: 4 Servings

This recipe can be made quickly

Soft poached chicken served in a creamy walnut sauce and sprinkled with chile or olive oil.

Ingredients:

- ½ teaspoon cayenne pepper
- 1 onion, chopped fine
- 2 cups walnuts, toasted
- 2 slices hearty white sandwich bread, crusts removed, torn into 1-inch pieces
- 2 tablespoons minced 3 cups chicken broth
- 3 garlic cloves, minced
- 3 tablespoons extra-virgin olive oil, plus extra for serving
- 4 (4- to 6-ounce) boneless, skinless chicken breasts, trimmed
- 4 teaspoons paprika
- Salt and pepper
- fresh parsley

Directions:

1. Pound thicker ends of chicken breasts between 2 sheets of plastic wrap to uniform ½-inch thickness. Pat chicken dry using paper towels and sprinkle with salt and pepper. Heat 1 tablespoon oil in 12-inch frying pan on moderate to high heat until just smoking. Place chicken in frying pan and cook until golden brown on first side, about 4 minutes. Flip chicken, put in broth, and bring to simmer. Decrease heat to moderate to low, cover, and cook until chicken registers 160 degrees, approximately eight minutes.
2. Move chicken to slicing board, allow to cool slightly, then shred into bite-size pieces using 2 forks. Move chicken to big container and set aside. Strain and reserve broth, discarding white foam.
3. Wipe frying pan clean using paper towels. Heat remaining 2 tablespoons oil in now-empty frying pan on moderate heat until it starts to shimmer. Put in onion and ½ teaspoon salt and cook till they become tender, approximately five minutes. Mix in paprika, garlic, and cayenne and cook until aromatic, approximately half a minute.
4. Process onion mixture, bread, walnuts, and 2½ cups reserved broth using a food processor until smooth, approximately half a

minute, scraping down sides of the container as required. Adjust sauce consistency with remaining reserved broth as required. (Sauce should be slightly thicker than heavy cream.) Put in sauce to chicken and toss to coat. Sprinkle with salt and pepper to taste. Move chicken to serving platter, drizzle with parsley, and drizzle with extra oil. Serve.

Spanish Pollo en pepitoria

Yield: 8 Servings

A classic chicken recipe from Spain!

Ingredients:

- ¼ teaspoon ground cinnamon
- ½ cup slivered almonds, toasted
- ⅔ cup dry sherry
- 1 (14.5-ounce) can whole peeled tomatoes, drained and chopped fine
- 1 bay leaf
- 1 cup chicken broth
- 1 onion, chopped fine
- 1 tablespoon extra-virgin olive oil
- 1½ teaspoons lemon 2 hard-cooked large eggs, yolks and whites separated, whites chopped fine
- 2 tablespoons chopped fresh parsley
- 3 garlic cloves, minced
- 8 (5- to 7-ounce) bone-in chicken thighs, trimmed
- Pinch saffron threads, crumbled
- Salt and pepper
- juice

Directions:

1. Place the oven rack in the centre of the oven and pre-heat your oven to 300 degrees. Pat chicken dry using paper towels and

sprinkle with salt and pepper. Heat oil in 12-inch frying pan on moderate to high heat until just smoking. Brown thighs, 5 to 6 minutes each side. Move thighs to plate and pour off all but 2 teaspoons fat from skillet.
2. Put in onion and ¼ teaspoon salt to fat left in frying pan and cook on moderate heat until just softened, approximately three minutes. Mix in two-thirds of garlic, bay leaf, and cinnamon and cook until aromatic, approximately one minute. Mix in sherry and cook, scraping up any browned bits, until sherry starts to thicken, approximately two minutes. Mix in broth and tomatoes and bring to simmer. Nestle thighs into skillet, cover, and move to oven. Cook until chicken registers 195 degrees, 45 to 50 minutes.
3. Using potholders, remove frying pan from oven. Being careful of hot frying pan handle, move thighs to serving platter, discard skin, and tent loosely with aluminium foil.
4. Discard bay leaf. Move ¾ cup cooking liquid, egg yolks, almonds, saffron, and remaining garlic to blender. Process until smooth, approximately two minutes, scraping down sides of jar as required. Return almond mixture to frying pan along with 1 tablespoon parsley and lemon juice. Bring to simmer on moderate heat and cook, beating often, until sauce has thickened, 3 to 5 minutes. Sprinkle with salt and pepper to taste. Spoon sauce over chicken and drizzle with remaining 1 tablespoon parsley and egg whites. Serve.

Classic chicken cacciatore

Yield: 8 Servings

A Classic Italian Chicken stew that includes earthy mushrooms, tomatoes, and red wine.

Ingredients:

- ½ cup chicken broth
- 1 (14.5-ounce) can diced tomatoes, drained

- 1 onion, chopped
- 1 Parmesan cheese rind (optional)
- 1 tablespoon extra-virgin olive oil
- 1½ cups dry red wine
- 1½ tablespoons all-purpose flour
- 2 teaspoons 2 teaspoons minced fresh thyme
- 4 garlic cloves, minced
- 6 ounces portobello mushroom caps, cut into ¾-inch pieces
- 8 (5- to 7-ounce) bone-in chicken thighs, trimmed
- Salt and pepper
- minced fresh sage

Directions:

1. Place the oven rack in the centre of the oven and pre-heat your oven to 300 degrees. Pat chicken dry using paper towels and sprinkle with salt and pepper. Heat oil in a Dutch oven on moderate to high heat until just smoking. Brown thighs, 5 to 6 minutes each side. Move thighs to plate and discard skin. Pour off all but 1 tablespoon fat from pot.
2. Put in onion, mushrooms, and ½ teaspoon salt to fat left in pot and cook, stirring intermittently, till they become tender and starting to brown, six to eight minutes. Mix in garlic and thyme and cook until aromatic, approximately half a minute. Mix in flour and cook for about sixty seconds. Slowly beat in wine, scraping up any browned bits and smoothing out any lumps.
3. Mix in broth, tomatoes, and cheese rind, if using, and bring to simmer. Nestle thighs into pot, cover, and move to oven. Cook until chicken registers 195 degrees, 35 to 40 minutes.
4. Remove pot from oven and move chicken to serving platter. Discard cheese rind, if using. Stir sage into sauce and sprinkle with salt and pepper to taste. Spoon sauce over chicken and serve.

Moroccan B'stilla

Yield: 8 Servings

A popular Moroccan dish, this recipe is basically a sweet and savory pie filled with soft simmered chicken.

Ingredients:

- ¼ cup dried currants
- ¼ cup shelled pistachios, toasted
- ¼ teaspoon orange ½ cup fresh parsley leaves
- ½ teaspoon ground cinnamon
- 1 tablespoon lime juice
- 3 shallots, sliced thin (½ cup)
- 5 tablespoons extra-virgin olive oil
- 6 tablespoons water
- 8 (5- to 7-ounce) bone-in chicken thighs, trimmed
- Salt and pepper
- blossom water

Directions:

1. Place oven racks in middle and lowest positions, place rimmed baking sheet on lower rack, and pre-heat your oven to 450 degrees.
2. Toss shallots with 1 tablespoon oil in a container. Cover and microwave until shallots become soft, approximately three minutes, stirring once halfway through microwaving. Place shallots in center of 12-inch square of aluminium foil. Cover with second 12-inch square of foil and fold edges together to create packet about 7 inches square; set aside.
3. Use a metal skewer to poke skin side of chicken thighs 10 to 12 times. Pat thighs dry using paper towels, rub skin with 1 tablespoon oil, and sprinkle with salt and pepper. Place thighs skin side down on hot sheet and place foil packet on upper rack. Roast chicken until skin side is starting to brown and chicken registers 160 degrees, 17 to 22 minutes, rotating sheet and

removing foil packet after 10 minutes. Take the chicken out of the oven and heat broiler.
4. Flip chicken skin side up and broil on upper rack until skin is crisp and thoroughly browned and chicken registers 175 degrees, approximately five minutes, rotating sheet as required for even browning. Move chicken to serving platter and allow to rest while preparing sauce.
5. Pulse shallots, parsley, water, currants, pistachios, lime juice, cinnamon, orange blossom water, and ¼ teaspoon salt using a food processor until thinly sliced, approximately ten pulses. While your food processor runs slowly drizzle in remaining 3 tablespoons oil and process until incorporated, scraping down sides of the container as required. Sprinkle with salt and pepper to taste. Serve chicken with sauce.

Tangy Roasted Chicken Thighs

Yield: 8 Servings

Ingredients:

- ¼ cup pitted oil-cured black olives, chopped
- ¼ cup water
- ¼ teaspoon ½ teaspoon ground fennel seeds
- ¾ cup fresh parsley leaves
- 1 anchovy fillet, rinsed
- 1 teaspoon grated orange zest
- 2 teaspoons red wine vinegar
- 3 shallots, sliced thin (½ cup)
- 5 tablespoons extra-virgin olive oil
- 8 (5- to 7-ounce) bone-in chicken thighs, trimmed
- Salt and pepper
- red pepper flakes

Directions:

1. Place oven racks in middle and lowest positions, place rimmed baking sheet on lower rack, and pre-heat your oven to 450 degrees.
2. Toss shallots with 1 tablespoon oil in a container. Cover and microwave until shallots have softened, approximately three minutes, stirring once halfway through microwaving. Place shallots in center of 12-inch square of aluminium foil. Cover with second 12-inch square of foil and fold edges together to create packet about 7 inches square; set aside.
3. Using metal skewer, poke skin side of chicken thighs 10 to 12 times. Pat thighs dry using paper towels, rub skin with 1 tablespoon oil, and sprinkle with salt and pepper. Place thighs skin side down on hot sheet and place foil packet on upper rack. Roast chicken until skin side is starting to brown and chicken registers 160 degrees, 17 to 22 minutes, rotating sheet and removing foil packet after 10 minutes. Take the chicken out of the oven and heat broiler.
4. Flip chicken skin side up and broil on upper rack until skin is crisp and thoroughly browned and chicken registers 175 degrees, approximately five minutes, rotating sheet as required for even browning. Move chicken to serving platter and allow to rest while preparing sauce.
5. Pulse shallots, parsley, olives, water, vinegar, anchovy, orange zest, fennel seeds, pepper flakes, and ¼ teaspoon salt using a food processor until thinly sliced, approximately ten pulses. While your food processor runs slowly drizzle in remaining 3 tablespoons oil and process until incorporated, scraping down sides of the container as required. Sprinkle with salt and pepper to taste. Serve chicken with sauce.

Za'atar-Coated Chicken

Yield: 4 Servings

Ingredients:

- ¼ preserved lemon, pulp and white pith removed, rind rinsed and minced (1 tablespoon)
- ½ teaspoon Dijon
- 1 (3½- to 4-pound) whole chicken, giblets discarded
- 1 tablespoon minced fresh mint
- 2 tablespoons za'atar
- 2 teaspoons white wine vinegar
- 5 tablespoons plus 1 teaspoon extra-virgin olive oil
- Salt and pepper
- mustard

Directions:

1. Place oven rack on the lowest position and pre-heat your oven to 450 degrees. Mix za'atar and 2 tablespoons oil in a small-sized container. With chicken breast side down, use kitchen shears to cut through bones on either side of backbone. Discard backbone and trim away excess fat and skin around neck. Flip chicken and tuck wingtips behind back. Press firmly on breastbone to flatten, then pound breast to be same thickness as legs and thighs. Pat chicken dry using paper towels and sprinkle with salt and pepper.
2. Heat 1 teaspoon oil in 12-inch oven-safe frying pan on moderate to high heat until just smoking. Place chicken skin side down in skillet, decrease the heat to medium, and place heavy pot on chicken to press it flat. Cook chicken until skin is crisp and browned, about 25 minutes. (If chicken is not crisp after 20 minutes, increase heat to moderate to high.)
3. Remove from the heat, remove pot and carefully flip chicken. Brush skin with za'atar mixture, move frying pan to oven, and roast until breast registers 160 degrees and thighs register 175 degrees, 10 to 20 minutes.
4. Move chicken to carving board and allow to rest for about ten minutes. In the meantime, beat mint, preserved lemon, vinegar, mustard, ⅛ teaspoon salt, and ⅛ teaspoon pepper together in a container until combined. Whisking continuously, slowly drizzle

in remaining 3 tablespoons oil until completely blended. Carve chicken and serve with dressing.

Italian alla Diavola

Yield: 4 Servings

This is a spicy grilled chicken recipe form Italy. Feel free to vary the amount of pepper flakes to your taste.

Ingredients:

- ¼ cup extra-virgin olive oil
- 1 (13 by 9-inch) disposable aluminium roasting pan (if using charcoal)
- 1 (3½- to 4-pound) whole chicken, giblets discarded
- 2 garlic heads, plus 4 cloves minced
- 2 teaspoons red pepper flakes
- 3 bay leaves
- LemSalt and pepper
- on wedges

Directions:

1. Mix garlic heads, bay leaves, and ½ cup salt in 1-gallon zipper-lock bag, crush gently with meat pounder, and move to large container. Mix in 2 quarts water to dissolve salt. With chicken breast side down, use kitchen shears to cut through bones on either side of backbone. Discard backbone and trim away excess fat and skin around neck. Flip chicken, press firmly on breastbone to flatten, then pound breast to be same thickness as legs and thighs. Immerse chicken in brine, cover, put inside your fridge for about one hour.
2. In the meantime, cook oil, minced garlic, pepper flakes, and 2 teaspoons pepper in small saucepan on moderate heat until aromatic, approximately three minutes. Let oil cool, then reserve 2 tablespoons for serving.

3. Remove chicken from brine and pat dry using paper towels. Gently loosen skin covering breast and thighs and rub remaining garlic-pepper oil underneath skin. Tuck wingtips behind back. **For a Charcoal Grill:** Open bottom vent completely and place disposable pan in center of grill. Light large chimney starter filled with charcoal briquettes (6 quarts). When top coals are partly covered with ash, pour into 2 even piles on either side of disposable pan. Set cooking grate in place, cover, and open lid vent fully. Heat grill until hot, approximately five minutes. **For a Gas Grill:** Turn all burners to high, cover, and heat grill until hot, about fifteen minutes. Turn all burners to moderate to low. (Adjust burners as required to maintain grill temperature of 350 degrees.)
4. Clean and oil cooking grate. Place chicken skin side down in center of grill (over pan if using charcoal). Cover and cook until skin is crisp, breast registers 160 degrees, and thighs register 175 degrees, 30 to 45 minutes.
5. Move chicken to carving board and allow to rest for 5 to 10 minutes. Carve chicken and serve with reserved garlic oil and lemon wedges.

Dressed & Grilled Chicken Kebabs

Yield: 4 to 6 Servings

Ingredients:

- ¼ cup extra-virgin olive oil
- ¼ cup plain yogurt
- ¼ cup thinly sliced red onion
- 1 pound cherry tomatoes, halved
- 1 tablespoon minced fresh oregano
- 1 teaspoon grated lemon zest plus 3 tablespoons juice
- 1½ pounds boneless, 3 garlic cloves, minced
- 4 ounces feta cheese, crumbled (1 cup)

- Salt and pepper
- skinless chicken breasts, trimmed and cut into 1-inch pieces

Directions:

1. Beat oil, lemon zest and juice, garlic, oregano, ½ teaspoon salt, and ½ teaspoon pepper together in medium bowl. Reserve half of oil mixture in second medium bowl. Put in tomatoes, feta, and onion to remaining oil mixture and toss to coat. Sprinkle with salt and pepper to taste and set aside for serving.
2. Beat yogurt into reserved oil mixture. Set aside half of yogurt dressing for serving. Put in chicken to remaining yogurt dressing and toss to coat. Thread chicken onto four 12-inch metal skewers.
3. **For a Charcoal Grill:** Open bottom vent fully. Light large chimney starter filled with charcoal briquettes (6 quarts). When top coals are partly covered with ash, pour uniformly over grill. Set cooking grate in place, cover, and open lid vent fully. Heat grill until hot, approximately five minutes. **For a Gas Grill:** Turn all burners to high, cover, and heat grill until hot, about fifteen minutes. Leave all burners on high.
4. Place skewers on grill and cook, turning occasionally, until chicken is thoroughly browned and registers 160 degrees, about 10 minutes. Using tongs, slide chicken off skewers onto serving platter. Serve chicken with salad and reserved dressing.

Greek Souvlaki

Yield: 4 to 6 Servings

A Grilled Chicken recipe from Greece!

Ingredients:

- ⅓ cup extra-virgin olive oil
- 1 cup 1 green bell pepper, quartered, stemmed, seeded, and each quarter cut into 4 pieces

- 1 small red onion, halved through root end, each half cut into 4 chunks
- 1 teaspoon dried oregano
- 1 teaspoon finely grated lemon zest plus ¼ cup juice (2 lemons)
- 1 teaspoon honey
- 1½ pounds boneless, skinless chicken breasts, trimmed and cut into 1-inch pieces
- 2 tablespoons minced fresh parsley
- 4–6 (8-inch) pita breads
- Salt and pepper
- Tzatziki

Directions:

1. Dissolve 2 tablespoons salt in 1 quart cold water in large container. Immerse chicken in brine, cover, put inside your fridge for half an hour. Mix oil, parsley, lemon zest and juice, honey, oregano, and ½ teaspoon pepper in medium bowl. Reserve ¼ cup oil mixture in a big container.
2. Remove chicken from brine and pat dry using paper towels. Toss chicken with remaining oil mixture. Thread 4 pieces of bell pepper, concave side up, onto one 12-inch metal skewer. Thread one-quarter of chicken onto skewer. Thread 2 chunks of onion onto skewer and place skewer on plate. Repeat skewering remaining chicken and vegetables on 3 more skewers. Lightly moisten 2 pita breads with water. Sandwich unmoistened pitas between moistened pitas and wrap stack tightly in lightly greased heavy-duty aluminium foil.
3. **For a Charcoal Grill:** Open bottom vent fully. Light large chimney starter mounded with charcoal briquettes (7 quarts). When top coals are partly covered with ash, pour uniformly over half of grill. Set cooking grate in place, cover, and open lid vent fully. Heat grill until hot, approximately five minutes. **For a Gas Grill:** Turn all burners to high, cover, and heat grill until hot, about fifteen minutes. Leave primary burner on high and turn off other burner(s).

4. Clean and oil cooking grate. Place skewers on hotter side of grill and cook, turning occasionally, until chicken and vegetables are thoroughly browned and chicken registers 160 degrees, fifteen to twenty minutes. Using tongs, slide chicken and vegetables off skewers into a container of reserved oil mixture. Toss gently, breaking up onion chunks. Cover loosely with foil and allow to sit while heating pitas.
5. Place packet of pitas on cooler side of grill and flip occasionally until heated through, approximately five minutes. Lay each warm pita on 12-inch square of foil. Lay out each pita with 2 tablespoons Tzatziki. Place one-quarter of chicken and vegetables in middle of each pita. Roll into cylindrical shape and serve.

French Bouillabaisse

Yield: 6 Servings

A Classic French chicken stew mix.

Ingredients:

- ¼ cup pastis or Pernod
- ¼ teaspoon cayenne pepper
- ¼ teaspoon saffron threads, crumbled
- ½ cup dry white wine
- 1 (14.5-ounce) can diced tomatoes, drained
- 1 (3-inch) strip orange zest
- 1 large leek, white and light green parts only, halved along the length, sliced thin, and washed thoroughly
- 1 small fennel bulb, stalks discarded, bulb halved, cored, and sliced thin
- 1 tablespoon all-purpose flour
- 1 tablespoon chopped 1 tablespoon tomato paste
- 12 ounces Yukon Gold potatoes, unpeeled, cut into ¾-inch pieces

- 2 tablespoons extra-virgin olive oil
- 3 cups chicken broth
- 3 pounds bone-in chicken pieces (split breasts cut in half, drumsticks, and/or thighs), trimmed
- 4 garlic cloves, minced
- Salt and pepper
- fresh tarragon or parsley

Directions:

1. Place oven racks in upper-middle and lowermost positions and pre-heat your oven to 375 degrees. Pat chicken dry using paper towels and sprinkle with salt and pepper. Heat oil in a Dutch oven on moderate to high heat until just smoking. Brown chicken well, five to ten minutes each side; move to plate.
2. Put in leek and fennel to fat left in pot and cook, stirring frequently, until starting to soften and turn translucent, about 4 minutes. Mix in garlic, tomato paste, flour, saffron, and cayenne and cook until aromatic, approximately half a minute. Slowly beat in broth, scraping up any browned bits and smoothing out any lumps. Mix in tomatoes, potatoes, wine, pastis, and orange zest. Bring to simmer and cook for about ten minutes.
3. Nestle chicken thighs and drumsticks into pot with skin above surface of liquid. Cook, uncovered, for about five minutes. Nestle breast pieces into pot, adjusting pieces as necessary to ensure that skin stays above surface of liquid. Move pot to upper rack and cook, uncovered, until breasts register 145 degrees and thighs/drumsticks register 160 degrees, 10 to 20 minutes.
4. Remove pot from oven and heat broiler. Return pot to oven and broil until chicken skin is crisp and breasts register 160 degrees and drumsticks/thighs register 175 degrees, 5 to 10 minutes (smaller pieces may cook faster than larger pieces; remove individual pieces as they reach correct temperature and return to pot before you serve).

5. Using large spoon, skim excess fat from surface of stew. Mix in tarragon and sprinkle with salt and pepper to taste. Serve with Rouille if you desire, in wide, shallow bowls.

ROUILLE

Yield: 1 cup

This recipe can be made quickly

Ⓥ *This is a Vegetarian Recipe* Ⓥ

Leftover Rouille will keep refrigerated for maximum seven days and can be used as a sauce for vegetables and fish.

- *Ingredients:*
- ¼ teaspoon cayenne pepper
- ¼ teaspoon saffron threads, crumbled
- ½ cup extra-virgin olive oil
- ½ cup vegetable oil
- 1 (3-inch) piece baguette, crusts removed, torn into 1-inch pieces (1 cup)
- 1 large egg yolk
- 2 small garlic cloves, minced
- 2 teaspoons Dijon mustard
- 3 tablespoons boiling water
- 4 teaspoons lemon juice
- Salt and pepper

Directions:

1. Mix boiling water and saffron in a moderate-sized container and allow to steep for about five minutes. Stir bread pieces and lemon juice into saffron-infused water and let soak for about five minutes. Using beat, mash soaked bread mixture until uniform paste forms, 1 to 2 minutes. Beat in egg yolk, mustard, garlic, and cayenne until smooth, approximately fifteen seconds.

2. Whisking continuously, slowly drizzle in vegetable oil until smooth mayonnaise-like consistency is reached, scraping down bowl as necessary. Slowly beat in olive oil gradually until smooth. Sprinkle with salt and pepper to taste.

North African Exotic Chicken Tagine

Yield: 8 Servings

Ingredients:

- ¼ teaspoon cayenne pepper
- ¼ teaspoon ground cinnamon
- ¼ teaspoon ground coriander
- ¼ teaspoon ground ginger
- ½ teaspoon ground cumin
- 1 (15-ounce) can chickpeas, rinsed
- 1 cup dried apricots, halved
- 1 large onion, halved and sliced ¼ inch thick
- 1 tablespoon honey
- 1¼ teaspoons paprika
- 2 carrots, peeled, halved along the length, and sliced ½ inch thick
- 2 cups chicken broth
- 2 tablespoons 2 tablespoons extra-virgin olive oil
- 3 (2-inch) strips lemon zest plus 3 tablespoons juice
- 4 pounds bone-in chicken pieces (split breasts cut in half, drumsticks, and/or thighs), trimmed
- 5 garlic cloves, minced
- Salt and pepper
- chopped fresh cilantro

Directions:

1. Mince 1 strip lemon zest and combine with 1 teaspoon garlic in a container; set aside.

2. Pat chicken dry using paper towels and sprinkle with salt and pepper. Heat oil in a Dutch oven on moderate to high heat until just smoking. Brown half of chicken well, five to ten minutes each side; move to large plate. Replicate the process with the rest of the chicken; move to plate. Pour off all but 1 tablespoon fat from pot.
3. Put in onion and remaining 2 lemon zest strips to fat left in pot and cook on moderate heat till they become tender, approximately five minutes. Mix in remaining garlic, paprika, cumin, cayenne, ginger, coriander, and cinnamon and cook until aromatic, approximately one minute. Mix in broth, scraping up any browned bits. Mix in carrots, chickpeas, and honey and bring to simmer.
4. Nestle chicken into pot along with any accumulated juices and bring to simmer. Decrease heat to moderate to low, cover, and cook until breasts register 160 degrees and drumsticks/thighs register 175 degrees, approximately twenty minutes for breasts and sixty minutes for thighs and drumsticks. (If using both types of chicken, simmer thighs and drumsticks for 40 minutes before adding breasts.)
5. Move chicken to a container, tent loosely with aluminium foil, and allow to rest while finishing sauce. Discard lemon zest. Using large spoon, skim excess fat from surface of sauce. Mix in apricots, return sauce to simmer on moderate heat, and cook until apricots are heated through, approximately five minutes. Return chicken and any accumulated juices to pot. Mix in cilantro, lemon juice, and garlic–lemon zest mixture. Sprinkle with salt and pepper to taste. Serve.

Glazed Roasted Quail

Yield: 4 Servings

Ingredients:

- 1 tablespoon minced fresh thyme

- 1 teaspoon ground 2 tablespoons extra-virgin olive oil
- 6 tablespoons pomegranate molasses
- 8 (5- to 7-ounce) whole quail, giblets discarded
- Salt and pepper
- cinnamon

Directions:

1. Place oven rack to upper-middle position and pre-heat your oven to 500 degrees. Set wire rack in aluminium foil–lined rimmed baking sheet and spray using vegetable oil spray. Dissolve ½ cup salt in 2 quarts water in large container. Immerse quail in brine put inside your fridge for 20 minutes.
2. Remove quail from brine, pat dry using paper towels, and season with pepper. Working with 1 quail at a time, make incision through meat of one drumstick, using tip of paring knife, about ½ inch from tip of drumstick bone. Cautiously insert other drumstick through incision so legs are tightly crossed. Tuck wingtips behind back.
3. Heat 1 tablespoon oil in 12-inch frying pan on moderate to high heat until just smoking. Brown 4 quail on all sides, about 4 minutes; move to prepared rack. Repeat with residual 1 tablespoon oil and remaining 4 quail.
4. Mix pomegranate molasses, thyme, cinnamon, and ⅛ teaspoon salt in a container. Brush quail evenly with half of pomegranate molasses mixture and roast for about five minutes. Brush quail with remaining pomegranate molasses mixture and continue to roast until thoroughly browned and breasts register 160 degrees and thighs register 175 degrees, 7 to 13 minutes. Move quail to serving platter and allow to rest for about five minutes. Serve.

Pork Recipes

Fiery Braised Greek Sausages

Yield: 4 to 6 Servings

Ingredients:

- ½ cup dry white wine
- ¾ cup chicken broth
- 1 (14.5-ounce) can diced tomatoes
- 1 onion, chopped
- 1 tablespoon minced 1 tablespoon tomato paste
- 1 teaspoon ground fennel
- 1½ pounds loukaniko sausage
- 2 jalapeño chiles, stemmed, seeded, and minced
- 2 tablespoons extra-virgin olive oil
- 2 teaspoons grated orange zest
- 3 garlic cloves, minced
- 4 bell peppers (red, yellow, and/or green), stemmed, seeded, and cut into 1½-inch pieces
- Salt and pepper
- fresh oregano

Directions:

1. Prick sausages with fork in several places. Heat 1 tablespoon oil in 12-inch non-stick frying pan on moderate to high heat until just smoking. Brown sausages well on all sides, approximately eight minutes. Move sausages to slicing board, allow to cool slighty, then cut into quarters.
2. Heat residual 1 tablespoon oil in now-empty frying pan on moderate heat until it starts to shimmer. Put in peppers, onion, jalapeños, ½ teaspoon salt, and ½ teaspoon pepper and cook until peppers are starting to soften, approximately five minutes. Mix in garlic, tomato paste, orange zest, and fennel and cook until aromatic, approximately one minute. Mix in wine, scraping up any browned bits.
3. Mix in tomatoes and their juice, broth, and sausages and any accumulated juices and bring to simmer. Cover, decrease the

heat to low, and simmer gently until sausages are cooked through, approximately five minutes.
4. Uncover, increase heat to medium, and cook until sauce has thickened slightly, about 10 minutes. Mix in oregano and sprinkle with salt and pepper to taste. Serve.

French-Style Sausage

Yield: 4 to 6 Servings

Ingredients:

- ½ cup dry white wine
- ½ cup Parmesan Bread Crumbs
- 1 (14.5-ounce) can diced tomatoes, drained with juice reserved
- 1 (15-ounce) can cannellini beans, rinsed
- 1 onion, chopped fine
- 1 pound hot or sweet Italian sausage
- 1½ cups chicken broth
- 12 ounces mustard greens, stemmed and cut into 2-inch pieces
- 2 tablespoons extra-virgin olive oil
- 2 tablespoons minced 2 tablespoons minced fresh thyme or 2 teaspoons dried
- 6 garlic cloves, minced
- Salt and pepper
- fresh parsley

Directions:

1. Prick sausages with fork in several places. Heat 1 tablespoon oil in a Dutch oven on moderate to high heat until just smoking. Brown sausages well on all sides, approximately eight minutes; move to plate.
2. Heat residual 1 tablespoon oil in now-empty pot on moderate heat until it starts to shimmer. Put in onion and ¼ teaspoon salt and cook till they become tender and lightly browned, 5 to 7 minutes. Mix in thyme and garlic and cook until aromatic,

approximately half a minute. Mix in wine and reserved tomato juice, scraping up any browned bits, and cook until nearly evaporated, approximately five minutes. Mix in broth, beans, and tomatoes and bring to simmer.
3. Mix in mustard greens and cook until slightly wilted, approximately one minute. Place sausages on top of greens. Decrease heat to low, cover, and cook until greens are wilted and reduced in volume by about half, about 10 minutes.
4. Uncover, increase heat to moderate to low, and continue to cook, stirring intermittently, until sausages are cooked through and greens are tender, about fifteen minutes. Remove from the heat, using back of spoon, mash portion of beans against side of pot to thicken sauce. Serve, sprinkling individual portions with bread crumbs and parsley.

Greek Braised Pork

Yield: 4 to 6 Servings

Ingredients:

- ½ cup chicken broth
- 1 (14.5-ounce) can diced tomatoes
- 1 bay leaf
- 1 cup dry white wine
- 2 garlic cloves, minced
- 2 pounds boneless pork butt roast, trimmed and cut into 1-inch pieces
- 2 pounds leeks, white and light green parts only, halved along the length, sliced 1 inch thick, and washed thoroughly
- 2 teaspoons cho3 tablespoons extra-virgin olive oil
- Salt and pepper
- Chopped fresh oregano

Directions:

1. Place oven rack to lower-middle position and pre-heat your oven to 325 degrees. Pat pork dry using paper towels and sprinkle with salt and pepper. Heat 1 tablespoon oil in a Dutch oven on moderate to high heat until just smoking. Brown half of pork on all sides, approximately eight minutes; move to a container. Repeat with 1 tablespoon oil and remaining pork; move to a container.
2. Put in remaining 1 tablespoon oil, leeks, ½ teaspoon salt, and ½ teaspoon pepper to fat left in pot and cook on moderate heat, stirring intermittently, till they become tender and lightly browned, 5 to 7 minutes. Mix in garlic and cook until aromatic, approximately half a minute. Mix in tomatoes and their juice, scraping up any browned bits, and cook until tomato liquid is nearly evaporated, 10 to 12 minutes.
3. Mix in wine, broth, bay leaf, and pork with any accumulated juices and bring to simmer. Cover, move pot to oven, and cook until pork becomes soft and falls apart when prodded with fork, 1 to 1½ hours. Discard bay leaf. Mix in oregano and sprinkle with salt and pepper to taste. Serve.

North African Spice Grilled Pork Skewers

Yield: 4 to 6 Servings

Ingredients:

- ¼ cup capers, rinsed
- ½ cup pitted kalamata olives, chopped
- ½ teaspoon ground cinnamon
- ½ teaspoon ground nutmeg
- 1 tablespoon grated lemon zest
- 1 tablespoon ground coriander
- 1½ pounds boneless country-style pork ribs, trimmed and cut into 1-inch pieces
- 2 onions, sliced into ½-inch-thick rounds
- 2 tablespoons honey

- 2 tablespoons minced 2 teaspoons ground cumin
- 3 tablespoons balsamic vinegar
- 5 garlic cloves, minced
- 6 tablespoons extra-virgin olive oil
- Salt and pepper
- fresh parsley

Directions:

1. Beat ¼ cup oil, garlic, lemon zest, coriander, cumin, 1½ teaspoons salt, ½ teaspoon pepper, nutmeg, and cinnamon together in medium bowl. Move 2 tablespoons marinade to small-sized container and set aside. Mix remaining marinade and pork in 1-gallon zipper-lock bag and toss to coat. Press out as much air as possible and seal bag. Refrigerate for minimum sixty minutes or maximum 2 hours, flipping bag every half an hour.
2. Beat honey into reserved marinade and microwave until aromatic, 15 to 30 seconds. Remove pork from bag and pat dry using paper towels. Thread pork tightly onto four 12-inch metal skewers. Thread onion rounds from side to side onto two 12-inch metal skewers, brush with 1 tablespoon oil, and sprinkle with salt and pepper.
3. **For a Charcoal Grill:** Open bottom vent fully. Light large chimney starter three-quarters filled with charcoal briquettes (4½ quarts). When top coals are partly covered with ash, pour uniformly over grill. Set cooking grate in place, cover, and open lid vent fully. Heat grill until hot, approximately five minutes. **For a Gas Grill:** Turn all burners to high, cover, and heat grill until hot, about fifteen minutes. Turn all burners to moderate to high.
4. Clean and oil cooking grate. Place pork and onion skewers on grill and cook (covered if using gas), turning skewers every 2 minutes and basting pork with honey mixture, until pork is browned and registers 140 degrees and onions are mildly charred and tender, 10 to fifteen minutes. Move pork and

onions to slicing board as they finish grilling and tent loosely with aluminium foil. Let pork rest while preparing relish.
5. Coarsely chop onions and combine with remaining 1 tablespoon oil, olives, capers, vinegar, and parsley. Sprinkle with salt and pepper to taste. Using tongs, slide pork off skewers onto serving platter. Serve pork with relish.

Spicy Pork Tenderloin

Yield: 6 Servings

Ingredients:

- ½ cup pitted kalamata olives, halved
- 1 pound cherry tomatoes, halved
- 1 tablespoon grated lemon zest
- 2 (12- to 16-ounce) pork tenderloins, trimmed
- 2 cups jarred whole baby artichoke hearts packed in water, quartered, rinsed, and patted dry
- 2 large fennel bulbs, stalks discarded, bulbs halved, cored, and sliced ½ inch thick
- 2 tablespoons minced 2 teaspoons herbes de Provence
- 3 tablespoons extra-virgin olive oil
- Salt and pepper
- fresh parsley

Directions:

1. Place oven rack to lower-middle position and pre-heat your oven to 450 degrees. Mix fennel and 2 tablespoons water in a container, cover, and microwave till they become tender, approximately five minutes. Drain fennel well, then toss with artichoke hearts, olives, and oil.
2. Pat tenderloins dry using paper towels, drizzle with herbes de Provence, and sprinkle with salt and pepper. Lay out vegetables in large roasting pan, then place tenderloins on top. Roast tenderloins and vegetables until pork registers 145 degrees,

about half an hour, turning tenderloins over halfway through roasting.
3. Move tenderloins to carving board, tent loosely with aluminium foil, and allow to rest for about ten minutes. In the meantime, stir tomatoes and lemon zest into vegetables and continue to roast until fennel becomes soft and tomatoes have softened, about 10 minutes. Mix in parsley and sprinkle with salt and pepper to taste. Slice pork into ½-inch-thick slices and serve with vegetables.

Lamb Recipes

Braised Lamb Shanks

Yield: 4 Servings

Ingredients:

- ¼ cup harissa
- 1 onion, chopped fine
- 1 tablespoon extra-virgin olive oil
- 1 tablespoon red wine vinegar
- 2 bay leaves
- 2 tablespoons minced 2 tablespoons tomato paste
- 2½ cups chicken broth
- 4 (10- to 12-ounce) lamb shanks, trimmed
- 4 bell peppers (red, orange, and/or yellow), stemmed, seeded, and cut into 1-inch pieces
- 4 garlic cloves, minced
- Salt and pepper
- fresh mint

Directions:

1. Place oven rack to lower-middle position and pre-heat your oven to 350 degrees. Pat shanks dry using paper towels and sprinkle with salt and pepper. Heat oil in a Dutch oven on moderate to high heat until just smoking. Brown shanks on all sides, eight to ten minutes; move to a container.
2. Put in onion, peppers, and ½ teaspoon salt to fat left in pot and cook on moderate heat till they become tender, approximately five minutes. Mix in 3 tablespoons harissa, tomato paste, and garlic and cook until aromatic, approximately half a minute. Mix in broth and bay leaves, scraping up any browned bits, and bring to simmer.
3. Nestle shanks into pot and return to simmer. Cover, move pot to oven, and cook until lamb becomes soft and fork slips easily in and out of meat and peppers begin to break down, 2 to 2½ hours, turning shanks halfway through cooking. Move shanks to a container, tent loosely with aluminium foil, and allow to rest while finishing sauce.
4. Strain braising liquid through fine-mesh strainer into fat separator; discard bay leaves and move solids to blender. Let braising liquid settle for about five minutes, then pour defatted liquid into blender with solids and process until smooth, approximately one minute.
5. Move sauce to now-empty pot and mix in vinegar and remaining 1 tablespoon harissa. Return shanks and any accumulated juices to pot, bring to mild simmer on moderate heat, and cook, spooning sauce over shanks occasionally, until heated through, approximately five minutes. Sprinkle with salt and pepper to taste. Move shanks to serving platter, spoon 1 cup sauce over top, and drizzle with mint. Serve, passing remaining sauce separately.

Braised Lamb Shoulder Chops

Yield: 4 Servings

Ingredients:

- ⅓ cup dry red wine
- 1 cup canned whole peeled tomatoes, chopped
- 1 small onion, chopped fine
- 2 small garlic cloves, minced
- 2 tablespoons 2 tablespoons extra-virgin olive oil
- 4 (8- to 12-ounce) lamb shoulder chops (round bone or blade), about ¾ inch thick, trimmed
- Salt and pepper
- minced fresh parsley

Directions:

1. Pat chops dry using paper towels and sprinkle with salt and pepper. Heat 1 tablespoon oil in 12-inch frying pan on moderate to high heat until just smoking. Brown chops, in batches if needed, 4 to 5 minutes each side; move to plate. Pour off fat from skillet.
2. Heat residual 1 tablespoon oil in now-empty frying pan on moderate heat until it starts to shimmer. Put in onion and cook till they become tender, approximately five minutes. Mix in garlic and cook until aromatic, approximately half a minute. Mix in wine, scraping up any browned bits. Bring to simmer and cook until reduced by half, 2 to 3 minutes. Mix in tomatoes.
3. Nestle chops into frying pan along with any accumulated juices and return to simmer. Decrease heat to low, cover, and simmer gently until chops are soft and fork slips easily in and out of meat, fifteen to twenty minutes. Move chops to serving platter, tent loosely with aluminium foil, and allow to rest while finishing sauce.
4. Stir parsley into sauce and simmer until sauce thickens, 2 to 3 minutes. Sprinkle with salt and pepper to taste. Spoon sauce over chops and serve.

Grilled Greek Gyro

Yield: 4 Servings

A Greek Grilled Lamb Sandwich.

Ingredients:

- ¼ teaspoon pepper
- ½ onion, chopped coarse
- ½ teaspoon salt
- 1 cup Tzatziki
- 1 large tomato, cored and sliced thin
- 1 pound ground lamb
- 1 tablespoon minced fresh oregano or 1 teaspoon dried
- 2 cups shredded iceberg lettuce
- 2 garlic cloves, minced
- 2 ounces feta 2 teaspoons extra-virgin olive oil
- 4 (8-inch) pita breads
- 4 teaspoons lemon juice
- cheese, crumbled (½ cup)

Directions:

1. Cut top quarter off each pita bread. Tear quarters into 1-inch pieces. (You should have ¾ cup pita pieces.) Lightly moisten 2 pita breads with water. Sandwich unmoistened pitas between moistened pitas and wrap stack tightly in lightly greased heavy-duty aluminium foil; set aside.
2. Process pita bread pieces, onion, oregano, lemon juice, garlic, salt, and pepper using a food processor until smooth paste forms, approximately half a minute; move to big container. Put in ground lamb and knead with your hands until thoroughly combined. Divide mixture into 12 equal portions. Shape each portion into ball, then gently flatten into round disk about ½ inch thick and 2½ inches in diameter.
3. **For a Charcoal Grill:** Open bottom vent fully. Light large chimney starter three-quarters filled with charcoal (4½ quarts). When top coals are partly covered with ash, pour uniformly over half of grill. Set cooking grate in place, cover, and open lid vent fully. Heat grill until hot, approximately five minutes. **For a Gas Grill:** Turn all burners to high, cover, and heat grill until hot,

about fifteen minutes. Turn primary burner to moderate to high and turn off other burner(s).
4. Clean and oil cooking grate. Place patties on hotter side of grill, cover (if using gas), and cook until thoroughly browned and crust forms, four to eight minutes each side. Move patties to paper towel–lined plate, cover loosely with foil, and allow to sit while heating pitas.
5. Place packet of pitas on cooler side of grill and flip occasionally until heated through, approximately five minutes. Using spoon, spread ¼ cup Tzatziki inside each warm pita. Divide patties evenly among pitas and fill each sandwich with tomato slices, ½ cup shredded lettuce, and 2 tablespoons feta. Serve instantly.

Grilled Lamb Kofte

Yield: 4 to 6 Servings

Ingredients:

- ⅛ teaspoon ground cinnamon
- ⅛ teaspoon ground nutmeg
- ¼ teaspoon ground cloves
- ¼ teaspoon ground coriander
- ⅓ cup minced fresh mint
- ⅓ cup minced fresh parsley
- ½ cup grated onion, drained
- ½ cup pine nuts
- ½ teaspoon pepper
- 1 (13 by 9-inch) disposable aluminium roasting pan (if using charcoal)
- 1 recipe Tahini-1 teaspoon ground cumin
- 1 teaspoon salt
- 1½ pounds ground lamb
- 1½ teaspoons hot smoked paprika
- 1½ teaspoons unflavored gelatin
- 4 garlic cloves, peeled and smashed

- Yogurt Sauce

Directions:

1. Process pine nuts, garlic, paprika, salt, cumin, pepper, coriander, cloves, nutmeg, and cinnamon using a food processor until coarse paste forms, 30 to 45 seconds; move to big container. Put in ground lamb, onion, parsley, mint, and gelatin and knead with your hands until thoroughly combined and mixture feels slightly sticky, approximately two minutes.
2. Divide mixture into 8 equal portions. Shape each portion into 5-inch-long cylinder about 1 inch in diameter. Using eight 12-inch metal skewers, thread 1 cylinder onto each skewer, pressing gently to stick. Move skewers to lightly greased baking sheet, cover up using plastic wrap, put inside your fridge for minimum sixty minutes or maximum 24 hours.
3. **For a Charcoal Grill:** Using kitchen shears, poke twelve ½-inch holes in bottom of disposable pan. Open bottom vent completely and place pan in center of grill. Light large chimney starter filled two-thirds with charcoal briquettes (4 quarts). When top coals are partly covered with ash, pour into pan. Set cooking grate in place, cover, and open lid vent fully. Heat grill until hot, approximately five minutes. **For a Gas Grill:** Turn all burners to high, cover, and heat grill until hot, about fifteen minutes. Leave all burners on high.
4. Clean and oil cooking grate. Place skewers on grill (directly over coals if using charcoal) at 45-degree angle to grate. Cook (covered if using gas) until browned and meat easily releases from grill, four to eight minutes. Flip skewers and carry on cooking until browned on second side and meat registers 160 degrees, about 6 minutes. Move skewers to serving platter and serve with Tahini-Yogurt Sauce.

Grilled Lamb Shish Kebabs

Yield: 4 to 6 Servings

Ingredients:

MARINADE

- ¼ teaspoon ½ teaspoon grated lemon zest plus 2 tablespoons juice
- 1 teaspoon salt
- 2 garlic cloves, peeled
- 2 teaspoons chopped fresh rosemary
- 6 tablespoons extra-virgin olive oil
- 7 large fresh mint leaves
- pepper

LAMB AND VEGETABLES

- 2 pounds boneless leg of lamb, pulled apart at seams, trimmed, and cut into 2-inch pieces
- 2 red onions, cut 2 red or green bell peppers, stemmed, seeded, and cut into 1½-inch pieces
- 2 zucchini or yellow summer squash, halved along the length and sliced 1 inch thick
- into 1-inch pieces, 3 layers thick

Directions:

1. **For The Marinade**: Process all ingredients using a food processor until smooth, approximately one minute, scraping down sides of the container as required. Move 3 tablespoons marinade to big container and set aside.
2. **For The Lamb And Vegetables:** Place remaining marinade and lamb in 1-gallon zipper-lock bag and toss to coat. Press out as much air as possible and seal bag. Refrigerate for minimum sixty minutes or maximum 2 hours, flipping bag every half an hour.
3. Put in zucchini, bell peppers, and onions to a container with reserved marinade and toss to coat. Cover and allow to sit at room temperature for minimum half an hour.
4. Remove lamb from bag and pat dry using paper towels. Thread lamb tightly onto two 12-inch metal skewers. In alternating

pattern of zucchini, bell pepper, and onion, thread vegetables onto four 12-inch metal skewers.
5. **For a Charcoal Grill:** Open bottom vent fully. Light large chimney starter mounded with charcoal briquettes (7 quarts). When top coals are partly covered with ash, pour uniformly over center of grill, leaving 2-inch gap between grill wall and charcoal. Set cooking grate in place, cover, and open lid vent fully. Heat grill until hot, approximately five minutes. **For a Gas Grill:** Turn all burners to high, cover, and heat grill until hot, about fifteen minutes. Leave primary burner on high and turn other burner(s) to moderate to low.
6. Clean and oil cooking grate. Place lamb skewers on grill (directly over coals if using charcoal or over hotter side of grill if using gas). Place vegetable skewers on grill (near edge of coals but still over coals if using charcoal or on cooler side of grill if using gas). Cook (covered if using gas), turning skewers every three to five minutes, until lamb is thoroughly browned and registers 120 to 125 degrees (for medium-rare), 10 to fifteen minutes. Move lamb skewers to serving platter, tent loosely with aluminium foil, and allow to rest while finishing vegetables.
7. Carry on cooking vegetable skewers until soft and mildly charred, 5 to 7 minutes; move to platter. Using tongs, slide lamb and vegetables off skewers onto platter. Serve.

Grilled Lamb Shoulder Chops

Yield: 4 to 6 Servings

Ingredients:

- ½ cup extra-virgin olive oil
- 1 small shallot, minced
- 1 teaspoon baking soda
- 1 teaspoon Dijon mustard
- 1½ pounds thick 2 garlic cloves, minced
- 2 tablespoons chopped fresh mint

- 2 teaspoons minced fresh oregano
- 3 tablespoons red wine vinegar
- 4 (8- to 12-ounce) lamb shoulder chops (blade or round bone), ¾ to 1 inch thick, trimmed
- Salt and pepper
- asparagus, trimmed

Directions:

1. Beat ¼ cup oil, vinegar, mint, shallot, mustard, ¼ teaspoon salt, and ⅛ teaspoon pepper together in a container; set aside for serving.
2. Beat remaining ¼ cup oil, garlic, oregano, baking soda, ½ teaspoon salt, and ½ teaspoon pepper together in a container. Place marinade and chops in 1-gallon zipper-lock bag and toss to coat. Press out as much air as possible and seal bag. Refrigerate for minimum half an hour or maximum 1 hour, flipping bag halfway through. Remove lamb and let excess marinade drip off but do not pat dry.
3. **For a Charcoal Grill:** Open bottom vent fully. Light large chimney starter filled with charcoal briquettes (6 quarts). When top coals are partly covered with ash, pour uniformly over grill. Set cooking grate in place, cover, and open lid vent fully. Heat grill until hot, approximately five minutes. **For a Gas Grill:** Turn all burners to high, cover, and heat grill until hot, about fifteen minutes. Leave all burners on high.
4. Clean and oil cooking grate. Place chops on grill and cook until thoroughly browned and meat registers 120 to 125 degrees (for medium-rare), 2 to 4 minutes each side. Move chops to serving platter, tent loosely with aluminium foil, and allow to rest while preparing asparagus.
5. Place asparagus on grill and cook, turning as required, until crisp-tender and lightly browned, approximately five minutes; move to platter with lamb. Sprinkle with vinaigrette and serve.

Lamb Meatballs

Yield: 4 Servings

Ingredients:

- ⅛ teaspoon ground cloves
- ½ teaspoon grated lemon zest plus ½ teaspoon juice
- ¾ teaspoon ground cinnamon
- 1 cup chicken 1 cup whole Greek yogurt
- 1 large egg yolk
- 1 pound ground lamb
- 1 teaspoon ground cumin
- 2 garlic cloves, minced
- 2 tablespoons extra-virgin olive oil
- 2 tablespoons water
- 3 tablespoons minced fresh mint
- 3 tablespoons panko bread crumbs
- 8 ounces leeks, white and light green parts only, chopped and washed thoroughly
- Salt and pepper
- broth

Directions:

1. Mash ⅓ cup yogurt, panko, and water together with fork in a big container to form paste. Put in ground lamb, 2 tablespoons mint, egg yolk, half of garlic, cumin, cinnamon, ¾ teaspoon salt, ⅛ teaspoon pepper, and cloves and knead with your hands until thoroughly combined. Pinch off and roll mixture into twelve 1½-inch meatballs.
2. Heat oil in 12-inch frying pan on moderate to high heat until just smoking. Brown meatballs on all sides, six to eight minutes; move to plate. Pour off all but 1 tablespoon fat from skillet.
3. Put in leeks and cook on moderate heat till they become tender and lightly browned, 5 to 7 minutes. Mix in lemon zest and remaining garlic and cook until aromatic, approximately half a

minute. Mix in broth, scraping up any browned bits, and bring to simmer.
4. Return meatballs to frying pan and bring to simmer. Decrease heat to moderate to low, cover, and simmer, turning meatballs occasionally, for about five minutes. Uncover and carry on cooking until liquid has reduced slightly, approximately two minutes.
5. Remove from the heat, move meatballs to serving platter and tent loosely with aluminium foil. Whisking continuously, slowly ladle approximately one cup hot liquid into remaining ⅔ cup yogurt in a container until combined. Stir yogurt mixture into frying pan along with lemon juice until combined. Sprinkle with salt and pepper to taste. Pour sauce over meatballs and drizzle with remaining 1 tablespoon mint. Serve.

Roast Butterflied Leg of Lamb

Yield: 8 to 10 Servings

Ingredients:

- ⅓ cup extra-virgin olive oil
- 1 (1-inch) piece ginger, peeled, sliced into ½-inch-thick rounds, and smashed
- 1 (3½- to 4-pound) butterflied leg of lamb
- 1 tablespoon coriander seeds
- 1 tablespoon cumin seeds
- 1 tablespoon mustard seeds
- 2 (2-inch) strips 3 bay leaves
- 3 shallots, sliced thin
- 4 garlic cloves, peeled and smashed
- Kosher salt
- lemon zest

Directions:

1. Place lamb on slicing board with fat cap facing down. Using sharp knife, trim any pockets of fat and connective tissue from underside of lamb. Flip lamb over, trim fat cap to between ⅛ and ¼ inch thick, and pound roast to even 1-inch thickness. Cut slits, spaced ½ inch apart, in fat cap in crosshatch pattern, being careful to cut down to but not into meat. Rub 1 tablespoon salt over entire roast and into slits. Let sit, uncovered, at room temperature for about one hour.
2. In the meantime, adjust oven rack to lower-middle position and second rack 4 to 5 inches from broiler element and pre-heat your oven to 250 degrees. Stir together oil, shallots, garlic, ginger, coriander seeds, cumin seeds, mustard seeds, bay leaves, and lemon zest in rimmed baking sheet and bake on lower rack until spices become soft and aromatic and shallots and garlic turn golden, about 1 hour. Remove sheet from oven and discard bay leaves.
3. Pat lamb dry using paper towels and move fat side up to sheet (directly on top of spices). Roast on lower rack until lamb registers 120 degrees, 20 minutes to half an hour. Remove sheet from oven and heat broiler. Broil lamb on upper rack until surface is thoroughly browned and charred in spots and lamb registers 125 degrees (for medium-rare), three to eight minutes.
4. Remove sheet from oven and move lamb to carving board (some spices will cling to bottom of roast). Tent loosely with aluminium foil and allow to rest for 20 minutes.
5. Slice lamb with grain into 3 equivalent pieces. Turn each piece and slice against grain into ¼-inch-thick slices. Serve.

Egg Recipes

Classic Greek Baked Eggs

Yield: 6 Servings

Ⓥ This is a Vegetarian Recipe Ⓥ

Ingredients:

- ¼ cup extra-virgin olive oil
- 1 teaspoon sugar
- 2 pounds cherry tomatoes
- 2 teaspoons tomato paste
- 3 slices French or Italian bread, cut into ½-inch pieces (4 cups)
- 5 teaspoons minced fresh oregano
- 6 garlic cloves, sliced thin
- 6 large eggs
- Salt and pepper
- 2 ounces feta cheese, crumbled (½ cup)

Directions:

1. Place two oven racks in your oven one just above, and one just below the middle position and pre-heat your oven to 450 degrees. Toss bread with 1 tablespoon oil in a big container and sprinkle with salt and pepper. Lay out bread into even layer in greased 13 by 9-inch baking dish; set aside.
2. Beat garlic, 1 tablespoon oil, 1 tablespoon oregano, tomato paste, 1½ teaspoons salt, sugar, and ¼ teaspoon pepper together in a big container. Put in tomatoes and toss to combine. Move tomato mixture to parchment paper–lined rimmed baking sheet and push tomatoes toward center of sheet. Scrape any remaining garlic and tomato paste from bowl into center of tomatoes; set bowl aside without washing.

3. Bake bread on upper rack and tomatoes on lower rack, stirring intermittently, until bread is golden and tomatoes start to become tender, about 10 minutes. Remove croutons from oven and allow to cool in dish. Continue to bake tomatoes until blistered and browned, about 10 minutes.
4. Put in tomatoes and 1 tablespoon oil to croutons, gently fold to combine, and smooth into even layer. Make 6 shallow indentations (about 2 inches wide) in surface of bread-tomato mixture using back of spoon. Crack 1 egg into each indentation and season eggs with salt and pepper.
5. Bake until whites are just starting to set but still have some movement when dish is shaken, 10 to 12 minutes. Move dish to wire rack, tent loosely with aluminium foil, and allow to sit for about five minutes. Sprinkle with feta and remaining 2 teaspoons oregano and drizzle with remaining 1 tablespoon oil. Serve instantly.

Crunchy Meaty Poached Eggs

Yield: 4 Servings

Ingredients:

- ¼ teaspoon cayenne pepper
- 1 onion, chopped fine
- 1 tablespoon 1 teaspoon ground coriander
- 1 teaspoon ground cumin
- 1½ pounds russet potatoes, peeled and cut into ½-inch pieces
- 1½ pounds Swiss chard, stems sliced ¼ inch thick, leaves sliced into ½-inch-wide strips
- 2 tablespoons extra-virgin olive oil
- 2 teaspoons paprika
- 3 garlic cloves, minced
- 4 large eggs
- 8 ounces ground lamb
- Salt and pepper

- minced fresh chives

Directions:

1. Toss potatoes with 1 tablespoon oil, ½ teaspoon salt, and ¼ teaspoon pepper in a container. Cover and microwave until potatoes are translucent around edges, seven to nine minutes, stirring halfway through microwaving; drain well.
2. Heat residual 1 tablespoon oil in 12-inch non-stick frying pan on moderate to high heat until it starts to shimmer. Put in chard stems and ¼ teaspoon salt and cook till they become tender and lightly browned, 5 to 7 minutes. Mix in chard leaves, 1 handful at a time, and cook until mostly wilted, about 4 minutes; move to a container with potatoes.
3. Cook lamb in now-empty frying pan on moderate to high heat, breaking up meat with wooden spoon, until starting to brown, approximately five minutes. Mix in onion and cook till they become tender and lightly browned, 5 to 7 minutes. Mix in garlic, paprika, cumin, coriander, and cayenne and cook until aromatic, approximately half a minute.
4. Mix in chard-potato mixture. Using back of spatula, gently pack chard-potato mixture into frying pan and cook, without stirring, for 2 minutes. Flip hash, 1 portion at a time, and lightly repack into skillet. Repeat flipping process every few minutes until potatoes are well browned, six to eight minutes.
5. Remove from the heat, make 4 shallow indentations (about 2 inches wide) in surface of hash using back of spoon, pushing hash up into center and around edges of frying pan (bottom of frying pan should be exposed in each divot). Crack 1 egg into each indentation and sprinkle with salt and pepper. Cover and cook over moderate to low heat until whites are just set and yolks are still runny, four to eight minutes. Sprinkle with chives and serve instantly.

Egyptian Eggah

Yield: 4 to 6 Servings

This recipe can be made quickly

Ingredients:

- ¼ cup minced ¼ teaspoon ground cinnamon
- 1 garlic clove, minced
- 1 pound leeks, whites and light green parts only, halved along the length, sliced thin, and washed thoroughly
- 1 teaspoon ground cumin
- 4 teaspoons extra-virgin olive oil
- 6 tablespoons water
- 8 large eggs
- 8 ounces (8 cups) baby spinach
- 8 ounces 90 percent lean ground beef
- Salt and pepper
- fresh cilantro

Directions:

1. Place spinach and ¼ cup water in a big container, cover, and microwave until spinach is wilted and decreased in volume by about half, approximately five minutes. Remove bowl from microwave and keep covered for about sixty seconds. Move spinach to colander and gently press to release liquid. Move spinach to slicing board and chop coarse. Return to colander and press again.
2. Heat 1 teaspoon oil in 10-inch non-stick frying pan on moderate heat until it starts to shimmer. Put in leeks and cook till they become tender, approximately five minutes. Put in ground beef and cook, breaking up meat with wooden spoon, until starting to brown, 5 to 7 minutes. Mix in garlic, cumin, cinnamon, ½ teaspoon salt, and ¼ teaspoon pepper and cook until aromatic, approximately half a minute. Mix in spinach until heated

through, approximately one minute; move to a container and allow to cool slightly.
3. Beat eggs, remaining 2 tablespoons water, ½ teaspoon salt, and ¼ teaspoon pepper together with fork in a big container until thoroughly combined and mixture is pure yellow; do not overbeat. Gently fold in spinach mixture and cilantro, making sure to scrape all of spinach mixture out of skillet.
4. Heat residual 1 tablespoon oil in now-empty frying pan on moderate to high heat until just smoking. Put in egg mixture and cook, shaking frying pan and folding mixture continuously for 15 seconds. Smooth top of egg mixture, decrease the heat to medium, cover, and cook, gently shaking frying pan every 30 seconds, until bottom is golden brown and top is lightly set, approximately three minutes.
5. Remove from the heat, run heat-resistant rubber spatula around edge of frying pan and shake frying pan gently to loosen eggah; it should slide around freely in skillet. Slide eggah onto large plate, then invert onto second large plate and slide back into frying pan browned side up. Tuck edges of eggah into frying pan using a rubber spatula. Carry on cooking on moderate heat, gently shaking frying pan every 30 seconds, until second side is golden brown, approximately two minutes. Slide eggah onto slicing board and allow to cool slightly. Slice and serve hot, warm, or at room temperature.

Fried Eggs with Sides

Yield: 8 Servings

(V) This is a Vegetarian Recipe (V)

Ingredients:

- ¼ cup plus 2 teaspoons extra-virgin olive oil
- 1 ounce Parmesan cheese, grated (½ cup)
- 1 tablespoon minced 1½ teaspoons cornstarch
- 2½ pounds Yukon Gold potatoes, peeled and shredded

- 8 large eggs
- Salt and pepper
- fresh chives

Directions:

1. Place potatoes in a big container and fill bowl with cold water. Using hands, swirl to remove excess starch, then drain, leaving potatoes in colander.
2. Wipe bowl dry. Place one-third of potatoes in center of clean dish towel. Gather towel ends together and twist tightly to squeeze out moisture. Move potatoes to now-empty bowl and repeat process with remaining potatoes in 2 batches.
3. Sprinkle cornstarch, 1 teaspoon salt, and pinch pepper over potatoes. Using hands or fork, toss ingredients together until thoroughly mixed.
4. Heat 2 tablespoons oil in 12-inch non-stick frying pan on moderate heat until it starts to shimmer. Put in potato mixture and spread into even layer. Cover and cook for 6 minutes. Uncover and, using spatula, gently press potatoes down to form round cake. Cook, occasionally pressing on potatoes to shape into uniform round cake, until bottom becomes deeply golden brown, eight to ten minutes.
5. Shake frying pan to loosen pancake and slide onto large plate. Put in 2 tablespoons oil to frying pan and swirl to coat. Invert potato pancake onto second plate and slide potato pancake, browned side up, back into skillet. Cook, occasionally pressing down on pancake, until bottom is well browned, eight to ten minutes. Move pancake to slicing board and set aside while preparing eggs.
6. Crack eggs into 2 small-sized containers (4 eggs per bowl) and sprinkle with salt and pepper. Wipe frying pan clean using paper towels. Heat remaining 2 teaspoons oil in now-empty frying pan on moderate heat until it starts to shimmer. Working quickly, pour 1 bowl of eggs in 1 side of frying pan and second bowl of eggs in other side. Cover and cook for 2 minutes.
7. Remove frying pan from heat and let sit, covered, approximately two minutes for runny yolks (white around edge

of yolk will be barely opaque), approximately three minutes for soft but set yolks, and about 4 minutes for medium-set yolks. Slide eggs onto individual plates. Sprinkle pancake with Parmesan and chives, cut into wedges, and serve with eggs.

Frittata 1: Broccoli-Feta

Yield: 6 Servings

This recipe can be made quickly

Ⓥ *This is a Vegetarian Recipe* Ⓥ

Ingredients:

- ⅓ cup whole milk
- ½ teaspoon grated lemon zest plus ½ teaspoon juice
- 1 tablespoon extra-virgin olive oil
- 12 large eggs
- 12 ounces broccoli florets, cut into ½-inch pieces (3½ to 4 cups)
- 3 tablespoons water
- Pinch red pepper flakes
- Salt
- 4 ounces feta cheese, crumbled into ½-inch pieces (1 cup)

Directions:

1. Place the oven rack in the centre of the oven and pre-heat your oven to 350 degrees. Beat eggs, milk, and ½ teaspoon salt together with fork in a container until thoroughly combined and mixture is pure yellow; do not overbeat.
2. Heat oil in 12-inch non-stick frying pan on moderate to high heat until it starts to shimmer. Put in broccoli, pepper flakes, and ¼ teaspoon salt and cook, stirring often, until broccoli is crisp-tender and spotty brown, seven to nine minutes. Put in water and lemon zest and juice and continue to cook, stirring

continuously, until broccoli is just soft and no water remains in skillet, approximately one minute.
3. Put in feta and egg mixture and, using heat-resistant rubber spatula, continuously and firmly scrape along bottom and sides of frying pan until large curds form and spatula begins to leave trail on bottom of frying pan but eggs are still very wet, approximately half a minute. Smooth curds into even layer and let cook without stirring for 30 seconds. Move frying pan to oven and bake until frittata is slightly puffy and surface bounces back when lightly pressed, 6 to 9 minutes. Using rubber spatula, loosen frittata from frying pan and move to slicing board. Allow to sit for about five minutes before slicing and serving.

Frittata 2: Asparagus and Goat Cheese

This recipe can be made quickly

Ⓥ *This is a Vegetarian Recipe* Ⓥ

This recipe works best with thin or standard-size asparagus spears.

Omit broccoli, pepper flakes, and water. Put in 1 pound asparagus, trimmed and cut into ¼-inch lengths, lemon zest and juice, ¼ teaspoon salt, and ¼ teaspoon pepper to oil in step 2; cook, stirring often, until asparagus is crisp-tender, three to five minutes. Continue with step 3, substituting 1 cup crumbled goat cheese for feta and adding 2 tablespoons chopped fresh mint with goat cheese and egg mixture.

Frittata 3: Mushroom and Pecorino Frittata

This recipe can be made quickly

Ⓥ *This is a Vegetarian Recipe* Ⓥ

Substitute 1 pound cremini mushrooms, stemmed and cut into ½-inch pieces, for broccoli and ¼ teaspoon pepper for red pepper flakes. Reduce water to 2 tablespoons and substitute 2 minced scallion whites, 1½ teaspoons minced fresh thyme, and 1 tablespoon sherry vinegar for lemon juice and zest. Substitute ¾ cup shredded Pecorino Romano for feta and put in 2 thinly sliced scallion greens with Pecorino and egg mixture.

Israeli Sabich Eggplant and Egg Sandwiches

Yield: 4 Servings

Ⓥ This is a Vegetarian Recipe Ⓥ

Sabich is an Israeli Eggplant and Egg sandwich.

Ingredients:

- ¼ cup thinly sliced red onion
- ¼ cup extra-virgin olive oil
- ¼ cup fresh parsley leaves
- ½ cup thinly sliced dill pickles
- ½ cup Green Zhoug
- ½ cup Tahini-Yogurt Sauce
- 1 cup hummus
- 1 garlic clove, minced
- 1 pound eggplant, sliced into ½-inch-thick rounds
- 1 tablespoon lemon juice
- 1 teaspoon ground 4 (8-inch) pita breads
- 6 hard-cooked large eggs, sliced thin
- 8 ounces cherry tomatoes, quartered
- Salt and pepper
- dried Aleppo pepper

Directions:

1. Lay out eggplant over a baking sheet lined using paper towels, drizzle both sides with 2 teaspoons salt, and allow to sit for half an hour.
2. Place oven rack 4 inches from broiler element and heat broiler. Comprehensively pat eggplant dry using paper towels, arrange on aluminium foil–lined rimmed baking sheet in one layer, and lightly brush both sides with 2 tablespoons oil. Broil eggplant until spotty brown, approximately five minutes each side.
3. Mix tomatoes, pickles, onion, parsley, lemon juice, garlic, and remaining 2 tablespoons oil in a container and sprinkle with salt and pepper to taste. Lay each pita on individual plate, spread with ¼ cup hummus, and top evenly with eggplant, tomato salad, and eggs. Sprinkle with Tahini-Yogurt Sauce and Green Zhoug and drizzle with Aleppo. Serve instantly.

Ratatouille with Poached Eggs

Yield: 4 Servings

This recipe can be made quickly

Ⓥ *This is a Vegetarian Recipe* Ⓥ

Ingredients:

- ¼ cup chopped fresh basil
- ¼ cup extra-virgin olive oil
- ½ cup chicken or vegetable broth
- 1 onion, chopped fine
- 1 ounce Parmesan 1 pound eggplant, cut into ¾-inch pieces
- 1 pound plum tomatoes, cored and cut into ½-inch pieces
- 1 pound zucchini, cut into ¾-inch pieces
- 4 garlic cloves, minced
- 4 large eggs
- Salt and pepper
- cheese, grated (½ cup)

Directions:

1. Heat 1 tablespoon oil in 12-inch non-stick frying pan on moderate to high heat until just smoking. Put in zucchini and cook until well browned, approximately five minutes; move to a container.
2. Put in eggplant, 2 tablespoons oil, and ¼ teaspoon salt to now-empty frying pan and cook on moderate to high heat until eggplant is browned, 5 to 7 minutes. Mix in onion and residual 1 tablespoon oil and cook until onion is softened, approximately five minutes. Mix in garlic and cook until aromatic, approximately half a minute. Mix in tomatoes and broth and simmer until vegetables become soft, 3 to 5 minutes. Mix in zucchini and any accumulated juice and sprinkle with salt and pepper to taste.
3. Remove from the heat, make 4 shallow indentations (about 2 inches wide) in surface of ratatouille using back of spoon. Crack 1 egg into each indentation and sprinkle with salt and pepper. Cover and cook over moderate to low heat until egg whites are just set and yolks are still runny, four to eight minutes. Sprinkle with basil and Parmesan and serve instantly.

Scrambled Eggs Mix 1

Yield: 6 to 8 Servings

✯This recipe can be made quickly ✯

Ingredients:

- ¼ teaspoon pepper
- ½ teaspoon salt
- 1 ounce Parmesan 12 large eggs
- 2 ounces thinly sliced prosciutto, chopped coarse
- 2 tablespoons water
- 3 tablespoons extra-virgin olive oil

- 8 ounces asparagus, trimmed and cut on bias into ¼-inch lengths
- cheese, grated (½ cup)

Directions:

1. Heat 1 tablespoon oil in 12-inch non-stick frying pan on moderate heat until it starts to shimmer. Put in asparagus and cook until crisp-tender and lightly browned, 2 to 4 minutes; move to a container and cover to keep warm.
2. Beat eggs, water, salt, and pepper together with fork in a container until thoroughly combined and mixture is pure yellow; do not overbeat.
3. Wipe frying pan clean using paper towels. Heat remaining 2 tablespoons oil in now-empty frying pan on moderate heat until it starts to shimmer. Put in egg mixture and, using heat-resistant rubber spatula, continuously and firmly scrape along bottom and sides of frying pan until eggs begin to clump and spatula leaves trail on bottom of skillet, 1½ to 2 minutes.
4. Decrease heat to low and gently but continuously fold eggs until clumped and slightly wet, 30 to 60 seconds. Remove from the heat, gently fold in asparagus, prosciutto, and Parmesan. Serve instantly.

Scrambled Eggs Mix 2

Yield: 6 to 8 Servings

✔ This recipe can be made quickly ✔

Ⓥ This is a Vegetarian Recipe Ⓥ

Ingredients:

- ½ cup plus 2 tablespoons water
- ½ onion, chopped fine
- 1 garlic clove, minced

- 12 large eggs
- 2 tablespoons chopped 2 tablespoons harissa, plus extra for serving
- 3 tablespoons extra-virgin olive oil
- 8 ounces cremini mushrooms, trimmed and halved if small or quartered if large
- 8 ounces red potatoes, unpeeled, cut into ½-inch pieces
- Salt and pepper
- fresh cilantro

Directions:

1. Heat 1 tablespoon oil in 12-inch non-stick frying pan on moderate heat until it starts to shimmer. Put in potatoes, mushrooms, onion, ½ cup water, and ¼ teaspoon salt. Cover and cook, stirring intermittently, until vegetables become soft, eight to ten minutes. Uncover and continue to cook, stirring intermittently, until liquid is evaporated and potatoes start to look golden brown, 3 to 5 minutes. Mix in garlic and cook until aromatic, approximately half a minute; move to a container and cover to keep warm.
2. Beat eggs, ¾ teaspoon salt, ¼ teaspoon pepper, and remaining 2 tablespoons water together with fork in a container until thoroughly combined and mixture is pure yellow; do not overbeat.
3. Wipe frying pan clean using paper towels. Heat remaining 2 tablespoons oil in now-empty frying pan on moderate heat until it starts to shimmer. Put in egg mixture and, using heat-resistant rubber spatula, continuously and firmly scrape along bottom and sides of frying pan until eggs begin to clump and spatula leaves trail on bottom of skillet, 1½ to 2 minutes.
4. Decrease heat to low and gently but continuously fold eggs until clumped and slightly wet, 30 to 60 seconds. Remove from the heat, gently fold in potato mixture. Sprinkle with harissa and drizzle with cilantro. Serve instantly, passing extra harissa separately.

Scrambled Eggs Mix 3

Yield: 6 to 8 Servings

Ⓥ *This is a Vegetarian Recipe* Ⓥ

Ingredients:

- ¾ teaspoon red pepper flakes
- 1 (14-ounce) can whole peeled tomatoes, drained with ¼ cup juice reserved, chopped coarse
- 1 bay leaf
- 1 large onion, chopped
- 1 teaspoon minced fresh thyme or ¼ teaspoon dried
- 12 large eggs
- 2 tablespoons 2 teaspoons paprika
- 2 teaspoons sherry vinegar
- 3 Cubanelle peppers, stemmed, seeded, and cut into ½-inch-wide strips
- 3 red bell peppers, stemmed, seeded, and cut into ½-inch-wide strips
- 3 tablespoons minced fresh parsley
- 4 garlic cloves, minced
- 5 tablespoons extra-virgin olive oil
- Salt and pepper
- water

Directions:

1. Heat 3 tablespoons oil in 12-inch non-stick frying pan on moderate heat until it starts to shimmer. Put in onion, bay leaf, and ½ teaspoon salt and cook until onion becomes tender and lightly browned, 5 to 7 minutes. Mix in garlic, paprika, thyme, and pepper flakes and cook until aromatic, approximately one minute. Put in bell peppers, Cubanelle peppers, and 1 teaspoon salt, cover, and cook, stirring intermittently, until peppers start to become tender, about 10 minutes.

2. Decrease heat to moderate to low. Put in tomatoes and reserved juice and cook, uncovered, stirring intermittently, until mixture seems to be dry and peppers are soft but not mushy, 10 to 12 minutes. Remove from the heat, discard bay leaf. Mix in 2 tablespoons parsley and vinegar and sprinkle with salt and pepper to taste; move to a container and cover to keep warm.
3. Beat eggs, water, ½ teaspoon salt, and ¼ teaspoon pepper together with fork in a container until thoroughly combined and mixture is pure yellow; do not overbeat.
4. Wipe frying pan clean using paper towels. Heat remaining 2 tablespoons oil in now-empty frying pan on moderate heat until it starts to shimmer. Put in egg mixture and, using heat-resistant rubber spatula, continuously and firmly scrape along bottom and sides of frying pan until eggs begin to clump and spatula leaves trail on bottom of skillet, 1½ to 2 minutes.
5. Decrease heat to low and gently but continuously fold eggs until clumped and slightly wet, 30 to 60 seconds. Remove from the heat, drizzle with remaining 1 tablespoon parsley and serve instantly with pepper mixture.

Spanish Tortilla

Yield: 6 Servings

Ⓥ This is a Vegetarian Recipe Ⓥ

Ingredients:

- ½ cup frozen ½ cup jarred roasted red peppers, rinsed, patted dry, and cut into ½-inch pieces
- 1 small onion, halved and sliced thin
- 1½ pounds Yukon Gold potatoes, peeled, quartered, and sliced ⅛ inch thick
- 6 tablespoons plus 1 teaspoon extra-virgin olive oil
- 8 large eggs
- Salt and pepper

- peas, thawed

Directions:

1. Toss potatoes and onion with ¼ cup oil, ½ teaspoon salt, and ¼ teaspoon pepper in a big container. Heat 2 tablespoons oil in 10-inch non-stick frying pan on moderate to high heat until it starts to shimmer. Put in potato mixture to frying pan and decrease the heat to moderate to low; set bowl aside without washing. Cover potatoes and cook, stirring every 5 minutes, until tender, about 25 minutes.
2. Beat eggs and ½ teaspoon salt together with fork in reserved bowl until thoroughly combined and mixture is pure yellow; do not overbeat. Gently fold in potato mixture, red peppers, and peas, making sure to scrape all of potato mixture out of skillet.
3. Heat remaining 1 teaspoon oil in now-empty frying pan on moderate to high heat until just smoking. Put in egg mixture and cook, shaking frying pan and folding mixture continuously for 15 seconds. Smooth top of egg mixture, decrease the heat to medium, cover, and cook, gently shaking frying pan every 30 seconds, until bottom is golden brown and top is lightly set, approximately two minutes.
4. Remove from the heat, run heat-resistant rubber spatula around edge of frying pan and shake frying pan gently to loosen tortilla; it should slide around freely in skillet. Slide tortilla onto large plate, then invert onto second large plate and slide back into frying pan browned side up. Tuck edges of tortilla into frying pan using a rubber spatula. Carry on cooking on moderate heat, gently shaking frying pan every 30 seconds, until second side is golden brown, approximately two minutes. Slide tortilla onto slicing board and allow to cool slightly. Slice and serve hot, warm, or at room temperature.

Traditional Greek Sfougato

Yield: 6 to 8 Servings

This recipe can be made quickly

Ⓥ *This is a Vegetarian Recipe* Ⓥ

Ingredients:

- ¼ cup minced fresh dill
- ¼ cup whole milk
- 1 tablespoon 1 tablespoon extra-virgin olive oil
- 2 garlic cloves, minced
- 4 ounces feta cheese, crumbled (1 cup)
- 4 zucchini, shredded
- 6 large eggs
- 8 scallions, sliced thin
- Salt and pepper
- chopped fresh oregano

Directions:

1. Place the oven rack in the centre of the oven and pre-heat your oven to 375 degrees. Toss zucchini with 1 teaspoon salt and allow to drain using a fine-mesh strainer for about ten minutes. Wrap zucchini in clean dish towel, squeeze out excess liquid, and set aside.
2. Heat oil in 12-inch non-stick frying pan on moderate heat until it starts to shimmer. Put in scallions and garlic and cook until scallions become soft, approximately two minutes. Mix in zucchini, cover, and cook until zucchini has released its liquid, four to eight minutes. Uncover and carry on cooking until zucchini is dry, approximately one minute; allow to cool slightly.
3. Beat eggs, milk, and ½ teaspoon pepper together with fork in a container until thoroughly combined and mixture is pure yellow; do not overbeat. Mix in zucchini mixture, feta, dill, and oregano until combined. Move mixture to greased 13 by 9-inch baking dish and bake until eggs are just set and edges are starting to brown, 20 minutes to half an hour. Serve warm or at room temperature.

Tunisian Shakshuka

Yield: 4 Servings

Ⓥ This is a Vegetarian Recipe Ⓥ

Ingredients:

- ⅛ teaspoon cayenne pepper
- ¼ cup water
- ⅓ cup chopped fresh cilantro
- 1 (14.5-ounce) can diced tomatoes
- 1 teaspoon ground cumin
- 1 teaspoon ground turmeric
- 1½ cups jarred piquillo peppers, chopped coarse
- 2 bay leaves
- 2 onions, chopped fine
- 2 ounces feta 2 teaspoons tomato paste
- 2 yellow bell peppers, stemmed, seeded, and cut into ¼-inch pieces
- 3 tablespoons extra-virgin olive oil
- 4 garlic cloves, minced
- 4 large eggs
- Salt and pepper
- cheese, crumbled (½ cup)

Directions:

1. Heat oil in 12-inch non-stick frying pan on moderate to high heat until it starts to shimmer. Put in onions and bell peppers and cook till they become tender and lightly browned, eight to ten minutes. Put in garlic, tomato paste, 1½ teaspoons salt, cumin, turmeric, ¼ teaspoon pepper, and cayenne. Cook, stirring often, until tomato paste begins to darken, approximately three minutes.

2. Mix in piquillo peppers, tomatoes and their juice, water, and bay leaves. Bring to simmer and cook, stirring intermittently, until sauce is slightly thickened, 10 to fifteen minutes.
3. Remove from the heat, discard bay leaves and mix in ¼ cup cilantro. Move 2 cups sauce to blender and process until smooth, about 60 seconds. Return puree to frying pan and bring sauce to simmer over moderate to low heat.
4. Remove from the heat, make 4 shallow indentations (about 2 inches wide) in surface of sauce using back of spoon. Crack 1 egg into each indentation and season eggs with salt and pepper. Cover and cook over moderate to low heat until egg whites are just set and yolks are still runny, four to eight minutes. Sprinkle with feta and remaining cilantro and serve instantly.

Breads

Catalan Red Pepper Coques

Yield: 4 coques, serving 6 to 8

Ⓥ *This is a Vegetarian Recipe* Ⓥ

A thin and crunchy flatbread.

Ingredients:

DOUGH

- ½ teaspoon instant or rapid-rise yeast
- 1⅓ cups ice water
- 1½ teaspoons 2 teaspoons sugar
- 3 cups (16½ ounces) bread flour
- 3 tablespoons extra-virgin olive oil
- salt

TOPPING

- ¼ cup pine nuts (optional)
- ¼ teaspoon red pepper flakes
- ½ cup extra-virgin olive oil
- 1 tablespoo1½ teaspoons salt
- 2 bay leaves
- 2 cups jarred roasted red peppers, patted dry and sliced thin
- 2 large onions, halved and sliced thin
- 3 garlic cloves, minced
- 3 tablespoons sherry vinegar
- 3 tablespoons sugar
- n minced fresh parsley

Directions:

1. **FOR THE DOUGH:** Pulse flour, sugar, and yeast using a food processor until combined, about 5 pulses. While your food processor runs slowly put in ice water and process until dough is just combined and no dry flour remains, about 10 seconds. Let dough rest for about ten minutes.
2. Put in oil and salt to dough and process until dough forms satiny, sticky ball that clears sides of bowl, 30 to 60 seconds. Move dough to slightly floured counter and knead using your hands to form smooth, round ball, approximately half a minute. Place dough seam side down in lightly greased big container or container, cover firmly using plastic wrap, put inside your fridge for minimum 24 hours or for maximum 3 days.
3. **FOR THE TOPPING:** Heat 3 tablespoons oil in 12-inch non-stick frying pan on moderate heat until it starts to shimmer. Mix in onions, red peppers, sugar, garlic, salt, pepper flakes, and bay leaves. Cover and cook, stirring intermittently, until onions become soft and have released their juice, about 10 minutes. Remove lid and continue to cook, stirring frequently, until onions start to look golden brown, 10 to fifteen minutes. Remove from the heat, discard bay leaves. Move onion mixture to a container, mix in vinegar, and allow to cool completely before using.
4. Press down on dough to deflate. Move dough to clean counter, divide into quarters, and cover loosely with greased plastic. Working with 1 piece of dough at a time (keep remaining pieces covered), form into rough ball by stretching dough around your thumbs and pinching edges together so that top is even.
5. Place ball seam side down on counter and, using your cupped hands, drag in small circles until dough feels taut and round. Space dough balls 3 inches apart, cover loosely with greased plastic, and allow to rest for about one hour.
6. Place two oven racks in your oven one just above, and one just below the middle position and pre-heat your oven to 500 degrees. Coat 2 rimmed baking sheets with 2 tablespoons oil each. Thoroughly coat 1 dough ball with flour and place on well-floured counter. Press and roll into 14 by 5-inch oval. Arrange oval on readied sheet, with long edge fitted snugly against 1

long side of sheet, and reshape as required. (If dough resists stretching, let it relax for 10 to 20 minutes before trying to stretch it again.) Repeat with the rest of the dough balls, arranging 2 ovals on each sheet, spaced ½ inch apart. Using fork, poke surface of dough 10 to 15 times.

7. Brush dough ovals with residual 1 tablespoon oil and bake until puffed, six to eight minutes, switching and rotating sheets halfway through baking.
8. Scatter onion mixture uniformly over flatbreads, from edge to edge, then drizzle with pine nuts, if using. Bake until topping is heated through and edges of flatbreads are deep golden brown and crisp, about fifteen minutes, switching and rotating sheets halfway through baking. Let flatbreads cool on sheets for about ten minutes, then move to slicing board using metal spatula. Sprinkle with parsley, slice, and serve.

French Socca

Yield: five 6-inch flatbreads, serving 4 to 6

This recipe can be made quickly

Ⓥ *This is a Vegetarian Recipe* Ⓥ

Ingredients:

- ½ teaspoon ground turmeric
- ½ teaspoon pepper
- ½ teaspoon salt
- 1½ cups (6¾ ounces) chickpea flour
- 1½ cups water
- 6 tablespoons plus 1 teaspoon extra-virgin olive oil

Directions:

1. Place the oven rack in the centre of the oven and pre-heat your oven to 200 degrees. Set wire rack in rimmed baking sheet and

place in oven. Beat chickpea flour, salt, pepper, and turmeric together in a container. Slowly beat in water and 3 tablespoons oil until combined and smooth.
2. Heat 2 teaspoons oil in 8-inch non-stick frying pan on moderate to high heat until it starts to shimmer. Put in ½ cup batter to skillet, tilting frying pan to coat bottom evenly. Decrease heat to medium and cook until crisp at edges and golden brown on bottom, 3 to 5 minutes. Flip socca and carry on cooking until second side is browned, 2 to 3 minutes. Move to wire rack in oven and repeat with remaining oil and batter. Slice and serve.

French Socca Variation 1

This recipe can be made quickly

(V) This is a Vegetarian Recipe (V)

Heat 1 tablespoon extra-virgin olive oil in 12-inch non-stick frying pan on moderate heat until it starts to shimmer. Put in 1 thinly sliced onion and cook till they become tender, approximately five minutes. Mix in 2 minced garlic cloves, ¾ teaspoon cumin, ¼ teaspoon salt, and ⅛ teaspoon allspice and cook until aromatic, approximately half a minute. Mix in 12 ounces Swiss chard, stemmed and chopped, and 3 tablespoons thinly sliced dried apricots and cook until chard is wilted, four to eight minutes. Remove from the heat, mix in 2 tablespoons thinly sliced toasted pistachios and 1 teaspoon white wine vinegar. Sprinkle with salt and pepper to taste. Top each cooked socca with ⅓ cup chard mixture before slicing and serving.

French Socca Variation 2

(V) This is a Vegetarian Recipe (V)

Substitute 1½ teaspoons minced fresh rosemary for turmeric in socca batter. Heat 1 tablespoon extra-virgin olive oil in 12-inch non-stick frying pan on high heat until it starts to shimmer. Put in 3 onions, halved and sliced thin, ½ teaspoon light brown sugar, and ¼ teaspoon salt and stir to coat. Cook, stirring intermittently, until onions start to become tender and release some moisture, approximately five minutes. Decrease heat to medium and continue to cook, stirring frequently, until onions are well caramelized, 30 to 35 minutes. (If onions are sizzling or scorching, reduce heat. If onions are not browning after fifteen to twenty minutes, increase heat.) Remove from the heat, mix in 1 teaspoon sherry vinegar and sprinkle with salt and pepper to taste. Top each cooked socca with 1 tablespoon grated Parmesan and scant ¼ cup onion mixture before slicing and serving.

Greek Pita Bread

Yield: eight 8-inch pitas

Ⓥ *This is a Vegetarian Recipe* Ⓥ

Ingredients:

- ¼ cup extra-virgin olive oil
- 1⅓ cups water, room temperature
- 2 teaspoons salt
- 2½ teaspoons 2½ teaspoons instant or rapid-rise yeast
- 3⅔ cups (20⅛ ounces) bread flour
- sugar

Directions:

1. Beat flour, yeast, and salt together in a container of stand mixer. Beat water, oil, and sugar together in 4-cup liquid measuring cup until sugar has dissolved.
2. Using dough hook on low speed, slowly put in water mixture to flour mixture and combine until cohesive dough starts to form and no dry flour remains, approximately two minutes, scraping down sides of the container as required. Increase speed to moderate to low and knead until dough is smooth and elastic and clears sides of bowl, approximately eight minutes.

3. Move dough to slightly floured counter and knead using your hands to form smooth, round ball, approximately half a minute. Place dough seam side down in lightly greased big container or container, cover firmly using plastic wrap, and let rise until doubled in size, 1 to 1½ hours.
4. Press down on dough to deflate. Move dough to slightly floured counter and divide into quarters, then cut each quarter into halves (about 4 ounces each); cover loosely with greased plastic.
5. Working with 1 piece of dough at a time (keep remaining pieces covered), form into rough ball by stretching dough around your thumbs and pinching edges together so that top is even.
6. Thoroughly coat 1 dough ball with flour and place on well-floured counter. Press and roll into 8-inch round of even thickness and cover loosely with greased plastic. (If dough resists stretching, let it relax for 10 to 20 minutes before trying to stretch it again.) Replicate the process with the rest of the balls. Let dough rounds rest for 20 minutes.
7. One hour before baking, adjust oven rack to lower-middle position, place baking stone on rack, and pre-heat your oven to 500 degrees. Gently move 2 dough rounds to well-floured pizza peel. Slide rounds onto stone and bake until single air pocket is just starting to form, approximately one minute.
8. Working quickly, flip pitas using metal spatula and continue to bake until light golden brown, 1 to 2 minutes. Move pitas to plate and cover with dish towel. Repeat with the rest of the dough rounds in 3 batches, allowing oven to reheat for about five minutes after each batch. Let pitas cool for about ten minutes before you serve.

Greek Spanakopita

Yield: Servings 10 to 12

Ⓥ *This is a Vegetarian Recipe* Ⓥ

A delicious Greek spinach and feta pie.

Ingredients:

FILLING

- ⅛ teaspo¼ cup minced fresh mint
- ¼ cup water
- ¼ teaspoon salt
- ½ teaspoon pepper
- ¾ cup whole-milk Greek yogurt
- 1 teaspoon grated lemon zest plus 1 tablespoon juice
- 1 teaspoon ground nutmeg
- 2 large eggs, lightly beaten
- 2 tablespoons minced fresh dill
- 20 ounces curly-leaf spinach, stemmed
- 3 garlic cloves, minced
- 4 scallions, sliced thin
- 8 ounces feta cheese, crumbled (2 cups)
- on cayenne pepper

PHYLLO LAYERS

- 1½ ounces Pecorino Romano cheese, grated (¾ cup)
- 2 teaspoons sesame 7 tablespoons extra-virgin olive oil
- 8 ounces (14 by 9-inch) phyllo, thawed
- seeds (optional)

Directions:

1. **FOR THE FILLING:** Place spinach and water in a container. Cover and microwave until spinach is wilted and volume is halved, approximately five minutes. Remove bowl from microwave and keep covered for about sixty seconds. Move spinach to colander and gently press to release liquid. Move spinach to slicing board and chop coarse. Return to colander and press again. Stir spinach and remaining ingredients in a container until thoroughly combined.

2. **FOR THE PHYLLO LAYERS:** Place oven rack to lower-middle position and pre-heat your oven to 425 degrees. Line rimmed baking sheet with parchment paper. Using pastry brush, lightly brush 14 by 9-inch rectangle in center of parchment with oil to cover area same size as phyllo. Lay 1 phyllo sheet on oiled parchment and brush thoroughly with oil. Repeat with 9 more phyllo sheets, brushing each with oil (you should have total of 10 layers of phyllo).
3. Lay out spinach mixture uniformly phyllo, leaving ¼-inch border on all sides. Cover spinach with 6 more phyllo sheets, brushing each with oil and sprinkling each with about 2 tablespoons Pecorino. Lay 2 more phyllo sheets on top, brushing each with oil (these layers should not be sprinkled with Pecorino).
4. Working from center outward, use palms of your hands to compress layers and press out any air pockets. Using sharp knife, score spanakopita through top 3 layers of phyllo into 24 equivalent pieces. Sprinkle with sesame seeds (if using). Bake until phyllo is golden and crisp, 20 minutes to half an hour. Let spanakopita cool on sheet for minimum 10 minutes or maximum 2 hours. Slide spanakopita, still on parchment, to slicing board. Cut into squares and serve.

Italian Rosemary Focaccia

Yield: two 9-inch round loaves, serving 6 to 8

(V) This is a Vegetarian Recipe (V)

A light and Airy Italian Bread

Ingredients:

SPONGE

- ¼ teaspoon instant ⅓ cup water, room temperature
- ½ cup (2½ ounces) all-purpose flour
- or rapid-rise yeast

DOUGH

- ¼ cup extra-virgin olive oil
- 1 teaspoon instant or rapid-rise yeast
- 1¼ cups water, room temperature
- 2 tablespoons chopped 2½ cups (12½ ounces) all-purpose flour
- Kosher salt
- fresh rosemary

Directions:

1. **FOR THE SPONGE**: Stir all ingredients together in a big container with wooden spoon until thoroughly mixed. Cover tightly using plastic wrap and allow to sit at room temperature until sponge has risen and begins to collapse, about 6 hours (sponge can sit at room temperature for maximum 24 hours).
2. **FOR THE DOUGH**: Stir flour, water, and yeast into sponge with wooden spoon until thoroughly mixed. Cover bowl tightly with plastic and let dough rest for about fifteen minutes.
3. Stir 2 teaspoons salt into dough with wooden spoon until thoroughly incorporated, approximately one minute. Cover bowl tightly with plastic and let dough rest for half an hour.
4. Using greased bowl scraper (or rubber spatula), fold dough over itself by gently lifting and folding edge of dough toward middle. Turn bowl 45 degrees and fold dough again; repeat turning bowl and folding dough 6 more times (total of 8 folds). Cover tightly with plastic and allow to rise for half an hour. Repeat folding and rising. Fold dough again, then cover bowl tightly with plastic and let dough rise until nearly doubled in size, half an hour to 1 hour.
5. One hour before baking, adjust oven rack to upper-middle position, place baking stone on rack, and pre-heat your oven to 500 degrees. Coat two 9-inch round cake pans with 2 tablespoons oil each. Sprinkle each pan with ½ teaspoon salt. Move dough to slightly floured counter and dust top with flour. Split the dough in half and cover loosely with greased plastic. Working with 1 piece of dough at a time (keep remaining piece

covered), shape into 5-inch round by gently tucking under edges.
6. Place dough rounds seam side up in prepared pans, coat bottoms and sides with oil, then flip rounds over. Cover loosely with greased plastic and let dough rest for about five minutes.
7. Using your fingertips, gently press each dough round into corners of pan, taking care not to tear dough. (If dough resists stretching, let it relax for 5 to 10 minutes before trying to stretch it again.) Using fork, poke surface of dough 25 to 30 times, popping any large bubbles. Sprinkle 1 tablespoon rosemary uniformly over top of each loaf, cover loosely with greased plastic, and let dough rest until slightly bubbly, about 10 minutes.
8. Place pans on baking stone and decrease oven temperature to 450 degrees. Bake until tops start to look golden brown, about half an hour, rotating pans halfway through baking. Let loaves cool in pans for about five minutes. Remove loaves from pans and move to wire rack. Brush tops with any oil remaining in pans and allow to cool for half an hour. Serve warm or at room temperature.

Italian Tart 1: Mushroom

Yield: one 9-inch tart, serving 4 to 6

Ⓥ This is a Vegetarian Recipe Ⓥ

Ingredients:

CRUST

- ⅓ cup ⅔ cup extra-virgin olive oil
- ¾ teaspoon salt
- 1 tablespoon sugar
- 1¾ cups (8¾ ounces) all-purpose flour

- water

FILLING

- 1 garlic clove, minced
- 1 ounce mozzarella cheese, shredded (¼ cup)
- 1 ounce Parmesan cheese, grated (½ cup)
- 1 pound white mushrooms, trimmed and sliced thin
- 2 tablespoons extra-virgin olive oil
- 2 teaspoons minced fresh thyme
- 4 ounces (½ cup) part-skim ricotta cheese
- Salt and pepper

Directions:

1. **FOR THE CRUST:** Place oven rack on the lowest position and pre-heat your oven to 350 degrees. Beat flour, sugar, and salt together in a container. Mix in oil and water with wooden spoon until large clumps of dough form and no dry flour remains.
2. Sprinkle walnut-size clumps of dough uniformly into bottom of 9-inch tart pan with removable bottom. Working outward from center, press dough into even layer, sealing any cracks. Working around edge, press dough firmly into corners with fingers. Go around edge once more, pressing dough up sides and into fluted ridges. Use thumb to level off top edge. Use excess dough to patch any holes.
3. Place pan on wire rack set in rimmed baking sheet and bake until crust is light golden brown and firm to touch, about 50 minutes, rotating pan halfway through baking. Let tart shell cool completely on sheet before filling.
4. **FOR THE FILLING:** Heat 1 tablespoon oil in 12-inch non-stick frying pan on moderate to high heat until it starts to shimmer. Put in mushrooms and ½ teaspoon salt and cook until dry and lightly browned, about fifteen minutes. Mix in thyme and garlic and cook until aromatic, approximately one minute.
5. Mix Parmesan, ricotta, mozzarella, and residual 1 tablespoon oil in a container and sprinkle with salt and pepper to taste. Lay

out ricotta mixture uniformly bottom of tart shell, then spoon mushroom mixture on top. Bake tart on sheet until heated through and starting to bubble around edges, 20 minutes to half an hour, rotating sheet halfway through baking.

6. Let tart cool on sheet for minimum 10 minutes or maximum 2 hours. Remove outer metal ring of tart pan, slide thin metal spatula between tart and pan bottom, and carefully slide tart onto serving platter. Sprinkle with basil and cut into wedges. Serve.

Italian Tart 2: Tomato

ⓥ This is a Vegetarian Recipe ⓥ

Omit mushroom mixture in step 5. Lay out 3 plum tomatoes, cored and sliced ¼ inch thick, on several layers of paper towels and drizzle with ½ teaspoon salt. Let tomatoes drain for half an hour, then blot dry using paper towels. Mix 2 tablespoons oil and 1 minced garlic clove in a small-sized container. After spreading ricotta mixture in tart shell, shingle tomatoes beautifully on top in concentric circles. Sprinkle with garlic-oil mixture and bake as directed.

Italian Tart 3: Zucchini

ⓥ This is a Vegetarian Recipe ⓥ

Omit mushroom mixture in step 5. Lay out 1 large zucchini, sliced into ¼-inch-thick rounds, on several layers of paper towels and drizzle with ½ teaspoon salt. Let zucchini drain for half an hour, then blot dry using paper towels. Mix 2 tablespoons oil and 1 minced garlic clove in a small-sized container. After spreading ricotta mixture in tart shell, shingle zucchini beautifully on top in concentric circles. Sprinkle with garlic-oil mixture and bake as directed.

Lahmacun

Yield: four 9-inch flatbreads, serving 4 to 6

Lahmacun is a meat pie common in Armenian and Turkish cuisines.

Ingredients:

DOUGH

- ¾ cup ice water
- ¾ teaspoon instant or rapid-rise yeast
- 1 teaspoon 1 teaspoon sugar
- 1¾ cups (9⅔ ounces) bread flour
- 2 tablespoons extra-virgin olive oil
- salt

TOPPING

- ¼ cup chopped fresh ½ teaspoon salt
- ⅔ cup coarsely chopped onion
- ¾ teaspoon ground allspice
- ¾ teaspoon smoked hot paprika
- 1 cup coarsely chopped red bell pepper
- 1 garlic clove, minced
- 1 tablespoon tomato paste
- 3 tablespoons Turkish hot pepper paste
- 4 ounces ground lamb
- parsley

Directions:

1. FOR THE DOUGH Pulse flour, sugar, and yeast using a food processor until combined, about 5 pulses. While your food processor runs slowly put in ice water and process until dough is just combined and no dry flour remains, about 10 seconds. Let dough rest for about ten minutes.

2. Put in oil and salt to dough and process until dough forms satiny, sticky ball that clears sides of bowl, 30 to 60 seconds. Move dough to slightly floured counter and knead using your hands to form smooth, round ball, approximately half a minute. Place dough seam side down in lightly greased big container or container, cover firmly using plastic wrap, put inside your fridge for minimum 24 hours or for maximum 3 days.
3. Press down on dough to deflate. Move dough to slightly floured counter, divide into quarters, and cover loosely with greased plastic. Working with 1 piece of dough at a time (keep remaining pieces covered), form into rough ball by stretching dough around your thumbs and pinching edges together so that top is even. Space balls 3 inches apart, cover loosely with greased plastic, and allow to rest for about one hour.
4. FOR THE TOPPING Process pepper paste, tomato paste, garlic, paprika, allspice, and salt in clean, dry workbowl until thoroughly mixed, approximately half a minute, scraping down sides of the container as required. Put in bell pepper and onion and pulse until finely ground, approximately ten pulses. Put in lamb and parsley and pulse until thoroughly mixed, approximately 8 pulses.
5. Place two oven racks in your oven one just above, and one just below the middle position and pre-heat your oven to 350 degrees. Grease 2 rimmed baking sheets. Thoroughly coat 1 dough ball with flour and place on well-floured counter. Press and roll into 9-inch round. Arrange round on readied sheet, with edges fitted snugly into 1 corner of sheet, and reshape as required. (If dough resists stretching, let it relax for 10 to 20 minutes before trying to stretch it again.) Repeat with the rest of the dough balls, arranging 2 rounds on each sheet in opposite corners.
6. Using back of spoon, spread one-quarter of topping in thin layer on surface of each dough round, leaving ¼-inch border around edge.
7. Bake until edges of flatbreads are set but still pale, 10 to 12 minutes, switching and rotating sheets halfway through baking. Remove flatbreads from oven and heat broiler.

8. Return 1 sheet to upper rack and broil until edges of flatbreads are crisp and spotty brown and filling is set, 2 to 4 minutes. Move flatbreads to wire rack with spatula and allow to cool for about five minutes before you serve. Repeat broiling with remaining flatbreads.

Lavash With Veggies Mix 1

Yield: two 12 by 9-inch flatbreads, serving 4 to 6

This recipe can be made quickly

Ⓥ This is a Vegetarian Recipe Ⓥ

Ingredients:

- ¼ teaspoon pepper
- ¼ teaspoon red pepper flakes
- ¼ teaspoon salt
- ½ cup pitted large brine-cured green olives, chopped
- 1 ounce Parmesan cheese1 tomato, cored and cut into ½-inch pieces
- 10 ounces frozen spinach, thawed and squeezed dry
- 2 (12 by 9-inch) lavash breads
- 2 tablespoons extra-virgin olive oil
- 3 garlic cloves, minced
- 4 ounces fontina cheese, shredded (1 cup)
- , grated (½ cup)

Directions:

1. Place two oven racks in your oven one just above, and one just below the middle position and pre-heat your oven to 475 degrees. Mix spinach, fontina, tomato, olives, garlic, pepper flakes, salt, and pepper in a container. Brush both sides of lavash with oil, lay on 2 baking sheets, and bake until golden

brown, about 4 minutes, flipping lavash halfway through baking.
2. Lay out spinach mixture uniformly each lavash and drizzle with Parmesan. Bake until cheese is melted and spotty brown, six to eight minutes, switching and rotating sheets halfway through baking. Slice and serve.

Lavash With Veggies Mix 2

This recipe can be made quickly

Ⓥ This is a Vegetarian Recipe Ⓥ

Omit spinach, tomato, and olives. Heat 2 tablespoons extra-virgin olive oil in 12-inch frying pan on moderate heat until it starts to shimmer. Put in 2 cups chopped cauliflower florets, 1 chopped fennel bulb, 3 tablespoons water, 1 teaspoon ground coriander, and ½ teaspoon salt. Cover and cook, stirring intermittently, until vegetables are tender, six to eight minutes; allow to cool slightly. Substitute 1 cup shredded whole-milk mozzarella cheese for fontina and combine with cauliflower mixture, garlic, and spices before topping lavash. Substitute ½ cup crumbled goat cheese for Parmesan. Sprinkle with 1 thinly sliced scallion before you serve.

Moroccan Chicken B'stilla

Yield: Servings 10 to 12

A delicious Moroccan Tart.

Ingredients:

- ¼ cup confectioners' sugar
- ½ cup extra-virgin olive oil
- ½ cup minced fresh cilantro
- ½ teaspoon ground turmeric

- ½ teaspoon paprika
- ½ teaspoon pepper
- ¾ teaspoon salt
- 1 onion, chopped fine
- 1 pound (14 by 9-inch) phyllo, thawed
- 1 tablespoon grated fresh ginger
- 1 tablespoon ground 1½ cups slivered almonds, toasted and chopped
- 1½ cups water
- 2 pounds boneless, skinless chicken thighs, trimmed
- 6 large eggs
- cinnamon

Directions:

1. Heat 1 tablespoon oil in 12-inch non-stick frying pan on moderate heat until it starts to shimmer. Put in onion and salt and cook till they become tender, approximately five minutes. Mix in ginger, pepper, turmeric, and paprika and cook until aromatic, approximately half a minute. Put in water and chicken and bring to simmer. Decrease heat to low, cover, and cook until chicken registers 175 degrees, fifteen to twenty minutes. Move chicken to slicing board, allow to cool slightly, then shred into bite-size pieces using 2 forks; move to big container.
2. Beat eggs together in a small-sized container. Bring cooking liquid to boil on high heat and cook until reduced to about 1 cup, about 10 minutes. Decrease heat to low. Whisking continuously, slowly pour eggs into broth and cook until mixture resembles loose scrambled eggs, six to eight minutes; move to a container with chicken. Mix in cilantro until combined. Wipe frying pan clean using paper towels and allow to cool fully.
3. Place the oven rack in the centre of the oven and pre-heat your oven to 375 degrees. Brush 1 phyllo sheet with oil and lay out on bottom of cooled frying pan with short side against side of pan. Some phyllo will overhang edge of skillet; leave in place. Turn frying pan 30 degrees. Brush second phyllo sheet with oil

and lay out on skillet, leaving any overhanging phyllo in place. Repeat turning and layering with 10 more phyllo sheets in pinwheel pattern, brushing each with oil, to cover entire circumference of frying pan (you should have total of 12 layers of phyllo).
4. Mix almonds, 3 tablespoons sugar, and 2 teaspoons cinnamon and drizzle over phyllo in skillet. Lay 2 phyllo sheets evenly across top of almond mixture and brush top with oil. Rotate frying pan 90 degrees and lay 2 more phyllo sheets evenly across top; do not brush with oil. Spoon chicken mixture into frying pan and spread into even layer.
5. Stack 5 phyllo sheets on counter and brush top with oil. Fold phyllo in half crosswise and brush top with oil. Lay phyllo stack on center of chicken mixture.
6. Fold overhanging phyllo over filling and phyllo stack, pleating phyllo every 2 to 3 inches, and press to seal. Brush top with oil and bake until phyllo is crisp and golden, 35 to 40 minutes.
7. Mix remaining 1 tablespoon sugar and remaining 1 teaspoon cinnamon in a small-sized container. Let b'stilla cool in frying pan for about fifteen minutes. Using rubber spatula, carefully slide b'stilla out onto slicing board. Dust top with cinnamon sugar, slice, and serve.

Palestinian Mushroom Musakhan

Yield: two 15 by 8-inch flatbreads, serving 4 to 6

Ⓥ This is a Vegetarian Recipe Ⓥ

Ingredients:

DOUGH

- ¾ teaspoon instant or rapid-rise yeast
- 1 cup (5½ ounces) bread flour

- 1¼ cups ice water
- 1½ cups (8¼ ounces) whole-wheat flour
- 1¾ teaspoons 2 tablespoons extra-virgin olive oil
- 2 teaspoons honey
- salt

TOPPINGS

- ⅛ teaspoon ground cardamom
- ¼ cup pine nuts
- ¼ teaspoon ground allspice
- ½ cup extra-virgin olive oil
- 1½ tablespoons ground sumac
- 2 pounds onions, halved and sliced ¼ inch thick
- 2 pounds portobello mushroom caps, gills removed, caps halved and sliced ½ inch thick
- 2 tablespoons 2 tablespoons minced fresh oregano or 2 teaspoons dried
- 2 teaspoons packed light brown sugar
- 4 garlic cloves, minced
- Salt and pepper
- minced fresh chives

Directions:

1. **FOR THE DOUGH:** Pulse whole-wheat flour, bread flour, honey, and yeast using a food processor until combined, about 5 pulses. While your food processor runs slowly put in ice water and process until dough is just combined and no dry flour remains, about 10 seconds. Let dough rest for about ten minutes.
2. Put in oil and salt to dough and process until dough forms satiny, sticky ball that clears sides of bowl, 30 to 60 seconds. Move dough to lightly oiled counter and knead using your hands to form smooth, round ball, approximately half a minute. Place dough seam side down in lightly greased big container or container, cover firmly using plastic wrap, put inside your fridge for minimum 18 hours or for maximum 2 days.

3. **FOR THE TOPPINGS:** Mix 1 tablespoon oil, oregano, garlic, sumac, allspice, and cardamom in a container. Heat 2 tablespoons oil in 12-inch non-stick frying pan on high heat until it starts to shimmer. Put in onions, sugar, and ½ teaspoon salt and stir to coat. Cook, stirring intermittently, until onions start to become tender and release some moisture, approximately five minutes. Decrease heat to medium and continue to cook, stirring frequently, until onions are well caramelized, 35 to 40 minutes. (If onions are sizzling or scorching, reduce heat. If onions are not browning after fifteen to twenty minutes, increase heat.) Push onions to sides of skillet. Put in oregano-garlic mixture to center and cook, mashing mixture into skillet, until aromatic, approximately half a minute. Stir oregano-garlic mixture into onions.
4. Move onion mixture to your food processor and pulse to jamlike consistency, about 5 pulses. Move to a container, mix in pine nuts, and sprinkle with salt and pepper to taste; allow to cool completely before using.
5. Wipe frying pan clean using paper towels. Heat 2 tablespoons oil in now-empty frying pan on moderate to high heat until it starts to shimmer. Put in half of mushrooms and ½ teaspoon salt and cook, stirring intermittently, until evenly browned, eight to ten minutes; move to different container. Repeat with 2 tablespoons oil, remaining mushrooms, and ½ teaspoon salt; move to a container and allow to cool completely before using.
6. One hour before baking, adjust oven rack 4 inches from broiler element, set baking stone on rack, and pre-heat your oven to 500 degrees. Press down on dough to deflate. Move dough to clean counter, divide in half, and cover loosely with greased plastic. Pat 1 piece of dough (keep remaining piece covered) into 4-inch round. Working around circumference of dough, fold edges toward center until ball forms.
7. Flip ball seam side down and, using your cupped hands, drag in small circles on counter until dough feels taut and round and all seams are secured on underside. (If dough sticks to your hands, lightly dust top of dough with flour.) Replicate the process with the rest of the piece of dough. Space dough balls 3 inches apart,

cover loosely with greased plastic, and allow to rest for about one hour.
8. Heat broiler for about ten minutes. In the meantime, heavily coat 1 dough ball with flour and place on well-floured counter. Press and roll into 12 by 8-inch oval. Move oval to well-floured pizza peel and stretch into 15 by 8-inch oval. (If dough resists stretching, let it relax for 10 to 20 minutes before trying to stretch it again.) Using fork, poke entire surface of oval 10 to 15 times.
9. Lay out half of onion mixture uniformly dough, edge to edge, and arrange half of mushrooms on top. Slide flatbread carefully onto baking stone and return oven to 500 degrees. Bake until bottom crust is evenly browned and edges are crisp, about 10 minutes, rotating flatbread halfway through baking. Move flatbread to wire rack and allow to cool for about five minutes. Sprinkle with 1½ teaspoons oil and drizzle with 1 tablespoon chives. Slice and serve.
10. Heat broiler for about ten minutes. Repeat with the rest of the dough and toppings, returning oven to 500 degrees when flatbread is placed on stone.

Phyllo Hand Pies

Yield: 15 triangles, serving 6 to 8

Ⓥ *This is a Vegetarian Recipe* Ⓥ

Ingredients:

FILLING

- ¼ cup pitted kalamata olives, chopped fine
- ½ cup dry white wine
- 1 large fennel bulb, stalks discarded, bulb halved, cored, and sliced thin
- 1 tablespoon extra-virgin olive oil
- 2 tablespoons chopped fresh oregano

- 2 teaspoons grated lemon zest plus 1 tablespoon juice
- 3 garlic cloves, minced
- 6 ounces goat cheese, crumbled (1½ cups)
- Salt and pepper

PIES

- ¼ cup extr10 (14 by 9-inch) phyllo sheets, thawed
- a-virgin olive oil

Directions:

1. **FOR THE FILLING:** Heat oil in 12-inch frying pan on moderate heat until it starts to shimmer. Put in fennel and cook till they become tender and lightly browned, eight to ten minutes. Mix in garlic and cook until aromatic, approximately half a minute. Mix in wine, cover, and cook for about five minutes. Uncover and carry on cooking until liquid has evaporated and fennel is very tender, 3 to 5 minutes.
2. Move fennel mixture to medium bowl and allow to cool to room temperature, about fifteen minutes. Gently mix in goat cheese, olives, oregano, and lemon zest and juice until combined. Sprinkle with salt and pepper to taste.
3. **FOR THE PIES:** Place oven rack to lower-middle position and pre-heat your oven to 375 degrees. Place 1 phyllo sheet on counter with long side parallel to counter edge, brush lightly with oil, then top with second phyllo sheet. Cut phyllo vertically into three 9 by 4⅔-inch strips. Place large 1 tablespoon filling on bottom left-hand corner of each strip. Fold up phyllo to form right-angle triangle, gently pressing on filling as required to create even layer. Continue folding up and over, as if folding a flag, to end of strip. Brush triangle with oil and place seam side down in parchment paper–lined rimmed baking sheet. Replicate the process with the rest of the phyllo sheets and filling to make 15 triangles.
4. Bake triangles until golden brown, 10 to fifteen minutes, rotating sheet halfway through baking. Let triangles cool on sheet for about five minutes. Serve.

Pissaladière

Yield: two 14 by 8-inch tarts, serving 4 to 6

Pissaladière is a pizza-like tart from Provence.

Ingredients:

DOUGH

- ½ teaspoon instant or rapid-rise yeast
- 1 tablespoon extra-virgin olive oil
- 1⅓ cups ice water
- 1½ teaspoons 2 teaspoons sugar
- 3 cups (16½ ounces) bread flour
- salt

TOPPINGS

- ¼ cup extra-virgin olive oil
- ½ cup pitted niçoise olives, chopped coarse
- ½ teaspoon pepper
- ½ teaspoon salt
- 1 tablespoon water
- 1 teaspoon fennel seeds
- 1 teaspoon packed brown sugar
- 2 pounds onions, halved and sliced ¼ inch thick
- 2 tablespoons 2 teaspoons minced fresh thyme
- 8 anchovy fillets, rinsed, patted dry, and chopped coarse, plus 12 fillets for garnish (optional)
- minced fresh parsley

Directions:

1. **FOR THE DOUGH**: Pulse flour, sugar, and yeast using a food processor until combined, about 5 pulses. While your food processor runs slowly put in ice water and process until dough

is just combined and no dry flour remains, about 10 seconds. Let dough rest for about ten minutes.
2. Put in oil and salt to dough and process until dough forms satiny, sticky ball that clears sides of bowl, 30 to 60 seconds. Move dough to slightly floured counter and knead using your hands to form smooth, round ball, approximately half a minute. Place dough seam side down in lightly greased big container or container, cover firmly using plastic wrap, put inside your fridge for minimum 24 hours or for maximum 3 days.
3. **FOR THE TOPPINGS:** Heat 2 tablespoons oil in 12-inch non-stick frying pan on moderate heat until it starts to shimmer. Mix in onions, sugar, and salt. Cover and cook, stirring intermittently, until onions become soft and have released their juice, about 10 minutes. Remove lid and continue to cook, stirring frequently, until onions start to look golden brown, 10 to fifteen minutes. Move onions to a container, mix in water, and allow to cool completely before using.
4. One hour before baking, adjust oven rack 4 inches from broiler element, set baking stone on rack, and pre-heat your oven to 500 degrees. Press down on dough to deflate. Move dough to clean counter, divide in half, and cover loosely with greased plastic. Pat 1 piece of dough (keep remaining piece covered) into 4-inch round. Working around circumference of dough, fold edges toward center until ball forms.
5. Flip ball seam side down and, using your cupped hands, drag in small circles on counter until dough feels taut and round and all seams are secured on underside. (If dough sticks to your hands, lightly dust top of dough with flour.) Replicate the process with the rest of the piece of dough. Space dough balls 3 inches apart, cover loosely with greased plastic, and allow to rest for about one hour.
6. Heat broiler for about ten minutes. In the meantime, heavily coat 1 dough ball with flour and place on well-floured counter. Press and roll into 14 by 8-inch oval. Move oval to well-floured pizza peel and reshape as required. (If dough resists stretching, let it relax for 10 to 20 minutes before trying to stretch it again.) Using fork, poke entire surface of oval 10 to 15 times.

7. Brush dough oval with 1 tablespoon oil, then drizzle evenly with ¼ cup olives, half of chopped anchovies, 1 teaspoon thyme, ½ teaspoon fennel seeds, and ¼ teaspoon pepper, leaving ½-inch border around edge. Arrange half of onions on top, followed by 6 whole anchovies, if using.
8. Slide flatbread carefully onto baking stone and return oven to 500 degrees. Bake until bottom crust is evenly browned and edges are crisp, 13 to fifteen minutes, rotating flatbread halfway through baking. Move flatbread to wire rack and allow to cool for about five minutes. Sprinkle with 1 tablespoon parsley, slice, and serve. Heat broiler for about ten minutes. Repeat with the rest of the dough, oil, and toppings, returning oven to 500 degrees when flatbread is placed on stone.

Pumpkin Borek

Yield: Servings 10 to 12

Ⓥ This is a Vegetarian Recipe Ⓥ

Borek is a delicious filled pastry popular throughout the eastern Mediterranean region.

Ingredients:

FILLING

- ½ cup chopped ½ teaspoon pepper
- 1 large onion, chopped
- 1 tablespoon extra-virgin olive oil
- 1 teaspoon grated fresh ginger
- 1½ cups dry white wine
- 1½ teaspoons salt
- 12 ounces halloumi cheese, grated (3 cups)
- 3 (15-ounce) cans unsweetened pumpkin puree
- 3 garlic cloves, minced
- 5 large eggs

- 8 ounces (1 cup) cottage cheese
- fresh mint

LAYERS

- ⅓ cup whole milk
- 1 large egg
- 2 pounds (14 by 9-inch) phyllo, thawed

Directions:

1. **FOR THE FILLING:** Heat oil in 10-inch frying pan on moderate to high heat until it starts to shimmer. Put in onion and salt and cook till they become tender, approximately five minutes. Mix in garlic, ginger, and pepper and cook until aromatic, approximately half a minute. Mix in wine, bring to simmer, and cook, stirring intermittently, until onion is very soft and mixture has reduced slightly and measures 1¼ cups, fifteen to twenty minutes.
2. Move onion mixture to your food processor and allow to cool slightly. Put in pumpkin and eggs and process until mixture is thoroughly combined and smooth, approximately three minutes, scraping down sides of the container as required. Mix halloumi, cottage cheese, and mint in different container.
3. **FOR THE LAYERS:** Place the oven rack in the centre of the oven and pre-heat your oven to 400 degrees. Beat milk and egg together in a container until combined. Trim 50 phyllo sheets to 12½ by 8½ inches.
4. Lay out 1 cup pumpkin filling on bottom of greased 13 by 9-inch baking dish. Lay 5 phyllo sheets in dish, brush with egg mixture, then top with 5 more phyllo sheets.
5. Brush phyllo with egg mixture, then spread 2⅓ cups pumpkin filling uniformly top. Lay 5 more phyllo sheets in dish, brush with egg mixture, then top with 5 more phyllo sheets.
6. Brush phyllo with egg mixture, then spread half of cheese mixture uniformly top. Lay 5 more phyllo sheets in dish, brush with egg mixture, then top with 5 more phyllo sheets.

7. Working from center outward, use palms of your hands to gently compress layers and press out any air pockets. Repeat layering in steps 5 and 6, then brush top with egg mixture.
8. Trim 10 phyllo sheets to 13 by 9 inches. Lay out remaining pumpkin filling uniformly phyllo layers. Lay 5 large phyllo sheets in dish, brush with egg mixture, then top with 5 more large phyllo sheets. Gently compress layers and wipe away excess filling that may have leaked out along sides of dish. Brush top with egg mixture and bake until borek registers 165 degrees and top is puffed and golden brown, 40 to 45 minutes. Allow it to cool for half an hour before you serve.

Turkish Pide

Yield: 6 pide, serving 6 to 8

(V) This is a Vegetarian Recipe (V)

A delicious canoe-shaped Turkish Flatbread.

Ingredients:

DOUGH

- ½ teaspoon instant or rapid-rise yeast
- 1 tablespoon extra-virgin olive oil
- 1⅓ cups ice water
- 1½ teaspoons 2 teaspoons sugar
- 3 cups (16½ ounces) bread flour
- salt

TOPPINGS

- ¼ teaspoon red pepper flakes
- ½ red bell pepper, chopped
- ½ teaspoon smoked paprika
- 1 (28-ounce) can whole peeled tomatoes
- 1 pound eggplant, cut into ½-inch pieces

- 3 garlic cloves, minced
- 5 tablespoons extra-virgin olive oil
- 6 ounces feta cheese6 tablespoons minced fresh mint
- Salt and pepper
- , crumbled (1½ cups)

Directions:

1. **FOR THE DOUGH:** Pulse flour, sugar, and yeast using a food processor until combined, about 5 pulses. While your food processor runs slowly put in ice water and process until dough is just combined and no dry flour remains, about 10 seconds. Let dough rest for about ten minutes.
2. Put in oil and salt to dough and process until dough forms satiny, sticky ball that clears sides of bowl, 30 to 60 seconds. Move dough to lightly oiled counter and knead using your hands to form smooth, round ball, approximately half a minute. Place dough seam side down in lightly greased big container or container, cover firmly using plastic wrap, put inside your fridge for minimum 24 hours or for maximum 3 days.
3. **FOR THE TOPPINGS:** Pulse tomatoes and their juice using a food processor until coarsely ground, about 12 pulses. Heat 2 tablespoons oil in 12-inch non-stick frying pan on moderate to high heat until it starts to shimmer. Put in eggplant, bell pepper, and ½ teaspoon salt and cook, stirring intermittently, till they become tender and starting to brown, 5 to 7 minutes. Mix in garlic, pepper flakes, and paprika and cook until aromatic, approximately half a minute.
4. Put in tomatoes, bring to simmer, and cook, stirring intermittently, until mixture is very thick and measures 3½ cups, about 10 minutes. Remove from the heat, mix in ¼ cup mint and sprinkle with salt and pepper to taste; allow to cool completely before using.
5. One hour before baking, adjust oven rack 4 inches from broiler element, set baking stone on rack, and pre-heat your oven to 500 degrees. Press down on dough to deflate. Move dough to clean counter and divide in half, then cut each half into thirds

(about 4¾ ounces each); cover loosely with greased plastic. Working with 1 piece of dough at a time (keep remaining pieces covered), form into rough ball by stretching dough around your thumbs and pinching edges together so that top is even. Space balls 3 inches apart, cover loosely with greased plastic, and allow to rest for about one hour.

6. Cut six 16 by 6-inch pieces of parchment paper. Thoroughly coat 1 dough ball with flour and place on well-floured counter. Press and roll into 14 by 5½-inch oval. Arrange oval on parchment rectangle and reshape as required. (If dough resists stretching, let it relax for 10 to 20 minutes before trying to stretch it again.) Repeat with 2 more dough balls and parchment rectangles.
7. Brush dough ovals with oil, then top each with ½ cup eggplant mixture and ¼ cup feta, leaving ¾-inch border around edges. Fold long edges of dough over filling to form canoe shape and pinch ends together to seal. Brush outer edges of dough with oil and move pide (still on parchment rectangles) to pizza peel.
8. Slide each parchment rectangle with pide onto baking stone, spacing pide at least 1 inch apart. Bake until crust is golden brown and edges are crisp, 10 to fifteen minutes. Move pide to wire rack, discard parchment, and allow to cool for about five minutes. Sprinkle with 1 tablespoon mint, slice, and serve. Replicate the process with the rest of the 3 dough balls, 3 parchment rectangles, oil, and toppings.

Za'atar Bread

Yield: one flatbread, serving 6 to 8

Ⓥ This is a Vegetarian Recipe Ⓥ

An Arabic flatbread covered with a thick coating of za'atar and olive oil.

Ingredients:

- ⅓ cup za'atar
- ½ cup plus 2 tablespoons extra-virgin olive oil

- 1⅓ cups ice water
- 2 teaspoons salt
- 2½ teaspoons instant or rapid-rise yeast
- 2½ teaspoons sugar
- 3½ cups (19¼ ounces) bread flour
- Coarse sea salt

Directions:

1. Pulse flour, yeast, and sugar using a food processor until combined, about 5 pulses. While your food processor runs slowly put in ice water and process until dough is just combined and no dry flour remains, about 10 seconds. Let dough rest for about ten minutes.
2. Put in 2 tablespoons oil and salt to dough and process until dough forms satiny, sticky ball that clears sides of bowl, 30 to 60 seconds. Move dough to slightly floured counter and knead using your hands to form smooth, round ball, approximately half a minute. Place dough seam side down in lightly greased big container or container, cover firmly using plastic wrap, put inside your fridge for minimum 24 hours or for maximum 3 days.
3. Remove dough from refrigerator and allow to sit at room temperature for about one hour. Coat rimmed baking sheet with 2 tablespoons oil. Gently press down on dough to deflate any large gas pockets. Move dough to readied sheet and, using your fingertips, press out to uniform thickness, taking care not to tear dough. (Dough may not fit snugly into corners.) Cover loosely with greased plastic and let dough rest for about one hour.
4. Place oven rack to lower-middle position and pre-heat your oven to 375 degrees. Using your fingertips, gently press dough into corners of sheet and dimple entire surface.
5. Mix remaining 6 tablespoons oil and za'atar in a container. Using back of spoon, spread oil mixture in a uniform layer on entire surface of dough to edge.

6. Bake until bottom crust is evenly browned and edges are crisp, 20 minutes to half an hour, rotating sheet halfway through baking. Let bread cool in sheet for about ten minutes, then move to slicing board with spatula. Sprinkle with sea salt, slice, and serve warm.

Pizzas

One of the most loved food in the world, pizzas can he delicious and nutritious if prepared at home!

Thin-Crust Pizza

Yield: two 13-inch pizzas, serving 4 to 6

Ⓥ This is a Vegetarian Recipe Ⓥ

Probably the most famous Italian flatbread in the world.

Ingredients:

DOUGH

- ½ teaspoon instant or rapid-rise yeast
- 1 tablespoon extra-virgin olive oil
- 1⅓ cups ice water
- 1½ teaspoons 2 teaspoons sugar
- 3 cups (16½ ounces) bread flour
- salt

SAUCE AND TOPPINGS

- ¼ teaspoon pepper
- ½ teaspoon salt
- 1 (28-ounce) can whole peeled tomatoes, drained with juice reserved
- 1 ounce Parmesan cheese, grated fine (½ cup)
- 1 tablespoon extra-virgin olive oil
- 1 teaspoon dried oregano
- 1 teaspoon red wine vinegar
- 2 garlic cloves, minced
- 8 ounces whole-milk mozzarella cheese, shredded (2 cups)

Directions:

1. **FOR THE DOUGH:** Pulse flour, sugar, and yeast using a food processor until combined, about 5 pulses. While your food processor runs slowly put in ice water and process until dough is just combined and no dry flour remains, about 10 seconds. Let dough rest for about ten minutes.
2. Put in oil and salt to dough and process until dough forms satiny, sticky ball that clears sides of bowl, 30 to 60 seconds. Move dough to lightly oiled counter and knead using your hands to form smooth, round ball, approximately half a minute. Place dough seam side down in lightly greased big container or container, cover firmly using plastic wrap, put inside your fridge for minimum 24 hours or for maximum 3 days.
3. **FOR THE SAUCE AND TOPPINGS:** Process tomatoes, oil, garlic, vinegar, oregano, salt, and pepper in clean, dry workbowl until smooth, approximately half a minute. Move mixture to 2-cup liquid measuring cup and put in reserved tomato juice until sauce measures 2 cups. Reserve 1 cup sauce; save for later rest of the sauce for another use.
4. One hour before baking, adjust oven rack 4 inches from broiler element, set baking stone on rack, and pre-heat your oven to 500 degrees. Press down on dough to deflate. Move dough to clean counter, divide in half, and cover loosely with greased plastic. Pat 1 piece of dough (keep remaining piece covered) into 4-inch round. Working around circumference of dough, fold edges toward center until ball forms.
5. Flip ball seam side down and, using your cupped hands, drag in small circles on counter until dough feels taut and round and all seams are secured on underside. (If dough sticks to your hands, lightly dust top of dough with flour.) Replicate the process with the rest of the piece of dough. Space dough balls 3 inches apart, cover loosely with greased plastic, and allow to rest for about one hour.
6. Heat broiler for about ten minutes. In the meantime, coat 1 dough ball heavily with flour and place on well-floured counter. Using your fingertips, gently flatten into 8-inch round, leaving 1 inch of outer edge slightly thicker than center. Use your hands

to gently stretch dough into 12-inch round, working along edge and giving disk quarter turns.

7. Move dough to well-floured pizza peel and stretch into 13-inch round. Using back of spoon or ladle, spread ½ cup tomato sauce in a uniform layer on surface of dough, leaving ¼-inch border around edge. Sprinkle ¼ cup Parmesan uniformly over sauce, followed by 1 cup mozzarella.
8. Slide pizza carefully onto baking stone and return oven to 500 degrees. Bake until crust is thoroughly browned and cheese is bubbly and partially browned, eight to ten minutes, rotating pizza halfway through baking. Move pizza to wire rack and allow to cool for about five minutes before slicing and serving. Heat broiler for about ten minutes. Repeat with the rest of the dough, sauce, and toppings, returning oven to 500 degrees when pizza is placed on stone.

Toppings For Thin-Crust Pizza

Mushroom and Fennel Pizza Topping

Ⓥ This is a Vegetarian Recipe Ⓥ

If desired, mince the fennel fronds and drizzle them over the pizza before you serve.

Toss 4 ounces cremini mushrooms, trimmed and sliced thin, and ½ fennel bulb, cored and sliced thin, with 1 tablespoon extra-virgin olive oil in a container and sprinkle with salt and pepper. Microwave until vegetables become soft and release liquid, 2 to 3 minutes. Drain vegetables, then toss with 2 teaspoons minced fresh thyme. Sprinkle uniformly over pizza before baking. Sprinkle white truffle oil, if desired, lightly over pizza before you serve. (Makes enough topping for 1 pizza.)

Olive, Caper, and Spicy Garlic Pizza Topping

Ⓥ This is a Vegetarian Recipe Ⓥ

Be sure to rinse the capers and anchovies, if using, or the pizza will be very salty.

Mix ⅓ cup pitted kalamata olives, halved, 2 tablespoons capers, rinsed and patted dry, 2 anchovy fillets, rinsed, patted dry, and chopped coarse (optional), 1 small minced garlic clove, 1 teaspoon extra-virgin olive oil, and ⅛ teaspoon red pepper flakes in a container. Sprinkle uniformly over pizza before baking. Sprinkle ¼ cup fresh parsley leaves over pizza before you serve. (Makes enough topping for 1 pizza.)

Prosciutto and Arugula Pizza Topping

This topping is added to the fully baked pizza before you serve. Don't dress the arugula too far in advance or it will turn soggy.

Toss 1 cup baby arugula with 2 teaspoons extra-virgin olive oil in a container and sprinkle with salt and pepper to taste. Sprinkle 2 ounces thinly sliced prosciutto, cut into 1-inch strips, and dressed arugula over pizza before you serve. Makes enough topping for 1 pizza.)

Whole-Wheat Crust Pizzas

Pizza 1: Feta, Figs, Honey

Yield: two 13-inch pizzas, serving 4 to 6

Ⓥ This is a Vegetarian Recipe Ⓥ

Ingredients:

DOUGH

- ¾ teaspoon instant or rapid-rise yeast
- 1 cup (5½ ounces) bread flour
- 1¼ cups ice water
- 1½ cups (8¼ ounces) whole-wheat flour
- 1¾ teaspoons 2 tablespoons extra-virgin olive oil
- 2 teaspoons honey
- salt

GARLIC OIL AND TOPPINGS

- ⅛ teaspoon salt
- ½ teaspoon dried thyme
- ½ teaspoon pepper
- 1 cup fresh basil leaves
- 2 garlic cloves, minced
- 2 tablespoons 2 tablespoons extra-virgin olive oil
- 4 ounces feta cheese, crumbled (1 cup)
- 8 ounces fresh figs, stemmed and quartered along the length (1½ cups)
- honey

Directions:

1. **FOR THE DOUGH**: Pulse whole-wheat flour, bread flour, honey, and yeast using a food processor until combined, about 5 pulses. While your food processor runs slowly put in ice water and process until dough is just combined and no dry flour remains, about 10 seconds. Let dough rest for about ten minutes.
2. Put in oil and salt to dough and process until dough forms satiny, sticky ball that clears sides of bowl, 45 to 60 seconds. Move dough to lightly oiled counter and knead using your hands to form smooth, round ball, approximately half a minute. Place dough seam side down in lightly greased big container or container, cover firmly using plastic wrap, put inside your fridge for minimum 18 hours or for maximum 2 days.
3. **FOR THE GARLIC OIL AND TOPPINGS**: Heat oil in 8-inch frying pan over moderate to low heat until it starts to shimmer. Put in

garlic, pepper, thyme, and salt and cook, stirring continuously, until aromatic, approximately half a minute. Move to a container and allow to cool completely before using.
4. One hour before baking, adjust oven rack 4 inches from broiler element, set baking stone on rack, and pre-heat your oven to 500 degrees. Press down on dough to deflate. Move dough to clean counter, divide in half, and cover loosely with greased plastic. Pat 1 piece of dough (keep remaining piece covered) into 4-inch round. Working around circumference of dough, fold edges toward center until ball forms.
5. Flip dough ball seam side down and, using your cupped hands, drag in small circles on counter until dough feels taut and round and all seams are secured on underside. (If dough sticks to your hands, lightly dust top of dough with flour.) Replicate the process with the rest of the piece of dough. Space dough balls 3 inches apart, cover loosely with greased plastic, and allow to rest for about one hour.
6. Heat broiler for about ten minutes. In the meantime, heavily coat 1 dough ball with flour and place on well-floured counter. Using your fingertips, gently flatten into 8-inch round, leaving 1 inch of outer edge slightly thicker than center. Use your hands to gently stretch dough into 12-inch round, working along edge and giving disk quarter turns.
7. Move dough to well-floured pizza peel and stretch into 13-inch round. Using back of spoon, spread half of garlic oil in a uniform layer on surface of dough, leaving ¼-inch border around edge. Layer ½ cup basil leaves over garlic oil. Sprinkle with ½ cup feta, followed by ¾ cup figs.
8. Slide pizza carefully onto baking stone and return oven to 500 degrees. Bake until crust is thoroughly browned and cheese is partially browned, eight to ten minutes, rotating pizza halfway through baking. Move pizza to wire rack and drizzle 1 tablespoon honey over surface. Allow it to cool for about five minutes before slicing and serving. Heat broiler for about ten minutes. Repeat with the rest of the dough, garlic oil, and toppings, returning oven to 500 degrees when pizza is placed on stone.

Pizza 2: Artichokes, Ricotta, Parmesan

Ⓥ This is a Vegetarian Recipe Ⓥ

While we prefer the flavor and texture of jarred whole baby artichokes, you can substitute 8 ounces of frozen artichoke hearts, thawed and patted dry, for the jarred.

For topping, omit honey and basil. Increase oil to 3 tablespoons, substitute ½ teaspoon dried oregano for thyme, and put in ⅛ teaspoon red pepper flakes to frying pan along with garlic in step 3. Toss 1¼ cups jarred whole baby artichokes packed in water, quartered, rinsed, and patted dry, with 1 tablespoon garlic oil and 1 tablespoon lemon juice. Mix ½ cup whole-milk ricotta, ¼ teaspoon lemon zest, ⅛ teaspoon salt, and pinch pepper in a container. Substitute ¼ cup grated Parmesan for feta and artichokes for figs. After baking, dollop half of ricotta mixture uniformly surface of each pizza and allow to cool for about five minutes.

Pizza 3: Pesto, Goat Cheese

Ⓥ This is a Vegetarian Recipe Ⓥ

For topping, omit figs and honey. Increase basil leaves to 2 cups and process with 7 tablespoons extra-virgin olive oil, ¼ cup pine nuts, 3 minced garlic cloves, and ½ teaspoon salt using a food processor until smooth, scraping down sides of the container as required, approximately one minute. Mix in ¼ cup finely grated Parmesan or Pecorino Romano cheese and sprinkle with salt and pepper to taste. Substitute pesto for garlic oil and basil leaves and ½ cup crumbled goat cheese for feta.

Fruit and Sweets

Almond Cake

Yield: Servings 12

Ingredients:

- ⅛ teaspoon baking soda
- ¼ teaspoon baking powder
- ½ cup extra-virgin ¾ cup (3¾ ounces) all-purpose flour
- ¾ teaspoon almond extract
- ¾ teaspoon salt
- 1 tablespoon plus ½ teaspoon grated lemon zest (2 lemons)
- 1¼ cups (8¾ ounces) plus 2 tablespoons sugar
- 1½ cups plus ⅓ cup blanched sliced almonds, toasted
- 4 large eggs
- olive oil

Directions:

1. Place the oven rack in the centre of the oven and pre-heat your oven to 300 degrees. Grease 9-inch round cake pan and line with parchment paper. Pulse 1½ cups almonds, flour, salt, baking powder, and baking soda using a food processor until almonds are finely ground, 10 to 15 pulses; move to a container.
2. Process eggs, 1¼ cups sugar, 1 tablespoon lemon zest, and almond extract in now-empty processor until pale yellow and frothy, approximately half a minute. While your food processor runs slowly put in oil gradually until incorporated, about 10 seconds. Put in almond mixture and pulse to combine, 4 to 5 pulses.

3. Move batter to prepared pan and smooth into even layer. Using your fingers, combine remaining 2 tablespoons sugar and remaining ½ teaspoon lemon zest in a small-sized container until aromatic, 5 to 10 seconds. Sprinkle top of cake evenly with remaining ⅓ cup almonds followed by sugar-zest mixture.
4. Bake until center of cake is set and bounces back when gently pressed and toothpick inserted in center comes out clean, 55 to 65 minutes, rotating pan after 40 minutes.
5. Let cake cool in pan on wire rack for about fifteen minutes. Run paring knife around sides of pan. Remove cake from pan, discarding parchment, and allow to cool completely on rack, about 2 hours. Serve.

Apricot Spoon Sweets

Yield: 4 cups

A syrup made from water, sugar, and honey turns fresh apricot wedges into a classic Greek sweet.

Ingredients:

- ¾ cup water
- 1 cup honey
- 1½ cups sugar
- 1½ pounds ripe but firm apricots, pitted and cut into ½-inch wedges
- 2 tablespoons lemon juice

Directions:

1. Bring sugar, honey, and water to boil in a Dutch oven on high heat and cook, stirring intermittently, until syrup measures 2 cups, about 10 minutes.
2. Put in apricots and lemon juice and return to boil. Decrease heat to moderate to low and simmer, stirring intermittently,

until apricots soften and release their juice, approximately five minutes. Remove pot from heat and allow to cool fully.
3. Move apricots and syrup to airtight container put inside your fridge for 24 hours before you serve. (Fruit will keep safely in a fridge for maximum seven days.)

Baklava

Yield: 32 to 40 pieces

Ingredients:

SUGAR SYRUP

- ⅛ teaspoon ⅓ cup honey
- ¾ cup water
- 1 cinnamon stick
- 1¼ cups (8¾ ounces) sugar
- 3 (2-inch) strips lemon zest plus 1 tablespoon juice
- 5 whole cloves
- salt

NUT FILLING

- ⅛ teaspoon ¼ teaspoon ground cloves
- 1 cup walnuts
- 1¼ teaspoons ground cinnamon
- 1¾ cups slivered almonds
- 2 tablespoons sugar
- salt

PASTRY

- 1 pound (14 5 tablespoons extra-virgin olive oil
- by 9-inch) phyllo, thawed

Directions:

1. **FOR THE SUGAR SYRUP:** Bring all ingredients to boil in small saucepan on moderate to high heat and cook, stirring intermittently, until sugar has dissolved, approximately five minutes. Move syrup to 2-cup liquid measuring cup and allow to cool to room temperature. Discard spices and zest; set aside.
2. **FOR THE NUT FILLING:** Pulse almonds using a food processor until very thinly sliced, about 20 pulses; move to medium bowl. Pulse walnuts using a food processor until very thinly sliced, about 15 pulses; move to a container with almonds and toss to combine. Measure out 1 tablespoon nuts and set aside for garnish. Put in sugar, cinnamon, cloves, and salt to nut mixture and toss well to combine.
3. **FOR THE PASTRY:** Place oven rack to lower-middle position and pre-heat your oven to 300 degrees. Lay 1 phyllo sheet in bottom of greased 13 by 9-inch baking pan and brush thoroughly with oil. Repeat with 7 more phyllo sheets, brushing each with oil (you should have total of 8 layers of phyllo).
4. Sprinkle 1 cup nut filling uniformly over phyllo. Cover nut filling with 6 more phyllo sheets, brushing each with oil, then drizzle with 1 cup nut filling. Repeat with 6 phyllo sheets, oil, and remaining 1 cup nut filling.
5. Cover nut filling with 8 more phyllo sheets, brushing each layer, except final layer, with oil. Working from center outward, use palms of your hands to compress layers and press out any air pockets. Spoon remaining oil (about 2 tablespoons) on top layer and brush to cover surface.
6. Using serrated knife with pointed tip, cut baklava into diamonds. Bake baklava until golden and crisp, about 1½ hours, rotating pan halfway through baking.
7. Immediately pour all but 2 tablespoons cooled syrup over cut lines (syrup will sizzle when it hits hot pan). Sprinkle remaining 2 tablespoons syrup over surface. Garnish center of each piece with pinch reserved ground nuts. Let baklava cool completely in pan, about three hours, then cover with aluminium foil and allow to sit at room temperature for about 8 hours before you serve.

Classic French Poached Pears

Yield: 6 to 8 Servings

Ingredients:

- ⅛ teaspoon salt
- ½ cinnamon stick
- ¾ cup sugar
- 1 (750-ml) bottle dry white wine
- 1 vanilla bean
- 3 sprigs fresh thyme
- 5 sprigs fresh mint
- 6 (2-inch) strips lemon zest
- 6 ripe but firm Bosc or Bartlett pears (8 ounces each), peeled, halved, and cored

Directions:

1. Cut vanilla bean in half along the length. Using tip of paring knife, scrape out seeds. Bring wine, sugar, lemon zest, mint sprigs, thyme sprigs, cinnamon stick, salt, and vanilla seeds and pod to boil in a big saucepan on high heat and cook, stirring intermittently, until sugar has dissolved, approximately five minutes.
2. Put in pears and return to boil. Decrease heat to moderate to low, cover, and simmer until pears are soft and toothpick slips easily in and out of pears, 10 to 20 minutes, gently turning pears over every 5 minutes.
3. Use a slotted spoon to move pears to shallow casserole dish. Bring syrup to simmer on moderate heat and cook, stirring intermittently, until slightly thickened and measures 1¼ to 1½ cups, about fifteen minutes. Strain syrup through fine-mesh strainer over pears; discard solids. Let pears cool to room temperature, then cover put inside your fridge until well chilled, minimum 2 hours or for maximum 3 days. Serve.

Classic Greek Lemon Rice Pudding

Yield: 8 Servings

Ingredients:

- ½ cinnamon stick
- ½ cup sugar
- ½ teaspoon salt
- 1 cup Arborio rice
- 1 vanilla bean
- 2 bay leaves
- 2 cups water
- 2 teaspoons 4½ cups whole milk, plus extra as required
- grated lemon zest

Directions:

1. Bring water to boil in a big saucepan on moderate to high heat. Mix in rice and salt. Decrease heat to low, cover, and simmer gently until water is almost fully absorbed, fifteen to twenty minutes.
2. Cut vanilla bean in half along the length. Using tip of paring knife, scrape out seeds. Stir vanilla bean and seeds, milk, sugar, cinnamon stick, and bay leaves into rice. Increase heat to moderate to high and bring to simmer. Cook, uncovered, stirring frequently, until rice is soft and pudding has thickened to consistency of yogurt, 35 to 45 minutes.
3. Remove from the heat, discard bay leaves, cinnamon stick, and vanilla bean. Mix in lemon zest. Move pudding to big container and allow to cool completely, about 2 hours. Stir pudding to loosen and regulate consistency with extra milk as required. Serve at room temperature or chilled.

Dried Fruit Compote

Yield: 6 Servings

Ingredients:

- ½ cup dried ¾ cup dried apricots
- 1¼ teaspoons ground coriander
- 2 (2-inch) strips lemon zest plus 1 tablespoon juice
- 2 cinnamon sticks
- 2 cups (12 ounces) dried Turkish or Calimyrna figs, stemmed
- 3 tablespoons honey
- 4 cups water
- cherries

Directions:

1. Bring water, honey, lemon zest and juice, cinnamon sticks, and coriander to boil in a big saucepan on moderate to high heat and cook, stirring intermittently, until honey has dissolved, approximately two minutes.
2. Mix in figs and apricots and return to boil. Decrease heat to moderate to low and simmer, stirring intermittently, until fruit is plump and tender, approximately half an hour.
3. Mix in cherries and cook until cherries are plump and tender, figs are just starting to break apart, and liquid becomes thick and syrupy, fifteen to twenty minutes. Remove from the heat, discard lemon zest and cinnamon sticks and let mixture cool slightly. Serve warm, at room temperature, or chilled.

Fruit & Wine Dessert

Yield: 6 to 8 Servings

This recipe can be made quickly

Ingredients:

- ¼ cup sugar, plus extra as required
- ¼ teaspoon grated lemon zest
- 1 cup chilled 1 pound nectarines, pitted and cut into ¼-inch wedges
- 1 tablespoon chopped fresh mint
- 1 tablespoon orange liqueur, such as Grand Marnier or triple sec
- 10 ounces (2 cups) blackberries or raspberries
- 10 ounces strawberries, hulled and quartered (2 cups)
- prosecco

Directions:

1. Gently toss blackberries, strawberries, nectarines, sugar, orange liqueur, mint, and lemon zest together in a big container. Allow to sit at room temperature, stirring intermittently, until fruit begins to release its juices, 10 to fifteen minutes.
2. Just before you serve, pour prosecco over fruit and season with extra sugar to taste. Serve.

Fruit and Nut Roasted Pears

Yield: 4 to 6 Servings

Ingredients:

- ⅛ teaspoon salt
- ¼ teaspoon ground cardamom
- ⅓ cup sugar
- ½ cup dried apricots, quartered
- 1 teaspoon lemon juice
- 1¼ cups dry white wine
- 2 tablespoons extra-virgin olive oil
- 4 ripe but firm Bosc or Bartlett pears (6 to 7 ounces each), peeled, halved, and cored
- ⅓ cup shelled pistachios, toasted and chopped

Directions:

1. Place the oven rack in the centre of the oven and pre-heat your oven to 450 degrees. Heat oil in 12-inch oven-safe frying pan on moderate to high heat until it starts to shimmer. Place pears cut side down in frying pan and cook, without moving them, until just starting to brown, 3 to 5 minutes.
2. Move frying pan to oven and roast pears for about fifteen minutes. Being careful of hot frying pan handle, flip pears and continue to roast until toothpick slips easily in and out of pears, 10 to fifteen minutes.
3. Using potholders, remove frying pan from oven and carefully move pears to serving platter. Put in wine, apricots, sugar, cardamom, and salt to now-empty frying pan and bring to simmer on moderate to high heat. Cook, beating to scrape up any browned bits, until sauce is reduced and has consistency of maple syrup, 7 to 10 minutes. Remove from the heat, mix in lemon juice. Pour sauce over pears and drizzle with pistachios. Serve.

Greek Pasteli

Yield: 32 bars

Ingredients:

- ¼ teaspoon ¾ cup honey
- 1¾ cups sesame seeds
- salt

Directions:

1. Place the oven rack in the centre of the oven and pre-heat your oven to 350 degrees. Make foil sling for 8-inch square baking pan by folding 2 long sheets of aluminium foil so each is 8 inches wide. Lay sheets of foil in pan perpendicular to each other, with extra foil hanging over edges of pan. Push foil into

corners and up sides of pan, smoothing foil flush to pan, then grease foil.
2. Lay out sesame seeds in a uniform layer in rimmed baking sheet and toast, stirring frequently, until golden, 10 to 12 minutes; instantly move to a container.
3. Heat honey in a big saucepan on moderate to high heat until bubbling. Decrease heat to moderate to low and cook, gently swirling pan occasionally, until honey is deep amber and registers 300 to 310 degrees, 4 to 5 minutes. Remove from the heat, mix in sesame seeds and salt until thoroughly combined.
4. Working quickly, carefully pour honey–sesame seed mixture into prepared pan and push into corners with greased rubber spatula. Allow to sit until cool enough to touch but still malleable, approximately five minutes. Using lightly greased fingers, gently press mixture into even layer. Allow it to cool until firm, approximately twenty minutes. (Do not let bars sit for longer than 20 minutes or they will be too hard to cut.)
5. Using foil overhang, lift bars out of pan and move to slicing board; discard foil. Cut into thirty-two 2 by 1-inch bars and move to wire rack. Let bars cool completely, about 1 hour, then move to airtight container. Allow to sit at room temperature until fully crisp, about 8 hours. Serve. (Bars can be stored safely at room temperature for up to 1 month.)

Honey Biscotti

Yield: Approximately 48 biscotti

Omit dried lavender if you don't have it. It should be easily available in spice store though.

Ingredients:

- ¼ teaspoon salt
- ½ teaspoon ½ teaspoon baking soda

- ⅔ cup (4⅔ ounces) sugar
- 1 tablespoon dried lavender (optional)
- 1 teaspoon baking powder
- 2 tablespoons grated orange zest
- 2¼ cups (11¼ ounces) all-purpose flour
- 3 large eggs
- 3 tablespoons honey
- vanilla extract

Directions:

1. Place the oven rack in the centre of the oven and pre-heat your oven to 350 degrees. Using ruler and pencil, draw two 13 by 2-inch rectangles, spaced 3 inches apart, on piece of parchment paper. Grease baking sheet and place parchment on it, marked side down.
2. Beat flour, baking powder, baking soda, and salt together in a small-sized container. In big container, beat sugar and eggs together until pale yellow. Beat in honey, orange zest, lavender, if using, and vanilla until combined. Using rubber spatula, mix in flour mixture until just combined.
3. Split the dough in half. Using floured hands, form each half into 13 by 2-inch rectangle, using lines on parchment as guide. Using rubber spatula mildly coated using vegetable oil spray, smooth tops and sides of loaves. Bake until loaves start to look golden and just starting to crack on top, about 35 minutes, rotating sheet halfway through baking.
4. Let loaves cool on sheet for about ten minutes, then move to slicing board. Reduce oven temperature to 325 degrees. Using serrated knife, slice each loaf on slight bias into ½-inch-thick slices.
5. Arrange cookies cut side down on sheet about ½ inch apart and bake until crisp and golden brown on both sides, about fifteen minutes, flipping cookies halfway through baking. Allow it to cool completely on wire rack before you serve. (Biscotti can be stored safely at room temperature for up to 1 month.)

Honey-Glazed Peaches

Yield: 6 Servings

✒ This recipe can be made quickly ✒

Ingredients:

- ¼ cup hazelnuts, toasted, skinned, and chopped coarse
- ¼ cup honey
- ¼ teaspoon salt
- ⅓ cup water
- 1 tablespoon extra-virgin olive oil
- 1 tablespoon sugar
- 2 tablespoons lemon juice
- 6 ripe but firm peaches, peeled, halved, and pitted

Directions:

1. Place oven rack 6 inches from broiler element and heat broiler. Mix lemon juice, sugar, and salt in a big container. Put in peaches and toss to combine, making sure to coat all sides with sugar mixture.
2. Arrange peaches cut side up in 12-inch broilersafe frying pan and spoon any remaining sugar mixture into peach cavities. Pour water around peaches in skillet. Broil until peaches are just starting to brown, 11 to fifteen minutes.
3. Mix honey and oil in a container and microwave until warm, approximately half a minute, then stir to combine. Using potholders, remove frying pan from oven. Being careful of hot frying pan handle, brush half of honey mixture on peaches. Return peaches to oven and continue to broil until spotty brown, 5 to 7 minutes.
4. Cautiously remove frying pan from oven, brush peaches with remaining honey mixture, and move to serving platter, leaving juice behind. Bring accumulated juice in frying pan to simmer on moderate heat and cook, beating frequently to combine,

until syrupy, approximately one minute. Pour syrup over peaches and drizzle with hazelnuts. Serve.

Icy Delight 1: Lemon

Yield: 1 quart, serving 8

Ingredients:

- ⅛ te1 cup (7 ounces) sugar
- 1 cup lemon juice (6 lemons)
- 2 tablespoons vodka (optional)
- 2¼ cups water, preferably spring water
- aspoon salt

Directions:

1. Beat all ingredients together in a container until sugar has dissolved. Pour mixture into 2 ice cube trays and freeze until solid, minimum three hours or for maximum 5 days.
2. Place medium bowl in freezer. Pulse half of ice cubes using a food processor until creamy and no large lumps remain, about 18 pulses. Move mixture to chilled bowl and return to freezer. Repeat pulsing remaining ice cubes; move to a container. Serve instantly.

Icy Delight 2: Minted Lemon

Bring 1 cup water, sugar, and salt to simmer in small saucepan on moderate to high heat, stirring intermittently. Remove from the heat, mix in ½ cup torn fresh mint leaves and allow to steep for about five minutes. Strain mixture through fine-mesh strainer into medium bowl. Mix in remaining 1¼ cups water, lemon juice, and vodka and allow to cool to room temperature, about fifteen minutes. Freeze and pulse ice cubes as directed.

Icy Delight 3: Orange

Reduce lemon juice to 2 tablespoons and sugar to ¾ cup. Put in ¾ cup orange juice (2 oranges) to mixture in step 1.

Italian Orange Polenta Cake

Yield: Servings 12

Ingredients:

- ⅓ cup (2⅓ ounces) packed brown sugar
- ½ teaspoon baking soda
- 1 cup (5 ounces) all-purpose flour
- 1 cup (7 ounces) granulated sugar
- 1 teaspoon baking powder
- 1½ cups (8¼ ounces) instant polenta
- 1½ cups whole milk
- 2 oranges plus 2 teaspoons grated orange zest
- 2 teaspoons 2 teaspoons cornstarch
- 3 large eggs
- 6 tablespoons extra-virgin olive oil
- Salt
- vanilla extract

Directions:

1. Place the oven rack in the centre of the oven and pre-heat your oven to 350 degrees. Lay out polenta in rimmed baking sheet and toast in oven until aromatic, about 10 minutes; move to big container. Mix in milk and orange zest and allow to sit until liquid is fully absorbed, about 10 minutes. Use your hands to break polenta into fine crumbs; set aside.
2. Grease 9-inch round cake pan, line with parchment paper, then grease parchment. Mix brown sugar, cornstarch, and ⅛ teaspoon salt in a small-sized container and drizzle evenly in bottom of prepared pan. Cut away peel and pith from oranges, then slice crosswise into ⅛-inch-thick slices. Arrange orange

slices in one layer over sugar mixture (some slices may overlap slightly).

3. Beat flour, baking powder, baking soda, and ½ teaspoon salt together in a container. Using stand mixer fitted with paddle attachment, beat eggs and granulated sugar together on medium speed until pale and tripled in volume, six to eight minutes. Reduce speed to low, slowly put in oil and vanilla, and beat until combined. Put in polenta crumbs and beat until combined. Put in flour mixture in 3 additions until combined, scraping down sides of the container as required. Give batter final stir by hand.
4. Pour batter over oranges in pan and spread into even layer. Bake until cake is golden brown and toothpick inserted into center comes out clean, 50 to 60 minutes, rotating pan halfway through baking.
5. Let cake cool in pan on wire rack for about fifteen minutes. Run paring knife around sides of pan. Place wire rack over pan and, holding rack tightly, invert cake onto rack and allow to sit until cake releases itself from pan, approximately one minute. Place rack over a baking sheet to catch drips. Remove pan; gently scrape off any orange slices stuck in pan and arrange on top of cake. Let cake cool completely, about 2 hours. Serve.

Italian Pignoli

Yield: Approximately 18 cookies

Classic Italian Cookies!

Ingredients:

- 1 cup pine 1⅓ cups (9⅓ ounces) sugar
- 1⅔ cups slivered almonds
- 2 large egg whites
- nuts

Directions:

1. Place two oven racks in your oven one just above, and one just below the middle position and pre-heat your oven to 375 degrees. Line 2 baking sheets with parchment paper.
2. Process almonds and sugar using a food processor until finely ground, approximately half a minute. Scrape down sides of the container and put in egg whites. Continue to process until smooth (dough will be wet), approximately half a minute; move mixture to a container. Place pine nuts in shallow dish.
3. Working with 1 scant tablespoon dough at a time, roll into balls, roll in pine nuts to coat, and space 2 inches apart on the readied sheets.
4. Bake cookies until light golden brown, 13 to fifteen minutes, switching and rotating sheets halfway through baking. Let cookies cool on sheets for about five minutes, then move to wire rack. Let cookies cool to room temperature before you serve. (Cookies can be stored in airtight container at room temperature for maximum 4 days.)

Italian Vinegar Strawberries

Yield: 6 Servings

✐This recipe can be made quickly✐

Ingredients:

- ¼ cup packed light brown sugar
- ⅓ cup balsamic vinegar
- ½ teaspoon lemon juice
- 2 pounds strawberries, hulled and sliced along the length ¼ inch thick (5 cups)
- 2 teaspoons granulated sugar
- Pinch pepper

Directions:

1. Bring vinegar, granulated sugar, and lemon juice to simmer in small saucepan on moderate heat and cook, stirring intermittently, until thickened and measures about 3 tablespoons, approximately three minutes. Move syrup to small-sized container and allow to cool fully.
2. Gently toss strawberries with brown sugar and pepper in a big container. Allow to sit at room temperature, stirring intermittently, until strawberries begin to release their juice, 10 to fifteen minutes. Pour syrup over strawberries and gently toss to combine. Serve.

Italian Zabaglione & Berry Mix

Yield: 4 Servings

Ingredients:

BERRY MIXTURE

- 11 ounces (2¼ cups) blackberries, blueberries, and/or raspberries
- 2 teaspoons granulated sugar
- 4 ounces strawberries, hulled and halved along the length if small or quartered if large (¾ cup)
- Pinch salt

ZABAGLIONE

- 2 teaspoons packed light brown sugar
- 3 large egg yolks
- 3 tablespoons 3 tablespoons dry white wine
- 3 tablespoons granulated sugar
- heavy cream, chilled

Directions:

1. **FOR THE BERRY MIXTURE:** Line rimmed baking sheet with aluminium foil. Toss berries, strawberries, sugar, and salt

together in a container. Divide berry mixture evenly among 4 shallow 6-ounce gratin dishes set in readied sheet; set aside.
2. **FOR THE ZABAGLIONE:** Beat egg yolks, 2 tablespoons plus 1 teaspoon granulated sugar, and wine together in a moderate-sized container until sugar has dissolved, approximately one minute. Set bowl over saucepan of barely simmering water and cook, beating continuously, until mixture is frothy. Carry on cooking, beating continuously, until mixture is slightly thickened, creamy, and glossy, 5 to 10 minutes (mixture will form loose mounds when dripped from beat). Remove bowl from saucepan and beat continuously for 30 seconds to cool slightly. Move bowl to refrigerator and chill until egg mixture is completely cool, about 10 minutes.
3. In the meantime, adjust oven rack 6 inches from broiler element and heat broiler. Mix brown sugar and remaining 2 teaspoons granulated sugar in a container.
4. Beat heavy cream in a big container until it holds soft peaks, 30 to 90 seconds. Using rubber spatula, gently fold whipped cream into cooled egg mixture. Spoon zabaglione over berries and drizzle sugar mixture uniformly top. Allow to sit at room temperature for about ten minutes, until sugar dissolves.
5. Broil gratins until sugar is bubbly and caramelized, 1 to 4 minutes. Serve instantly.

Lemon Yogurt Mousse

Yield: 6 Servings

Ingredients:

BLUEBERRY SAUCE

- 2 tablespoons sugar
- 2 tablespoons water
- 4 ounces (¾ cup) blueberries
- Pinch salt

MOUSSE

- ⅛ teaspoon salt
- ¼ cup heavy cream
- ¼ teaspoon cream of tartar
- ½ cup whole Greek yogurt
- ¾ teaspoon unflavored gelatin
- 1 teaspoon vanilla extract
- 1½ teaspoons grated lemon zest plus 3 tablespoons juice
- 3 large egg whites
- 3 tablespoons water
- 6 tablespoons (2⅔ ounces) sugar

Directions:

1. **FOR THE BLUEBERRY SAUCE:** Bring blueberries, sugar, water, and salt to simmer in moderate-sized saucepan on moderate heat. Cook, stirring intermittently, until sugar has dissolved and fruit is heated through, 2 to 4 minutes.
2. Move mixture to blender and process until smooth, approximately half a minute. Strain puree through fine-mesh strainer, pressing on solids to extract as much puree as possible (you should have about ½ cup). Spoon sauce evenly into six 4-ounce ramekins put inside your fridge until chilled, approximately twenty minutes.
3. **FOR THE MOUSSE:** Sprinkle gelatin over water in a container and allow to sit until gelatin softens, approximately five minutes. In a different container, beat yogurt, heavy cream, lemon zest and juice, vanilla, and salt together until smooth.
4. Beat egg whites, cream of tartar, and sugar together in a container of stand mixer. Set bowl over saucepan of barely simmering water and cook, beating continuously, until mixture has tripled in volume and registers about 160 degrees, 5 to 10 minutes.
5. Remove from the heat, quickly beat in hydrated gelatin until dissolved. Move bowl to stand mixer fitted with beat attachment and whip on medium-high speed until stiff, shiny

peaks form, four to eight minutes. Put in yogurt mixture and continue to whip until just combined, 30 to 60 seconds.
6. Divide mousse evenly among chilled ramekins, cover firmly using plastic wrap, put inside your fridge until chilled and set, 6 to 8 hours. Serve chilled.

Lemon-Anise Biscotti

Yield: Approximately 48 biscotti

Ingredients:

- ¼ teaspoon salt
- ¼ teaspoon vanilla 1 cup (7 ounces) sugar
- 1 tablespoon anise seeds
- 1 tablespoon grated lemon zest
- 1 teaspoon baking powder
- 2 cups (10 ounces) all-purpose flour
- 2 large eggs
- extract

Directions:

1. Place the oven rack in the centre of the oven and pre-heat your oven to 350 degrees. Using ruler and pencil, draw two 13 by 2-inch rectangles, spaced 3 inches apart, on piece of parchment paper. Grease baking sheet and place parchment on it, marked side down.
2. Beat flour, baking powder, and salt together in a small-sized container. In big container, beat sugar and eggs together until pale yellow. Beat in lemon zest, anise seeds, and vanilla until combined. Using rubber spatula, mix in flour mixture until just combined.
3. Split the dough in half. Using floured hands, form each half into 13 by 2-inch rectangle, using lines on parchment as guide. Using rubber spatula mildly coated using vegetable oil spray, smooth tops and sides of loaves. Bake until loaves start to look golden

and just starting to crack on top, about 35 minutes, rotating sheet halfway through baking.
4. Let loaves cool on sheet for about ten minutes, then move to slicing board. Reduce oven temperature to 325 degrees. Using serrated knife, slice each loaf on slight bias into ½-inch-thick slices.
5. Arrange cookies cut side down on sheet about ½ inch apart and bake until crisp and golden brown on both sides, about fifteen minutes, flipping cookies halfway through baking. Allow it to cool completely on wire rack before you serve. (Biscotti can be stored safely at room temperature for up to 1 month.)

Mediterranean Berry Mix

Yield: 4 to 6 Servings

This recipe can be made quickly

Ingredients:

- ½ teaspoon pepper
- 1 tablespoon lime 10 ounces (2 cups) blackberries
- 10 ounces strawberries, hulled and quartered (2 cups)
- 2 tablespoons chopped fresh basil
- 3 peaches, halved, pitted, and cut into ½-inch pieces
- 4 teaspoons sugar
- juice, plus extra for seasoning

Directions:

1. Mix sugar, basil, and pepper in a big container. Using rubber spatula, press mixture into side of the container until sugar becomes damp, approximately half a minute. Put in peaches, blackberries, and strawberries and gently toss to combine.
2. Allow to sit at room temperature, stirring intermittently, until fruit releases its juices, 15 to half an hour. Mix in lime juice and season with extra lime juice to taste. Serve.

Poached Peaches and Cherries

Yield: 6 Servings

⁄This recipe can be made quickly ⁄

Poached fruit is a popular Mediterranean dessert.

Ingredients:

- ½ cinnamon stick
- 1 cup sugar1 pound fresh sweet cherries, pitted and halved
- 1 pound ripe but firm peaches, peeled, halved, pitted, and sliced ¼ inch thick
- 2 cups dry red wine
- 2 whole cloves
-

Directions:

1. Mix cherries, peaches, cinnamon stick, and cloves in a big container. Bring red wine and sugar to boil in small saucepan on high heat and cook, stirring intermittently, until sugar has dissolved, approximately five minutes.
2. Pour syrup over fruit, cover, and allow to cool to room temperature. Discard cinnamon stick and cloves. Serve.

Raspberry Sorbet

Yield: 1 quart, serving 8

Ingredients:

- ⅛ teaspoon salt
- ¼ cup light ½ cup (3½ ounces) plus 2 tablespoons sugar

- 1 cup water
- 1 teaspoon low- or no-sugar-needed fruit pectin
- 1¼ pounds (4 cups) fresh or frozen raspberries
- corn syrup

Directions:

1. Heat water, pectin, and salt in moderate-sized saucepan on moderate to high heat, stirring intermittently, until pectin has fully dissolved, approximately five minutes. Remove saucepan from heat and let mixture cool slightly, about 10 minutes.
2. Process raspberries, sugar, corn syrup, and cooled water mixture using a blender or food processor until smooth, approximately half a minute. Strain mixture through fine-mesh strainer, pressing on solids to extract as much liquid as possible. Move 1 cup mixture to small-sized container and place remaining mixture in a big container. Cover both bowls using plastic wrap. Place big container in refrigerator and small-sized container in freezer and chill for minimum 4 hours or for maximum 24 hours. (Small bowl of base will freeze solid.)
3. Remove mixtures from refrigerator and freezer. Scrape frozen base from small-sized container into big container of base. Stir occasionally until frozen base has fully dissolved. Move mixture to ice cream machine and churn until mixture has consistency of thick milkshake and color lightens, 15 to 25 minutes.
4. Move sorbet to airtight container, pressing firmly to remove any air pockets, and freeze until firm, minimum 2 hours or for maximum 5 days. Let sorbet sit at room temperature for about five minutes before you serve.

Semolina Pudding

Yield: 6 to 8 Servings

Ingredients:

- ⅛ teaspoon saffron threads, crumbled

- ⅛ teaspoon salt
- ½ cup slivered almonds, toasted and chopped
- ½ cup sugar
- ½ teaspoon ground cardamom
- ¾ cup fine semolina flour
- 1 tablespoon extra-virgin olive oil
- 3 ounces pitted 4½ cups whole milk, plus extra as required
- dates, sliced thin (½ cup)

Directions:

1. Heat oil in 12-inch frying pan on moderate heat until it starts to shimmer. Put in semolina and cook, stirring intermittently, until aromatic, 3 to 5 minutes; move to a container.
2. Bring milk, sugar, cardamom, saffron, and salt to simmer in a big saucepan on moderate heat. Whisking continuously, slowly put in semolina, 1 tablespoon at a time, and cook until mixture thickens slightly and begins to bubble, approximately three minutes. Remove saucepan from heat, cover, and let pudding rest for half an hour.
3. Stir pudding to loosen and regulate consistency with extra warm milk as required. Sprinkle individual portions with almonds and dates before you serve.

Sicilian Fig Phyllo Cookies

Yield: Approximately 24 cookies

Ingredients:

SUGAR SYRUP

- ¼ cup granulated sugar
- 2 (2-inch2 tablespoons honey
- 2 tablespoons water
-) strips orange zest plus 2 tablespoons juice

FIG FILLING

- ½ cup granulated sugar
- ½ cup walnuts, toasted and chopped coarse
- ½ teaspoon anise seeds
- ¾ cup water
- 1 tablespoon 1 teaspoon orange zest
- 1½ cups (9 ounces) dried figs, stemmed and halved
- dry sherry

PASTRY

- ¼ cup extra-virgin olive oil
- 2 tablespoons confectioners' 6 (14 by 9-inch) phyllo sheets, thawed
- sugar

Directions:

1. **FOR THE SUGAR SYRUP:** Bring all ingredients to boil in small saucepan on moderate to high heat and cook, stirring intermittently, until sugar has dissolved, approximately two minutes. Decrease heat to moderate to low and simmer until syrup becomes thick and slightly reduced, approximately three minutes. Discard zest and move syrup to a container; set aside.
2. **FOR THE FIG FILLING:** Bring figs, water, sugar, orange zest, and anise seeds to simmer in now-empty saucepan on moderate heat and cook until thickened and syrupy, approximately five minutes. Let mixture cool to room temperature, about 1 hour.
3. Process fig mixture using a food processor until paste forms, approximately fifteen seconds. Scrape down sides of bowl, put in walnuts and sherry, and pulse until walnuts are thinly sliced, approximately ten pulses. Move fig-walnut mixture to zipper-lock bag and snip off 1 corner to create 1-inch opening.
4. **FOR THE PASTRY:** Place the oven rack in the centre of the oven and pre-heat your oven to 375 degrees. Line rimmed baking sheet with parchment paper. Place 1 phyllo sheet on counter with long side parallel to counter edge, brush lightly with oil, then dust with 1 teaspoon sugar. Repeat with 2 more phyllo

sheets, brushing each with oil and dusting with 1 teaspoon sugar (you should have total of 3 layers of phyllo).
5. Pipe half of filling along bottom edge of phyllo, leaving 1½-inch border along edge. Fold bottom edge of phyllo over filling, then continue rolling phyllo away from you into firm cylinder. With cylinder seam side down, use serrated knife to cut cylinder into 12 equivalent pieces. Arrange cookies on readied sheet, spaced 1½ inches apart. Replicate the process with the rest of the 3 phyllo sheets, oil, and filling and arrange on sheet.
6. Bake cookies until light golden brown, fifteen to twenty minutes, rotating sheet halfway through baking. Sprinkle warm cookies with syrup and allow to cool for about five minutes. Move cookies to wire rack and allow to cool completely before you serve. (Cookies can be stored safely at room temperature for up to 4 days.)

Spanish Olive Oil–Yogurt Cake

Yield: Servings 12

Ingredients:

CAKE

- 1 cup plain 1 tablespoon baking powder
- 1 teaspoon salt
- 1¼ cups (8¾ ounces) granulated sugar
- 1¼ cups extra-virgin olive oil
- 3 cups (15 ounces) all-purpose flour
- 4 large eggs
- whole-milk yogurt

LEMON GLAZE

- 1 tablespoon plain whole-milk yogurt
- 2–3 tablespoons lemon juice
- 2 cups (8 ounces) confectioners' sugar

Directions:

1. **FOR THE CAKE:** Place oven rack to lower-middle position and pre-heat your oven to 350 degrees. Grease 12-cup non-stick Bundt pan. Beat flour, baking powder, and salt together in a container. In separate big container, beat sugar and eggs together until sugar is mostly dissolved and mixture is pale and frothy, approximately one minute. Beat in oil and yogurt until combined. Using rubber spatula, mix in flour mixture until combined and no dry flour remains.
2. Pour batter into prepared pan, smooth top, and gently tap pan on counter to settle batter. Bake until cake is golden brown and wooden skewer inserted into center comes out clean, 40 to 45 minutes, rotating pan halfway through baking.
3. **FOR THE LEMON GLAZE:** Beat 2 tablespoons lemon juice, yogurt, and confectioners' sugar together in a container until smooth, adding more lemon juice gradually as required until glaze is thick but still pourable (mixture should leave faint trail across bottom of mixing bowl when drizzled from beat). Let cake cool in pan for about ten minutes, then gently turn cake out onto wire rack. Sprinkle half of glaze over warm cake and allow to cool for about one hour. Sprinkle remaining glaze over cake and allow to cool completely, about 2 hours. Serve.

Spicey Biscotti

Yield: Approximately 48 biscotti

Ingredients:

- ¼ teaspoon ground ginger
- ¼ teaspoon ground white pepper
- ¼ teaspoon salt
- ½ teaspoon baking soda
- ½ teaspoon ground cinnamon
- ½ teaspoon ground cloves

- ½ teaspoon vanilla 1 cup (7 ounces) sugar
- 1 teaspoon baking powder
- 2 large eggs plus 2 large yolks
- 2¼ cups (11¼ ounces) all-purpose flour
- extract

Directions:

1. Place the oven rack in the centre of the oven and pre-heat your oven to 350 degrees. Using ruler and pencil, draw two 13 by 2-inch rectangles, spaced 3 inches apart, on piece of parchment paper. Grease baking sheet and place parchment on it, marked side down.
2. Beat flour, baking powder, baking soda, cloves, cinnamon, ginger, salt, and pepper together in a small-sized container. In big container, beat sugar and eggs and egg yolks together until pale yellow. Beat in vanilla until combined. Using rubber spatula, mix in flour mixture until just combined.
3. Split the dough in half. Using floured hands, form each half into 13 by 2-inch rectangle, using lines on parchment as guide. Using rubber spatula mildly coated using vegetable oil spray, smooth tops and sides of loaves. Bake until loaves start to look golden and just starting to crack on top, about 35 minutes, rotating sheet halfway through baking.
4. Let loaves cool on sheet for about ten minutes, then move to slicing board. Reduce oven temperature to 325 degrees. Using serrated knife, slice each loaf on slight bias into ½-inch-thick slices.
5. Arrange cookies cut side down on sheet about ½ inch apart and bake until crisp and golden brown on both sides, about fifteen minutes, flipping cookies halfway through baking. Allow it to cool completely on wire rack before you serve. (Biscotti can be stored safely at room temperature for up to 1 month.)

Sweet Fruit Salad

Yield: 4 to 6 Servings

This recipe can be made quickly

Ingredients:

- ¼ teaspoon vanilla extract
- 1 tablespoon minced fresh mint
- 2 plums, halved, pitted, and cut into ½-inch pieces
- 3 cups cantaloupe, cut into ½-inch pieces
- 4 teaspoons sugar
- 8 ounces fresh sweet cherries, pitted and halved
- 1 tablespoon lime juice, plus extra for seasoning

Directions:

1. Mix sugar and mint in a big container. Using rubber spatula, press mixture into side of the container until sugar becomes damp, approximately half a minute. Put in cantaloupe, plums, cherries, and vanilla and gently toss to combine.
2. Allow to sit at room temperature, stirring intermittently, until fruit releases its juices, 15 to half an hour. Mix in lime juice and season with extra lime juice to taste. Serve.

Sweet Warm Figs

Yield: 4 to 6 Servings

This recipe can be made quickly

Ingredients:

- 1½ ounces goat cheese
- 16 walnut halves, toasted
- 3 tablespoons honey8 fresh figs, halved along the length

Directions:

1. Place the oven rack in the centre of the oven and pre-heat your oven to 500 degrees. Spoon heaping ½ teaspoon goat cheese onto each fig half and lay out on parchment paper–lined rimmed baking sheet. Bake figs until heated through, about 4 minutes; move to serving platter.
2. Place 1 walnut half on top of each fig half and drizzle with honey. Serve.

Turkish Stuffed Apricots

Yield: 6 Servings

Ingredients:

- ¼ cup sugar
- ½ cup plain Greek yogurt
- ½ teaspoon grated lemon zest plus 1 tablespoon juice
- ½ teaspoon rose water
- 2 bay leaves
- 2 cups water
- 24 whole dried apricots
- 4 green cardamom pods, cracked
- Salt
- ¼ cup shelled pistachios, toasted and chopped fine

Directions:

1. Mix yogurt, 1 teaspoon sugar, rose water, lemon zest, and pinch salt in a small-sized container. Refrigerate filling until ready to use.
2. Bring water, cardamom pods, bay leaves, lemon juice, and remaining sugar to simmer in small saucepan over moderate to low heat and cook, stirring intermittently, until sugar has dissolved, approximately two minutes. Mix in apricots, return to

simmer, and cook, stirring intermittently, until plump and tender, about half an hour. Use a slotted spoon to move apricots to plate and allow to cool to room temperature.
3. Discard cardamom pods and bay leaves. Bring syrup to boil on high heat and cook, stirring intermittently, until thickened and measures about 3 tablespoons, four to eight minutes; allow to cool to room temperature.
4. Place pistachios in shallow dish. Place filling in small zipper-lock bag and snip off 1 corner to create ½-inch opening. Pipe filling evenly into opening of each apricot and dip exposed filling into pistachios; move to serving platter. Sprinkle apricots with syrup and serve.

Endnote

Thank you for being my most valued customer. If you enjoyed this book, don't forget to leave a review on amazon! I hope this book helps you achieve your fitness and wellness goals. Good Luck!